Gonadal Steroids and Brain Function

Experimental Brain Research Supplementum 3

Gonadal Steroids and Brain Function

IUPS-Satellite-Symposium
Berlin, July 10–11, 1980

Edited by
W. Wuttke and R. Horowski

With 136 Figures and 10 Tables

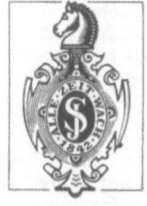

Springer-Verlag Berlin Heidelberg New York 1981

Professor Dr. Wolfgang Wuttke
Max-Planck-Institut für biophysikalische Chemie
Abt. Neurobiologie
Postfach 968
3400 Göttingen

Dr. Reinhard Horowski
Department Klinische Neuropsychopharmakologie
Postfach 650 311
1000 Berlin 65

ISBN 978-3-540-10606-7   ISBN 978-3-642-45525-4   (eBook)
DOI 10.1007/978-3-642-45525-4

Library of Congress Cataloging in Publication Data.
Main entry under title:
Gonadal steroids and brain function.
(Experimental brain research. Supplement ; 3)
Includes bibliographical references and index. 1 Hormones, Sex--Physiological
effect. 2. Brain. 3. Gonads. 4. Neuroendocrinology. I. Wuttke, W. II. Horowski,
R. (Reinhard), 1944--. III. International Union of Physiological Sciences. IV.
Series. [DNLM: 1. Gonads--Congresses. 2. Steroids--Physiology--Congresses. 2.
Brain--Physiology--Congresses. Gonadotropins--Secretion--Congresses. WL 300
G635 1980]
QP572.S4G66 599.05'6 81-1677 AACR2
ISBN 978-3-540-10606-7

2125/3321-543210

Contents

VI

Poster Presentations

List of Senior Contributors

BALL, P., Institut für Biochemische Endokrinologie, Arbeitsgruppe für Klinische Endokrinologie, Medizinische Hochschule Lübeck, 2400 Lübeck, FRG

BARRACLOUGH, C.A., Dept. of Physiology, School of Medicine, University of Maryland, Baltimore, MD 21201, USA

BAUER, K., Max-Volmer Institut, Abt. Biochemie, TU Berlin, Franklinstr. 29, 1000 Berlin 10, FRG

BECKER, D., Institute for Psychology, Univ. Göttingen, 3400 Göttingen, FRG

BLAKE, C.A., Department of Anatomy, University of Nebraska Medical Center, Omaha, NE, USA

BREUER, H., Institut für Klinische Biochemie, Universität Bonn, 5300 Bonn, FRG

DE COTTE, D.M., Department of Physiology, St. George's Hospital Medical School, London SW17, U.K.

DÖCKE, F., Institute of Experimental Endocrinology, Humboldt University, Berlin, GDR

DÖRNER, G. Institute of Experimental Endrocrinology, Humboldt University, Berlin, GDR

DONOVAN, B.T., Department of Physiology, Institute of Psychiatry, De Crespigny Par, London SE5 8AF, U.K.

DÜKER, E., Max-Planck-Institute for Biophysical Chemistry, 3400 Göttingen, FRG

FENSKE, M., Institut f. Tierzucht u. Haustiergenetik, Universität Göttingen, 3400 Göttingen, FRG

GETHMANN, U., Kliniken für Frauenheilkunde und Geburtshilfe, Medizinische Hochschule Lübeck, 2400 Lübeck, FRG

GHRAF, R., Institut für Physiologische Chemie, Fachbereich Theoretische Medizin, Universitätsklinikum Essen, 4300 Essen, FRG

GILMORE D.P., Institute of Physiology, University of Glasgow, U.K.

GORSKI, R.A., Department of Anatomy of the Brain Research Institute UCLA School of Medicine, Los Angeles, CA 90024, USA

HANCKE, J.L., Dept. Clinical Endocrinology, Medical School, 3000 Hannover, FRG

HIEMKE, C., Institut für Physiologische Chemie, Universitätsklinikum Essen, 4300 Essen, FRG

v. HOLST, D., Lehrstuhl für Tierphysiologie, Universität Bayreuth, 8580 Bayreuth, FRG

HOROWSKI, R., Research Laboratories of Schering AG, 1000 Berlin, FRG

JUNGBLUT, P.W., Max-Planck-Institut für experimentelle Endokrinologie, POB 61 03 09, 3000 Hannover 61, FRG

KAWAKAMI, M., Department of Physiology, Yokohama City University School of Medicine, Yokohama, Japan

KELLY, M.J., Department of Physiology, University of Pittsburgh, School of Medicine, Pittsburgh, PA 15261, USA

KIRCHHOFF, J., Institut für Physiologische Chemie, Fachbereich Theoretische Medizin, Universitätsklinikum Essen, Hufelandstr. 55, 4300 Essen, FRG

KNOBIL, E., Department of Physiology, University of Pittsburgh, School of Medicine, Pittsburgh, PA 15261, USA

KNUPPEN, R., Institut für Biochemische Endokrinologie der Medizinischen Hochschule Lübeck, Ratzeburger Allee 160, 2400 Lübeck, FRG

KOW, L.-M., The Rockefeller University, York Avenue & 66th Street, New York, NY 10021, USA

LADOSKY, W., Departamento de Fisiologia e Farmacologia Universidade Federal de Pernambuco, Recife, Brasil

LINTON, E.A., Department of Biochemical Endocrinology, Chelsea Hospital for Women, Dovehouse Street, London SW3 6LT, U.K.

MANSKY, T., Max-Planck-Institute for Biophysical Chemistry, 3400 Göttingen, FRG

McCANN, S.M., Department of Physiology, Southwestern Medical School, University of Texas, Dallas, TX, USA

McEWEN, B.S., The Rockefeller University, New York, NY 10021, USA

MEITES, J., Department of Physiology, Neuroendocrine Research Laboratory, Michigan State University, East Lansing, Michigan, MI 48824, USA

MOTTA M., Department of Endocrinology, University of Milano, 21, Via Andrea del Sarto, 20129 Milano, Italy

NESBITT, K., Department of Physiology, St. George's Hospital Medical School, London, U.K.

NEUMANN F., Research Laboratories of SCHERING AG, 1000 Berlin, FRG

PARVIZI, N., Insitut für Tierzucht und Tierverhalten, FAL, Mariensee, 3057 Neustadt 1, FRG

RUBERG M., Unité 159 de Neuroendocrinologie, Centre Paul Broca de l'INSERM, 2ter rue d'Alésia, 75014 Paris, France

SAR, M., Department of Anatomy, University of North Carolina, Chapel Hill, NC 27514, USA

SAWYER C.H., Department of Anatomy and Brain Research Institute, UCLA School of Medicine, Los Angeles, CA 90024, USA

STUMPF, W.E., Department of Pharmacology, University of North Carolina, Chapel Hill, NC 27514, USA

WEINDL, A., Neurologische Klinik der Technischen Universität München, 8000 München, FRG

WUTTKE, W., Max-Planck-Institute for Biophysical Chemistry, 3400 Göttingen, FRG

Acknowledgements

The editors wish to express their gratitude to all persons who helped making the symposium and this book a success. In particular the assistance of Mrs. A. Scholz, R. Schley and H. Heinze (Schering) and of S. Schlette (Max-Planck-Institute for Biophysical Chemistry) is acknowledged. The patience of Mrs. B. Bartsch to type and of Dr. J. Ondo (visiting Professor Univ. South Carolina Med. School) to proofread all manuscripts was also of invaluable help. This symposium was only possible due to the financial generosity of the German Research Society, the Senator für Wirtschaft (Berlin) and the Schering Company. The fast processing of this book by the Springer-Company is encouraging to continue this inexpensive Symposium-Series in EXPERIMENTAL BRAIN RESEARCH.

W. Wuttke (Göttingen)
R. Horowski (Berlin)

The Morphology of LRH and Oxytocin Neurons

A. Weindl and M.V. Sofroniew, München

Peptidergic neurons are involved in the regulation of gonadal steroids. The adenohypophyseal gonadotropic hormones luteinizing hormone (LH) and follicle stimulating hormone (FSH) are under the control of the decapeptide luteinizing hormone releasing hormone (LH–RH or LRH) produced by hypothalamic secretory neurons.

Other peptidergic neurons of the hypothalamus which are involved in reproductive functions and which also appear to be sensitive to gonadal steroids are neurons producing oxytocin. Oxytocin, an octapeptide produced in magnocellular perikarya of the supraoptic and paraventricular nucleus and transported within axons to the fenestrated capillaries of the neural lobe causes uterine contraction at term, and milk ejection. The secretion of oxytocin and its associated neurophysin (neurophysin I or estrogen–stimulated neurophysin) is influenced by estrogens (Robinson, 1978).

In this communication the morphology and distribution of neurons producing LRH and oxytocin, and their fiber connections to the hypophysis as well as to non–hypophyseal target areas in the brain of several mammals will be presented.

1. Material and Methods

Brains of tree shrews (Tupaia belangeri), a prosimian, and of rabbits fixed by perfusion with Bouin's solution were embedded in paraffin–paraplast and sectioned serially in the frontal, sagittal and horizontal plane. Details of the tissue preparation and of the unlabeled antibody enzyme immunohistochemical method used to

1

visualize LRH, oxytocin and neurophysin, as well as of the specificity tests of the antisera have been described previously (Sofroniew
et al., 1979).

2.   Observations

Perikarya containing LRH are widely distributed in the anterior
hypothalamic/preoptic area of tupaia and rabbit. LRH perikaya often
are bipolar or multipolar giving rise to two or several processes.
Fig. 1 shows a LRH perikaryon in the anterior hypothalamic area of
the rabbit.   Two cell processes leave the perikaryon in opposite
directions and have different calibers.   The thin fiber directed
caudally resembles an axon, the large fiber directed rostrally
resembles a dendrite when compared to Golgi-impregnated neurons.
        The main target of LRH fibers are the fenestrated portal
capillaries of the external zone of the median eminence (Fig. 2a,b).
In the external zone, LRH terminals are distributed laterally.
Furthermore, LRH fibers are found in the stalk and proximal part of
the neural lobe (Fig. 2c). In the preoptic region, LRH fibers run
dorso-ventrally in the lamina terminalis and terminate at fenestrated
capillaries of the organum vasculosum of the lamina terminalis
(Fig. 3) where as in median eminence and neural lobe the blood-
brain barrier for peptides and proteins is not present (Weindl and
Joynt, 1972).   In the subfornical organ, only a few LRH fibers
terminate at capillaries (Krisch and Leonhardt, 1980; Weindl and
Sofroniew, 1980), whereas no LRH fibers or cells are found in the
area postrema and pineal organ, additional circumventricular organs
lacking a blood-brain barrier.
        In addition to vascular targets, LRH fibers are directed to
neural targets inside and outside the hypothalamus (Fig. 8) where
they form axosomatic contacts with other neurons. Areas where LRH
fibers are found are: the mamillary and retromamillary area of the
hypothalamus, the septum, the dorsal thalamus, the habenular
region, the posterior commissure (Weindl and Sofroniew, 1980), the
periaqueductal grey of the mesencephalon, the inferior colliculi
(Fig. 5), the fasciculus retroflexus and the ventral hippocampus
(Fig. 4).   In the pigeon where groups of LRH perikarya are located

2

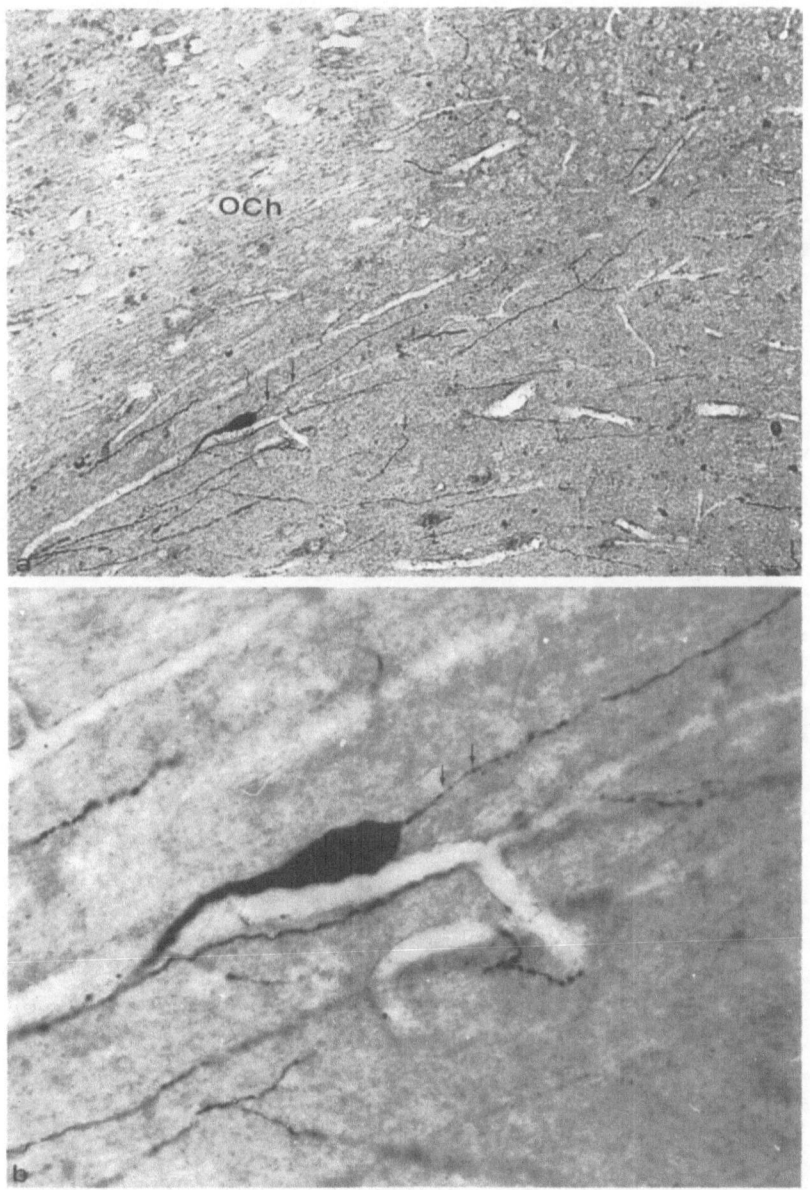

Figure 1a,b: Rabbit.   Horizontal section through the anterior hypothalamus near the optic chiasm (OCh).   LRH immunoperoxidase reaction. a.
Survey. 133x.   b. Detail of a. 350x. LRH perikaryon having two processes
of different diameters.   The rostrally directed thick fiber resembles a
dendrite, the caudally directed thin fiber (↓) resembles an axon

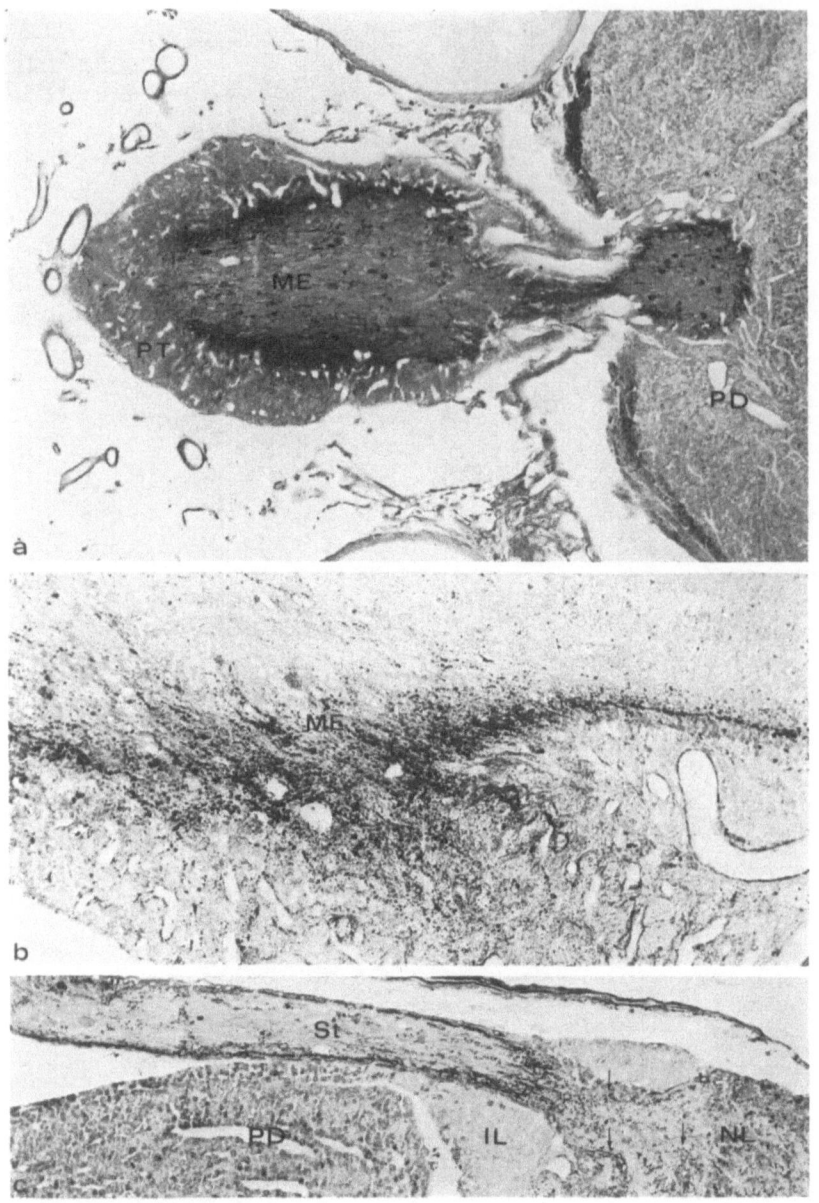

Figure 2a-c: Tupaia belangeri. Horizontal (a) and sagittal sections through the median eminence (b) and neurohypophyseal stalk (c). LRH immunoperoxidase reaction. LRH fibers terminate laterally in the external zone of the median eminence (ME) at portal capillaries in the vicinity of the pars tuberalis (PT) of the adenohypophysis (a,b). Other LRH fibers (↓) continue into the stalk (St) and proximal part of the neural lobe (NL). IL intermediate lobe. PD pars distalis. a. 53x. b. 133x. c. 53x

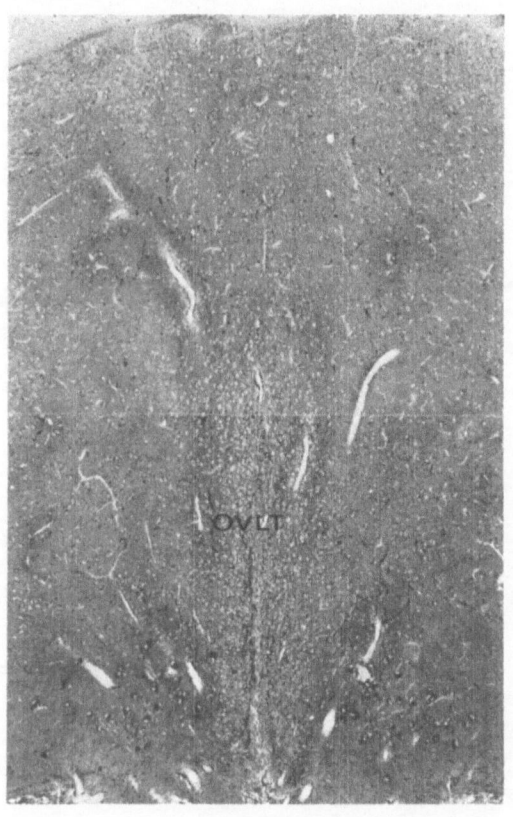

Figure 3: Tupaia belangeri. Frontal section through the preoptic area and organum vasculosum of the lamina terminalis (OVLT). LRH immuno-peroxidase reation. LRH perikarya are located near the OVLT. LRH fibers are present in the preoptic area and the OVLT. 54x

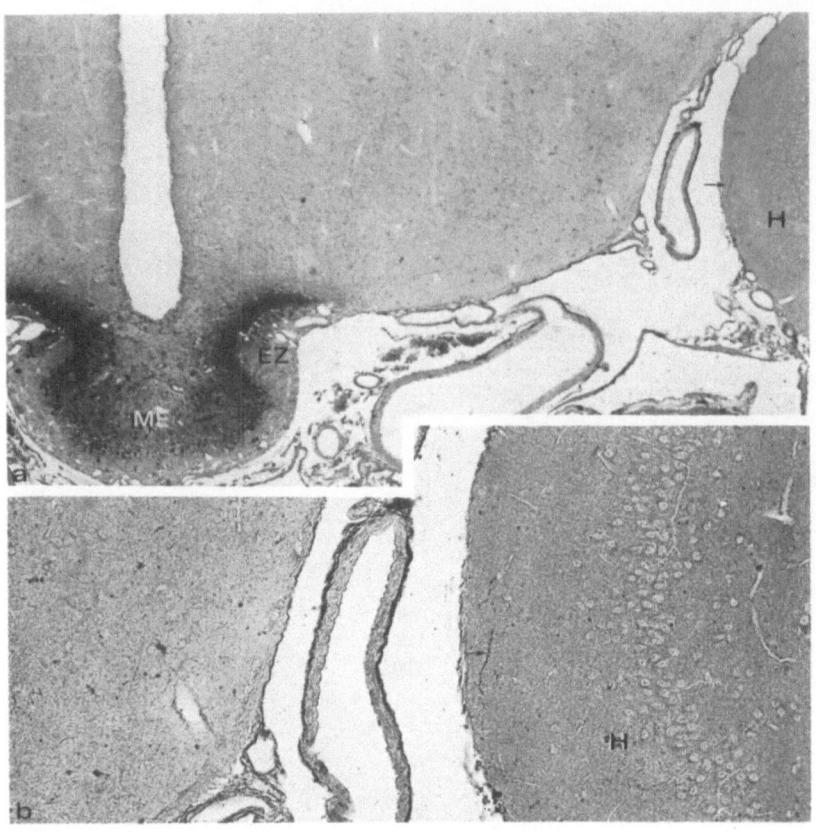

Figure 4a,b: Tupaia. Frontal section through median eminence, hypothalamus and neighbouring ventral hippocampus. LRH immunoperoxidase reaction. LRH fibers terminate in the lateral parts of the external zone
(EZ) of the median eminence (ME). Extrahypothalamic LRH fibers are
present in the ventral hippocampus (→). a. Survey. 53x. b. Detail of a.
133x

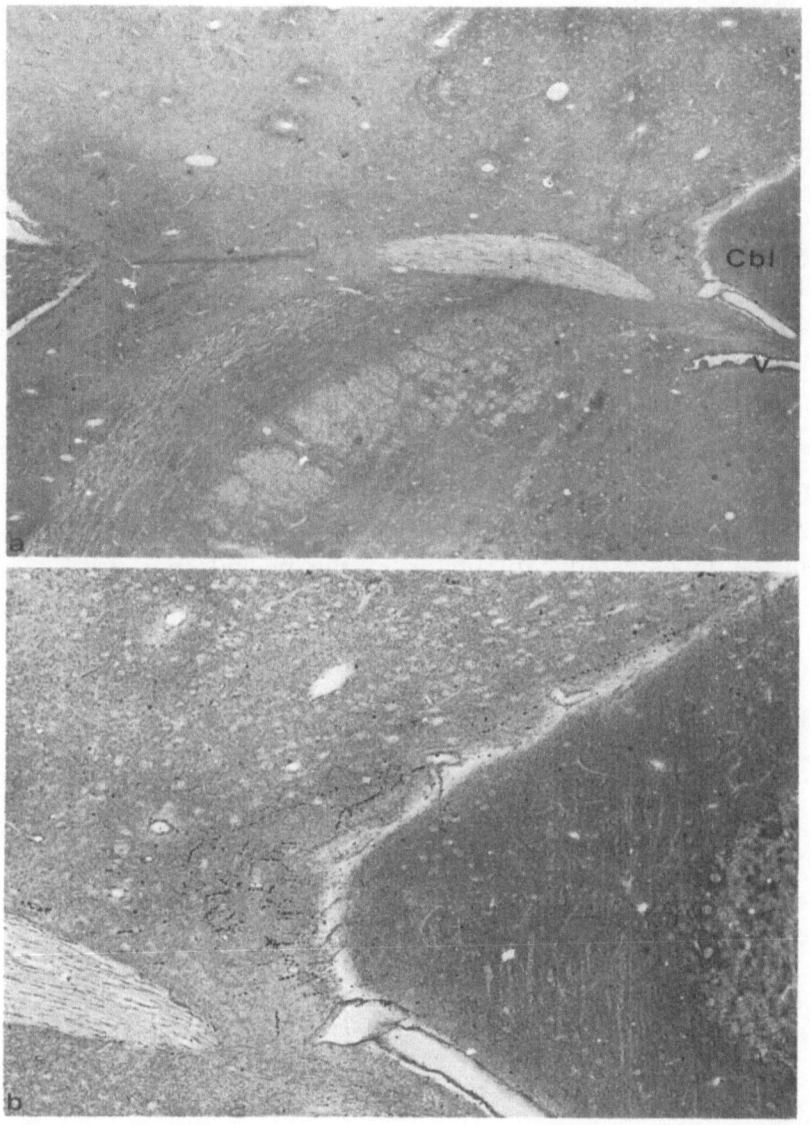

Figure 5a,b: Tupaia. Frontal section at the transition caudal mesencephalon – pons. LRH immunoperoxidase reaction. LRH fibers are present
near the surface of the inferior colliculus. Cbl Cerebellum. V ventricle. a. Survey. 54x. b. Detail of a. 136x

in the anterior and central part of the hypothalamus, LRH fibers
also form dense fields of axosomatic contacts with a group of neurons
in the dorso-caudal medulla oblongata (personal observation). Oxytocin and its associated neurophysin are produced in magnocellular
perikarya of the supraoptic and paraventricular nucleus and the
internuclear zone.   In the tupaia the supraoptic nucleus contains a
high number of vasopressin and only few oxytocin perikarya.   In the
paraventricular nucleus oxytocin perikarya are located medially
along the walls of the third ventricle, and vasopressin perikarya
are located laterally.   Oxytocin as well as vasopressin perikarya
are found in the internuclear zone.   Many magnocellular perikarya
are multipolar (Fig. 6) and give rise to processes which often
branch.   Oxytocin and neurophysin containing processes are directed
ventrocaudally to traverse the infundibulum in the internal zone and
to terminate at the fenestrated capillaries of the neural lobe.

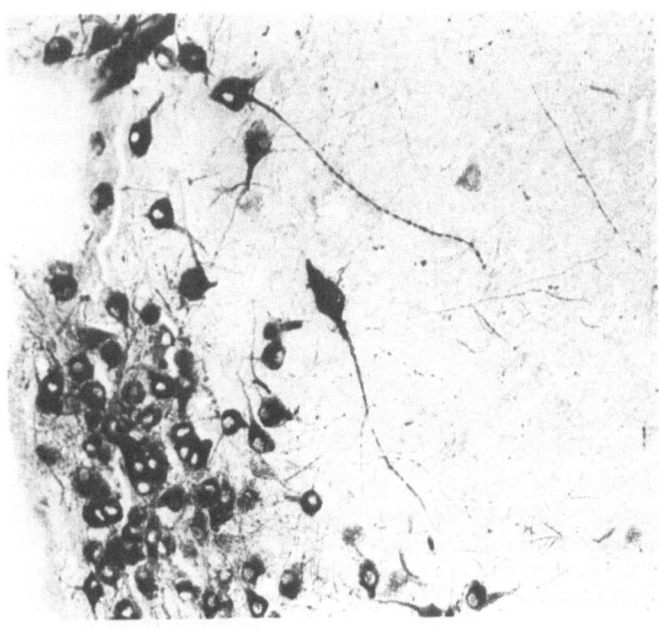

Figure 6:   Rabbit.   Sagittal section through the periventricular portion
of the paraventricular nucleus.   Neurophysin immunoperoxidase reaction.
Several magnocellular perikarya are multipolar giving rise to processes
which branch. 136x

Many oxytocin perikarya in the paraventricular nucleus and the neighbouring perifornical group send extrahypothalamic fibers in caudal direction to the caudal medulla oblongata and the spinal cord (Fig. 9). Bilateral bundles run ventrally and laterally through the substantia nigra and above the cerebral peduncles through the ventral pons and medulla oblongata towards the spinal cord. In the mesencephalon, fibers from these bundles bend dorsally and run caudally under the floor of the fourth ventricle. Fibers bending dorsally in the caudal medulla oblongata from the bundles terminate at dendrites and somata of the nucleus of the solitary tract and the dorsal nucleus of the vagus and the commissural nucleus where they form dense fields of contacts (Fig. 7). Other fibers terminate in the lateral reticular nucleus. Fibers continuing caudally are mainly distributed around the central canal, in the dorsal horn and in the intermediolateral area of the spinal cord.

3. Discussion

Barry (1979) who has surveyed numerous mammalian species using the immunofluorescence technique found LRH perikarya in the pre-optic/anterior hypothalamic area. Only in the human (Barry, 1977) and rhesus monkey (Weindl and Sofroniew, 1980) additional LRH perikarya are present in the mediobasal hypothalamus.

Some reports of LRH perikarya in the arcuate nucleus region of the rat and other non-primate mammals (Silverman and Krey, 1976) need yet to be confirmed by other laboratories since the antiserum used had cross-reactivity with ACTH due to a prior immunization of the same animal against ACTH (Clayton and Hoffman, 1979). Perikarya immunoreactive with antiserum to ACTH are regularly found in the area of the arcuate nucleus of the rat (Sofroniew, 1979), tupaia (Weindl and Sofroniew, 1980) and human (Bugnon et al., 1979). The same perikarya are immunoreactive with antisera to beta-endorphin (Bloom et al., 1978), alpha-MSH (Watson et al., 1977) and beta-lipotropin (Nilaver et al., 1979).

LRH fibers contacting portal capillaries in the external zone of the median eminence terminate laterally in the rat (Hökfelt et al., 1978), guinea pig (Silverman and Krey, 1976) and tupaia (Weindl

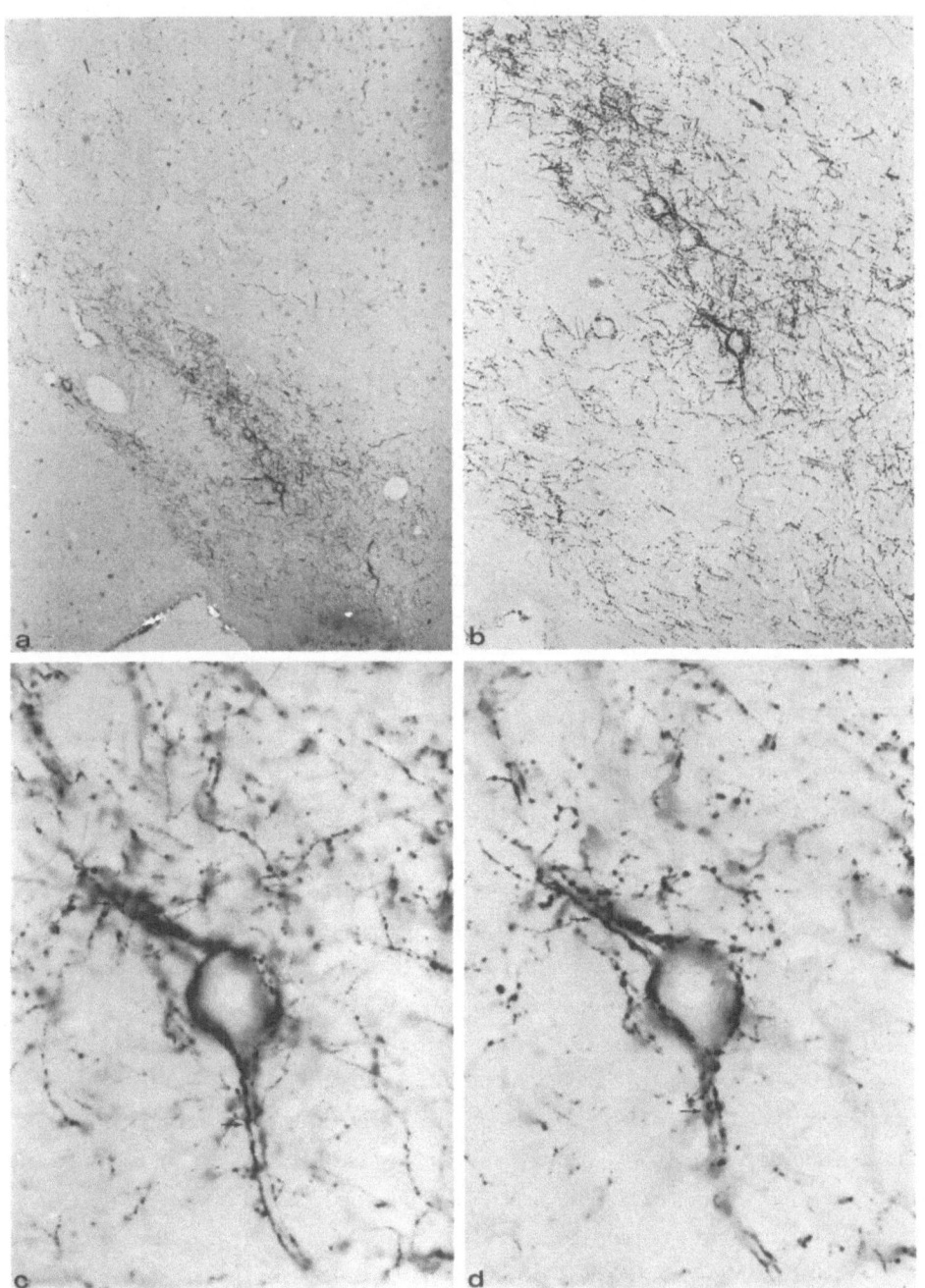

Figure 7a-d: Rabbit. Horizontal section through the area of the nucleus of the solitary tract in the caudal brain stem. Neurophysin immunoperoxidase reaction. Neurophysin fibers form dense fields of contacts on target neurons (→). a. Survey. 54x. b. Detail of a. 163x. c,d. Details of b, photographed at different planes of focus. Neurophysin terminals form bouton-like axosomatic and axodendritic contacts on a target neurons. 410x

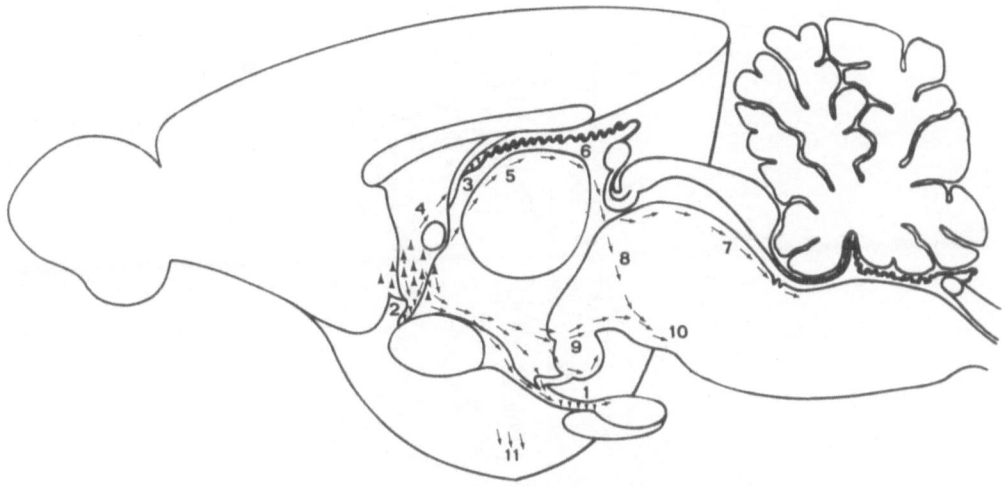

Figure 8: Distribution of LRH perikarya (▲) and fibers in the sagittally sectioned tupaia brain. From perikarya located in the preoptic/anterior hypothalamic area fibers descend to the median eminence where they terminate at portal vessels (▼) and to the rostral portion of the neural lobe (1). Other neuro-hemal target areas where LRH fibers terminate are the fenestrated capillaries of the organum vasculosum of the lamina terminalis (2) and the subfornical organ (3). LRH fibers are present in the septum (4), dorsal thalamus (5), epithalamus (6), and mesencephalic and rhombencephalic brain stem (7). LRH fibers project through the fasciculus retroflexus (8) to the interpeduncular nucleus (10). Other LRH fibers project from the preoptic/anterior hypothalamic area ventrally to the mamillary region (9) and to the interpeduncular nucleus. LRH fibers are also present in the ventral hippocampus (11)

11

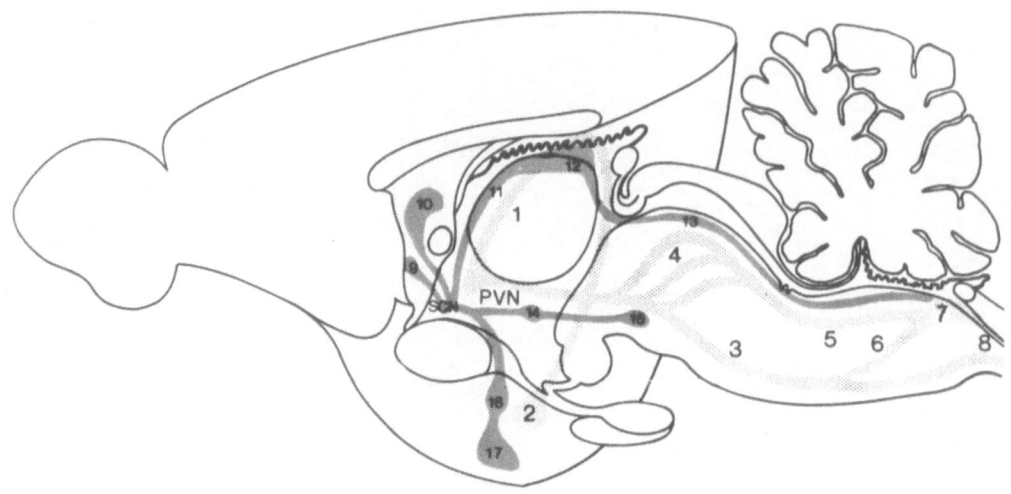

Figure 9: Extrahypothalamic projections of fibers containing neurohypophyseal peptides in the sagitally sectioned tupaia brain. From magnocellular perikarya located mainly in and in the vicinity of the paraventricular nucleus (PVN) vasopressin and neurophysin fibers project through the stria terminalis (1) to the central nucleus of the amygdala (2). Fibers directed caudally containing neurophysin and mainly oxytocin project ventrally (3) and laterally to brain stem and spinal cord (8). Fibers bending dorsally in the mesencephalon (4) run dorsocaudally (5) within the brain stem. Fibers of the ventral bundles bend dorsally (6) in the lower brainstem, form dense fields of contacts in the nucleus of the solitary tract, dorsal nucleus of the vagus and commissural nucleus (7) and continue to the spinal cord (8) where they are present around the central canal, in the dorsal horn and in the intermediolateral nucleus. From parvocellular vasopressin and neurophysin containing neurons of the suprachiasmatic nucleus (SCN) small caliber fibers project rostrally to the nucleus of the diagonal tract (9), lateral septum (10), dorsally to the mediodorsal thalamus (11), lateral habenular nuclei (12) and mesencephalic and rhombencephalic central gray (13), caudally to the posterior hypothalamus (14) and interpeduncular nucleus (15), and ventrolaterally to the medial amygdala (16) and ventral hippocampus (17)

and Sofroniew, 1980) while somatostatin fibers termiante more medially (Hökfelt et al., 1978; Weindl and Sofroniew, 1980). This regional distribution of the terminals corresponds to the lateral location of LRH perikarya in the preoptic/anterior hypothalamic area and to the medial periventricular location of somatostatin perikarya in the anterior hypothalamic nucleus. In the narrow space between LRH terminals and portal surface, dopamine terminals are present (Hökfelt et al., 1978). An interaction between dopamine (Fuxe et al., 1976) and enkephalin fibers (Rotsztejn, 1980) with LRH fibers may be

12

important for the release of LRH into the adenohypophyseal portal vessels and the regulation of gonadotropin secretion.

Another major target of LRH fibers is the organum vasculosum of the lamina terminalis (Barry, 1980). Although several structural similarities with the median eminence such as an inner and outer network of fenestrated capillary loops suggest a similar function, a portal drainage could not yet be proven for the OVLT. Palkovits et al. (1978) have proposed that LRH transported in fibers from perikarya in the preoptic region is released into the permeable capillaries of the OVLT and is carried back within blood vessels to LRH perikarya in the median preoptic nucleus. A physiological role for this hypothesized backflow remains unclear. A vascular drainage of LRH to the median eminence and anterior pituitary is unlikely. The blood vessel which connects the OVLT with the infundibular region is an artery deriving from the internal carotid artery (Weindl and Sofroniew, 1978). The secretion of LRH into the systemic circulation would result in a very high dilution and very low concentration at possible peripheral targets.

LRH fibers found inside and outside the hypothalamus which are not directed to vascular targets terminate at groups of neurons mainly in the limbic system (septum, ventral hippocampus), diencephalon (dorsal thalamus, habenula), and mesencephalon. Recently projections of LRH fibers to the frontal telencephalon and olfactory bulb and to the pial surface of the hamster brain were described by Jennes and Stumpf (1980). LRH immunoreactivity in fibers of the nervus terminalis which may have a function in regulating blood flow in the olfactory mucosa, and in cells of the ganglion terminale have been reported in the fetal and adult guinea pig (Schwanzel-Fukuda and Silverman, 1980). LRH fibers contacting neurons may be important in modulating the electrical activity of neurons influencing sexual behaviour as suggested from electrophysiological (Moss and Dudley, 1980) and behavioural studies (Pfaff, 1973). Neurons with specific receptors for gonadal steroids were demonstrated by autoradiographic (Pfaff, 1968; Stumpf, 1968) and electrophysiological techniques (Moss and Dudley, 1980) in areas which are interconnected with the region where LRH perikarya are located. Whether LRH neurons themselves have receptors for gonadal steroids needs to be demonstrated by improvements of a combined immunohistochemical autoradiographic technique (Morrell et al., 1980).

Oxytocin and vasopressin as well as their associated neuro-physins are produced in separate magnocellular neurons. According to Gainer et al. (1977), oxytocin (M.W. 1000), neurophysin (M.W. 10000) and various other peptide fragments are cleaved in the perikarya from a larger precursor molecule (M.W. 25000). In contrast to the precursor of vasopressin, the precursor of oxytocin does not have a glycopeptide component (Gainer, personal communication). The supraoptic nucleus contains more vasopressin than oxytocin perikarya in the tupaia and in the guinea pig (Sofroniew et al., 1979). In the human supraoptic nucleus most neurophysin perikarya contain vasopressin and very few perikarya contain oxytocin (Dierickx and Vandesande, 1977). In the para-ventricular nucleus vasopressin perikarya are located laterally and oxytocin perikarya medially. In the guinea pig, oxytocin perikarya of the periventricular division of the paraventricular nucleus are found along the caudal surface of the anterior commissure, in the triangular nucleus of the septum and in the immediate vicinity of the OVLT (Sofroniew et al., 1979). Vasopressin fibers deriving from the paraventricular nucleus terminate at portal capillaries of the extern-al zone of the median eminence; they appear to be involved in the vasopressin-mediated stimulation of ACTH release (Sofroniew et al., 1977).

In contrast, only few oxytocin fibers terminate at the portal capillaries of the external zone.

Although vasopressin is also found in neurophysin containing parvocellular neurons of the suprachiasmatic nucleus and their fine caliber projections to neurons in the lateral septum, lateral habenula, mesencephalic grey, interpeduncular nucleus, medial amygdala and ventral hippocamupus (Sofroniew and Weindl, 1978), oxytocin is present only in magnocellular neurons and their processes.

Extrahypothalamic neurophysin (Swanson and McKellar, 1979) and oxytocin containing fibers which originate from perikarya in the paraventricular nucleus and the perifornical area (Buijs, 1978) project caudally to the medulla oblongata and to the spinal cord. In the region of the nucleus of the solitary tract, of the dorsal nucleus of the vagus and of the commissural nucleus of the medulla oblongata, and in the dorsal horn and in the intermediolateral

14

division of the spinal cord, the fibers form contacts with the soma or the processes of target neurons. The functions of these extensive projections are not yet clear. On the basis of functions ascribed to the areas innervated, several possibilities may be considered.

The nucleus of the solitary tract, the dorsal nucleus of the vagus, the lateral horn of the spinal cord and several other areas are involved in autonomic functions such as cardiovascular reflexes (Cohen and Cabot, 1979; Weindl and Sofroniew, 1980; Sofroniew and Weindl, 1981).

The projections to the dorsal horn where several other neuro-peptides such as somatostatin, substance P, TRH and enkephalin can be demonstrated immunohistochemically (Hökfelt et al., 1978) may modulate sensory input such as pain (see Sofroniew and Weindl, 1981).

Since sensory inputs such as tactile stimuli are important for eliciting reflexes essential to reproductive functions (e.g. lordosis behaviour, milk ejection), the question arises whether some of the oxytocin projections play a role in the regulation of reproductive functions at the spinal cord level. Additional functions of oxytocin which has attracted much less interest than vasopressin are still unkown.

Acknowledgement

Supported by DFG grant WE 608/6.

References

Barry J (1977) Immunofluorescence study of LRF neurons in man. Cell Tiss Res 181:1-14.
Barry H (1979) Immunohistochemistry of luteinizing hormone-releasing-hormon-producing neurons of the vertebrates. In: Bourne and Danielli (eds) Internat. Review of Cytology, Vol. 60, Academic Press, New York, pp.179-221.
Barry J (1980) Immunofluorescence study of LRH-producing neurons in prosimians (Tupaia and Galago). Cell Tiss Res 206:355-365.
Bloom F, Battenberg E, Rossier J, Ling N, Guillemin R (1978) Neurons containing β-endorphin in rat brain exist separately from those containing enkephalin: Immunohistochemical studies. Proc Nat Acad Sci 75:1591-1595.
Bugnon C, Bloch B, Lenys D, Fellmann D (1979) Infundibular neurons of the human hypothalamus simultaneously reactive with antisera against en-

dorphins, ACTH, MSH, and β-LPH. Cell Tiss Res 199:177-196.

Buijs RM (1978) Intra- and extrahypothalamic vasopressin and oxytocin pathways in the rat. Cell Tiss Res 192:423-435.

Clayton CJ, Hoffman GE (1979) Immunohistochemical evidence for anti-LHRH and anti-ACTH activity in the "F"-antiserum Am J Anat 155:139-145.

Cohen DH, Cabot JH (1979) Toward a cardiovascular neurobiology. Trends in Neurosciences 3:273-276.

Dierickx K, Vandesande F (1977) Immunocytochemical localization of vaso-pressinergic and oxytocinergic neurons in the human hypothalamus. Cell Tiss Res 184:15-27.

Fuxe K, Hökfelt T, Löfström A, Johannsson O, Agnati L, Everitt B, Goldstein M, Jeffcoate S, White N, Eneroth P, Gustafsson J-A, Scott P (1976) On the role of neurotransmitters and hypothalamic hormones and their interactions in hypothalamic and extrahypothalamic control of pituitary function and sexual behavior. In: Naftolin F, Ryan KJ, Davies J (eds) Subcellular mechanisms in reproductive neuroendo-crinology. Elsevier, Amsterdam, pp.193-246.

Gainer H, Sarne K, Brownstein MJ (1977) Biosynthesis and axonal transport of rat neurohypophysial proteins and peptides. J Cell Biol 73:366-381.

Hökfelt T, Elde R, Fuxe K, Johannsson O, Ljungdahl A, Goldstein M, Luft R, Effendic S, Nilsson G, Terenius L, Ganten D, Jeffcoate S, Rehfeld J, Said S, Perez de la Mora M, Passani L, Tapia R, Teran L, Palacios R (1978) Aminergic and peptidergic pathways in the nervous system with special reference to the hypothalamus. In: Reichlin S, Baldessarine RJ, Martin JB (eds) The hypothalamus. Raven Press, New York, pp.69-135.

Jennes L, Stumpf WE (1980) LHRH-systems in the brain of the golden hamster. Cell Tiss Res 209:239-256.

Krisch B, Leonhardt H (1980) Luliberin and somatostatin fiber-terminals in the subfornical organ of the rat. Cell Tiss·Res 210:33-46.

Nilaver G, Zimmerman EA, Defendini R, Liotta AS, Krieger DT, Brownstein MJ (1979) Adrenocorticotropin and β-lipotropin in the hypothalamus. Localization in the same arcuate neurons by sequential immunocyto-chemcial procedures. J Cell Biol 81:50-58.

Moss RL, Dudley CA (1980) Neurophysiology and behavioral effects of neuropeptides. In: Wuttke W, Weindl A, Voigt K-H, Dries R-R (eds) Brain and pituitary peptides. Ferring Symp. Munich 1979. Karger, Basel, pp.168-175.

Morrell JI, Rhodes CH, Pfaff DW (1980) Modern neuroanatomical approaches to neuroendocrine control systems. In: Müller EE (ed) Neuroactive drugs in endocrinology. Elsevier/North Holland Biomedical Press, pp.3-18.

Palkovits M, Mezey E, Ambach G, Kivovicz P (1978) Neural and vascular connections between the organum vasculosum laminae terminalis and preoptic nuclei. In: Scott DE, Kozlowski GP, Weindl A (eds) Brain - Endocrine Interaction III; Neural hormones and reproduction. Karger, Basel, pp.117-137.

Pfaff D (1968) Autoradiographic localization of radioactivity in rat brain after injection of tritiated sex hormones Science 161:1355-1356.

Pfaff DW (1973) Luteinizing hormone releasing factor (LRF) potentiates lordosis behavior in hypophysectomized ovariectomized female rats. Science 182:1148-1149.

Robinson AG (1978) Neurophysins an aid to understanding the structure and function of the neurophysins. In: Ganong WF and Martini L (eds) Frontiers in Neuroendocrinology. Vol. 5, Raven Press, New York, pp.35-59.

Rotsztejn WH (1980) Neuromodulation in neuroendocrinology. Trends in Neurosciences 3:67–70.

Schwanzel-Fukuda M, Silvermann AJ (1980) The nervus terminalis of guinea pig: A new luteinizing hormone (LHRH) neuronal system. J Comp Neurol 191:213–225.

Silverman AJ, Krey LC (1976) The luteinizing hormon-releasing hormone (LH-RH) neuronal networks of the guinea pig brain. I. Intra- and extrahypothalamic projections. Brain Res 157:233–246.

Sofroniew MV (1979) Immunoreactive β-endorphin and ACTH in the same neurons of the hypothalamic arcuate nucleus in the rat. Am J Anat 154:283–289.

Sofroniew MV, Weindl A (1978) Projections from the parvocellular vaso-pressin- and neurophysin containing neurons in the suprachiasmatic nucleus. Am J Anat 153:391–430.

Sofroniew MV, Weindl A (1981) Central nervous system distribution of vasopressin, oxytocin and neurophysin. In: Martinez jr JL, Jensen RA, Messing RB, Rigter H, McGaugh JL (eds) Endogenous peptides and learning and memory processes. Academic Press, New York, in press.

Sofroniew MV, Weindl A, Schinko I, Wetzstein R (1979) The distribution of vasopressin-, oxytocin-, and neurophysin-producing neurons in the guinea pig brain. I. The classical hypothalamo-neurohypophyseal system. Cell Tiss Res 196:367–384.

Sofroniew MV, Weindl A, Wetzstein R (1977) Immunoperoxidase staining of vasopressin in the rat median eminence following adrenalectomy and steroid substitution. Acta endocrinol Suppl 212:93.

Stumpf WE (1968) Estrogen-concentrating neurons: Topography in the hypothalamus by dry-mount autoradiography. Science 162:1001–1003.

Swanson LW, McKellar S (1979) The distribution of oxytocin- and neuro-physin-stained fibers in the spinal cord of the rat and monkey. J Comp Neurol 188:87–106.

Watson SJ, Barchas JD, Li CH (1978) β-Lipotropin localization of cells and axons in rat brain by immunocytochemistry. Proc Nat Acad Sci 74:5155–5158.

Weindl A, Joynt RJ (1972) The median eminence as a circumventricular organ. In: Knigge KM, Scott DE, Weindl A (eds) Brain-endocrine interaction: Median eminence structure and function. Karger, Basel, pp.281–297.

Weindl A, Sofroniew MV (1978) Neurohormones and circumventricular organs. An immunohistochemical investigation. In: Scott DE, Kozlowski GP, Weindl A (eds) Brain-endocrine interaction III. Neural hormones and reproduction. Karger Basel, pp.117–137.

Weindl A, Sofroniew MV (1980a) Immunohistochemical localization of hypo-thalamic peptide hormones in neural target areas. In: Wuttke W, Weindl A, Voigt K-H, Dries R-R (eds) Brain and pituitary peptides, pp.97–109.

Weindl A, Sofroniew MV (1980b) Relation of neuropeptides to circum-ventricular organs. In: Martin JB, Bick K, Reichlin S (eds) Neurosecretion and brain peptides. Implications for brain function and neurological disease. Raven Press, New York, in press.

Weindl A, Sofroniew MV (1980c) Funktionelle Anatomie neuroendokriner Systeme. In: Buchborn E (ed) Proceedings of the German Society of Internal Medicine. J.F. Bergmann, München, in press.

Anatomical Relationships Between Estrogen Target Sites and Peptidergic-Aminergic Neurons: Multiple Activation of Heterogeneous Systems (MAHS)

W.E. Stumpf and M. Sar, Chapel Hill

Sites of hormone production and action in the brain can be defined through the use of histochemical techniques, such as formaldehyde induced fluorescence of catechol- and indolamines, autoradiography with radioactively labeled substances, and immunohistochemistry with specific antibodies. The term hormonearchitecture has been introduced – in analogy to cyto-, chemo-, and angio-architecture – for the anatomical distribution and relationships of sites of production and action of chemical messengers (Stumpf, 1975). The word hormone is understood in its widest sense to include multipotential messengers such as norepinephrine and serotonin, being distributed by blood, cerebrospinal fluid, or diffusion through tissue. Advancement of hormone architectonics of the brain is linked to development of techniques. Localization of steroid hormone target sites at the cellular and subcellular light microscopic level became possible through the introduction of the dry-mount and thaw-mount autoradiographic techniques (Stumpf and Roth, 1966; Stumpf and Sar, 1975a). Procedures applied by others, such as apposition techniques, embedding in paraffin or resin, or double fixation of frozen sections, were unsuccessful.

The topographical pattern of distribution of estrogen target neurons was defined first in the rat diencephalon (Stumpf, 1968), lower brain stem (Stumpf, 1970; Stumpf and Sar, 1975b), telencephalon and spinal cord (Stumpf 1970), and confirmed in part by others. Phylogenetic studies demonstrated the presence of estrogen target sites in the brain of representatives of all vertebrate classes (Kim et al., 1978; Stumpf and Sar, 1978a). Ontogenetic studies revealed the existence of nuclear target sites in the brain of 2-day neonatal rats (Sheridan et al., 1974), 16-day fetal mice (Stumpf and Sar, 1978b), and 10-day chicken embryo (Martinze-Vargas et al., 1975). Results from competition studies in our laboratory and chemical characterization of radioactivity from brain extracts in several other laboratories suggest that the radioactivity which is concentrated and retained in cell nuclei after injection of ^{3}H estradiol and ^{3}H diethylstilbestrol, is specific for estrogen.

We have provided evidence that all steroid hormones have target sites in neural tissues and in the adenohypophysis. In addition to estrogens, this includes androgens (Sar and Stumpf, 1972), progestagens (Sar and Stumpf, 1973), gluco- and mineralcorticosteroids (Stumpf and Sar, 1979), as well as $1,25 (OH)_2$ vitamin D_3 (Stumpf et al., 1979; Sar et al., 1980).

As early as 1968, we proposed that steroid hormones are activators of target neurons (Stumpf, 1968) based on evidence derived from their nuclear concentration in neurons and genomic actions. We also suggested that the negative feedback, generally perceived as a direct action of gonadal steroids, is a primary stimulatory feedback and that inhibitory effects are mediated through the steroid stimulated production of messengers, in turn mediating a secondary inhibitory effect (Stumpf, 1970; Stumpf and Sar, 1973).

As we shall see, this line of thinking appears to be correct. Evidence is now accumulating that, for instance, estrogen stimulates turnover of neural messengers related to pituitary LH release. In order to prove that steroid hormones act directly on neurohormone producing cells, efforts were made in our laboratory to provide simultaneous demonstrations of two hormones in the same histological section. If successful, this would resolve the question, whether or not steroid hormones concentrate in nuclei of catecholamine and peptide producing cells. Also, it would provide clues as to which neurohormones innervate a given population of steroid hormone target cells. Close anatomical correlation and direct interactions between peptidergic-aminergic neurons and steroid hormones were expected to exist from topographical overlap of hormone target and production sites (Stumpf and Sar, 1977). However, demonstrative proof was required.

1. Combined Autoradiography of Steroid Hormones and Formaldehyde-induced Fluorescence of Catecholamines

Four to six µm freeze-dried sections, obtained from the brains of animals which were injected with tritiated steroid hormones, were treated with paraformaldehyde vapor, photographically exposed and processed. Radioactivity, related to steroids, and fluorescence, related to catecholamines, were both preserved in these unembedded sections (Grant and Stumpf, 1975). With this approach (Fig. 1) it was found that dopaminergic neurons in the arcuate-periventricular nucleus of the rat hypothalamus concentrate ^{3}H estradiol in their nuclei, as do catecholamine neurons in the pons in the locus ceruleus, the subceruleal region and in an area ventral to the

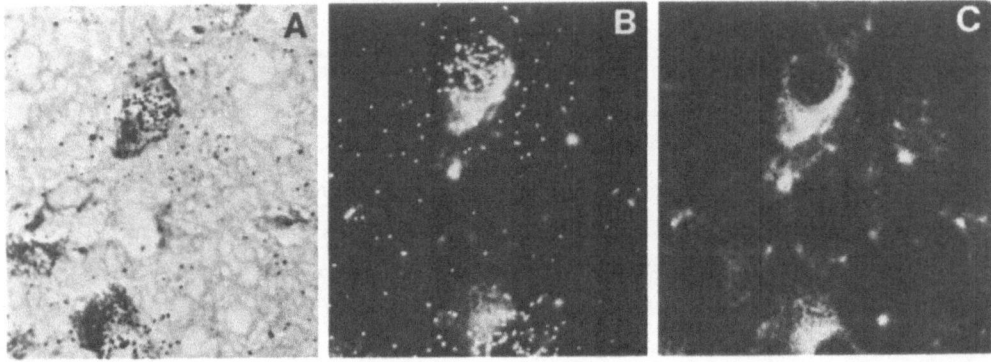

Figure 1: Combined autoradiogram after ^{3}H estradiol-17β injection with formaldehyde induced fluorescence for catecholamines. Neurons of the rat nucleus reticularis lateralis region show nuclear concentration of radio-activity with transmitted light (A and B) and fluorescence in perikarya with ultraviolet light (B and C). Note combination of nuclear radio-activity and cytoplasmic fluorescence in B. From Heritage et al., 1979

pedunculus cerebellaris superior, and in the medulla in and adjacent to the nucleus reticularis lateralis and in the nucleus tractus solitarii (Heritage et al., 1977). Recently, these results were confirmed with antibodies to dopamine-β-hydroxylase as an indicator for catecholamine neurons (see Sar and Stumpf, this volume).

When the androgen ^{3}H-dihydrotestosterone was used, nuclear concentration of radioactivity and catecholamine fluorescence in the same neuron were found in dopaminergic cells in the arcuate-peri-

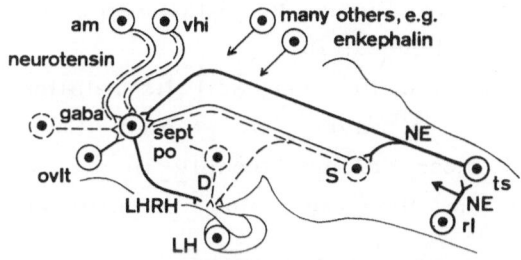

Figure 2: Multiple activation of heterogeneous system (MAHS) by estrogen for regulation of LHRH-LH secretion. Evidence suggests that estrogen genomically activates specific target neuron groups for production and secretion of specific messengers. Catecholaminergic estrogen target neurons (NE) in the nucleus reticularis lateralis (rl) and nucleus tractus solitarii (ts) stimulate septal-preoptic (sept-pt) LHRH producing neurons for initiation of the ovulatory LHRH peak. Certain LHRH neurons are probably also directly activated by estrogen. The release of LHRH stimulates gonadotropes, which are also estrogen target cells and activated by estrogen for LH secretion ("positive feedback"). Simultaneous estrogen activation of dopaminergic (D) and serotoninergic (S) estrogen target neurons may lead to messenger production and release with inhibitory effects on LHRH neurons or gonadotropes. Such secondary inhibitory mechanisms may be a basis for "negative feedback". Estrogen activation of certain GABAergic, neurotensinergic, enkephalinergic and other neuronal systems probably is also involved. Regional quantitative differences in nuclear estrogen binding - in part incurred by the steroidal milieu - may reflect differential sensitivities and responses regarding time of release and tissue levels of messengers. For messengers, such as serotonin, which exert both stimulatory (solid line) and at other times inhibitory (dashed line) actions, changes of membrane receptors may be involved. Among the many afferents, entered are those from the amygdala (am), the vascular organ of the lamina terminalis (OVLT), and the ventral hippocampus (vhi)

ventricular nucleus, as well as in catecholaminergic cells in the pons, in the locus ceruleus and in the subceruleal area, at the lateral corner of the fourth ventricle, in the substantia grisea, in the nucleus parabrachialis medialis and near the nucleus olivarius superior, while no such relationship could be observed in catecholamine neurons in the medulla oblongata, contrary to results obtained with ^{3}H-estradiol (Heritage et al., 1980).

In many of the brain regions which accumulate target neurons for sex steroids a close network of catecholamine fibers is found (Heritage et al., 1980). This suggests an interesting dual or multiple action of the same steroid hormone on certain of its target cells, which are innervated by messenger producing cells, themselves target cells for the same hormone. In Figure 2, relationships are depicted as suggested by results from above studies.

Effects of estrogen on catecholamine turnover and its relationship to the preovulatory LHRH–LH surge have been studied (Honma and Wuttke, 1980). The results of those studies strongly suggest an important role of catecholamines in the regulation of pituitary functions.

Connections between catecholamine neurons in the medulla and hypothalamic nuclei have been demonstrated (Ricardo and Koh, 1978; Day et al., 1980). Conflicting reports about the effectiveness of lesions of the ventral noradrenergic bundle (Hancke and Wuttke, 1979) do not contradict the concept that connections between the hindbrain and forebrain are essential for the trigger of ovulation.

Figure 2 depicts schematically our concept about the activation of multiple messenger systems by estrogen, which influence LHRH–LH release. There is supportive evidence published in the literature for the involvement of serotonin (Al Satli, 1979; Parker et al., 1979), GABA (Ondo, 1974; Earley and Leonard, 1978), enkephalin (Dupont et al., 1980) and many others.

2. Combined Autoradiography of Steroid Hormones and Immunohistochemistry of Antibodies

Autoradiograms prepared after the dry-mount or thaw-mount procedure may be used for immunohistochemistry in order to obtain in the same preparation information from both approaches (Sar and Stumpf, 1979; Sar and Stumpf, 1980). At the end of autoradiographic exposure, the autoradiogram is histologically fixed before being photographically processed. The developed autoradiogram is then treated with antibodies according to a modified bridge technique, described earlier by Sar and Stumpf (1980; and in this volume). With this combination technique it could be demonstrated that neurophysin immunoreactive cells concentrate estrogen in their nuclei (Fig. 3). Accordingly, a relationship can be proposed for the neurophysin systems with other estrogen activated messenger systems (Fig. 4) as it has been indicated for the LHRH release system.

Secretion of neurophysin and its associated hormones vasopressin and oxytocin is stimulated by estrogen (Crowley et al.,

22

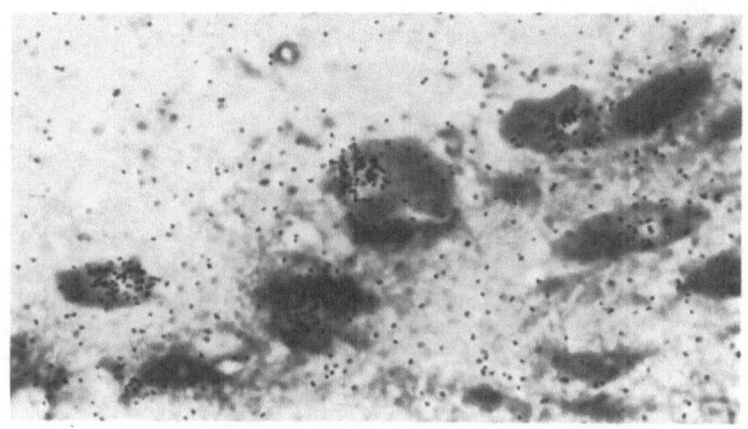

Figure 3:   Combined autoradiogram after ^{3}H estradiol-17β injection with immunohistochemistry using antiserum Neurophysin I. Magnocellular neurons in rat anterior hypothalamus show nuclear concentration of radioactivity and cytoplasmic staining with antibody.   From Sar and Stumpf, 1981.

1978), probably through both direct (Sar and Stumpf, 1980; Yukitake, 1978) and indirect stimulation. The latter involves catecholamines (Crowley et al., 1978). Involvement of other messengers is suggested, but remains to be established.   Since vasopressinergic and oxytociner- gic neurons form separate systems (Vandesande and Dierickx, 1975), an analysis of the individual systems will be required in order to define their relationships to the proposed and other messenger systems.

Enkephalinergic neurons (Sar et al., 1978) and estrogen target neurons overlap topographically in the hypothalamic paraventricular and supraoptic nucleus, lateral preoptic region, nucleus (n.) peri- fornicalis, n. amygdaloideus medialis and centralis, n. para- brachialis lateralis, n. tractus solitarii, n. reticularis lateralis, n. raphes magnus, locus ceruleus and subceruleus, spinal cord substantia gelatinosa, cerebellar Golgy type II cells and others. Support through results from physiological studies is forthcoming. Estrogen treatment increases Met-enkephalin levels in globus pallidus, n. interstitialis striae terminalis, medial and lateral pre- optic nuclei and periaqueductal gray, while a decrease in the n. amygdaloideus centralis was found, assessed by radioimmunoassay (Dupont et al., 1980).

β-endorphin is present, as assessed by radioimmunoassay, in

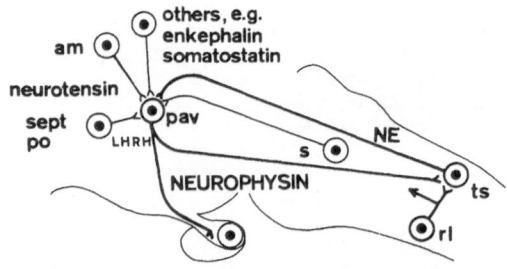

Figure 4: The principle of differential multiple activation of heterogeneous systems (MAHS) by estrogen applies to the secretion of neurophysin and its related peptides, as it does to the secretion of LHRH
(Fig. 2) and probably enkephalin, neurotensin and others. Estrogen
directly activates neurophysin neurons in the paraventricular nucleus
(pav) (Sar and Stumpf, 1980). In addition, it is proposed that estrogen
activates specific target–neuron groups which influence neurophysin
secretion. This is supported by incomplete evidence. As shown in figure
2 for LHRH, catecholaminergic estrogen target neurons (NE) in the lower
brainstem project to estrogen target neurons in the paraventricular
nucleus. Similarly, serotoninergic estrogen target neurons (S) in the
raphe nuclei, estrogen target neurons in the septal-preoptic region
(sept–pt), the medial amygdala (am), and elsewhere, are likely to modulate functions of neurons in the paraventricular nucleus through genomic
activation of secretion of chemical messengers. Since estrogen binding
varies among different target neuron groups, production and release of
individual messengers probably follows individual time–dose responses
which are likely to be dependent on estrogen blood levels and the
hormonal milieu. Differential modulation of cell functions and numbers of
receptors caused, for instance, by estrogen-progestagen actions, may
account for changes in time related secretory patterns. Only a few of the
neurophysin projections are indicated here, including an apparent feed-
back-loop to the catecholaminergic estrogen target neurons in the
medulla, nucleus tractus solitarii (ts) and, perhaps, the nucleus
reticularis lateralis (rl). Estrogen activation of pituicytes, also
target cells for estradiol, may play some role in hormonal release

the medial preoptic nucleus, the n. interstitialis striae terminalis
and the periaqueductal gray (Dupont et al., 1980). In all of these
sites estrogen target neurons are concentrated.

Somatostatin immunoreactive perikarya (Finley et al., 1981)
overlap in their anatomical distribution with estrogen target cells in
the n. olfactorius anterior, n. septi lateralis, n. periventricularis
hypothalami, zona incerta, certain amygdaloid nuclei, midbrain
periaqueductal gray, n. parabrachialis lateralis, n. tractus solitarii, n. reticularis lateralis, n. reticularis gigantocellularis dorsalis and ventralis (pars α) and others.

Neurotensin immunoreactive cell bodies (Uhl et al., 1979, Kahn
et al., 1980) overlap in their topographical distribution with

24

estrogen target neurons in amygdaloidal sites of origin of the stria terminalis. The stria terminalis is a major link of sex steroid hormone target sites in the brain (Stumpf, 1975) and reported to transport neurotensin amygdalofugally (Uhl et al., 1979). Nuclear groups include the n. amgydaloideus medialis and centralis, n. preopticus medialis and lateralis, n. periventricularis hypothalami, n. perifornicalis, n. paraventricularis, n. arcuatus hypothalami, ventral tegmental area, periaqueductal gray, n. raphes dorsalis, locus ceruleus, n. parabrachialis medialis and lateralis, n. tractus solitarii and substantia gelatinosa.

3. Conclusions

From the topographical distribution of estrogen target neurons it is expected that many of the brain messenger systems can be chemically addressed by this steroid hormone. The relationships outlined for the LHRH as well as oxytocin release regulation (Figs. 2 and 4) appear paradigmatic and lead us to propose the principle of multiple activation of heterogeneous systems (MAHS) by steroid hormones. Thus, simultaneously different neuronal circuits may be activated in a purposeful manner. The degree of this activation most likely is dependent on blood and tissue levels of steroid hormones and the number of binding (receptor) sites in the steroid hormone target cells. Since the number of binding sites in a given target cell is believed to correlate with its capability to respond, a certain blood level of steroid hormone can be expected to lead to a differential activation of various brain target cell populations. Considerable differences in nuclear estrogen concentration for different neuronal cell populations have been described, which may provide a basis for the proposed differential activation.

Hormonal preconditions of the animal, which can lead to estrogen or progestagen related stimulation or suppression of hormone receptors – probably in a non-uniform fashion as demonstrated for the uterus (Stumpf and Sar, 1976) and pituitary (Keefer et al., 1976) – are expected to modulate steroid hormone effects. During the course of steroid hormone action, a quantitative and differential receptor shift, as indicated above for the uterus, can be expected to

occur in certain neuronal target cell populations, through which an
initial positive feedback action may subsequently be converted into a
negative feedback action or vice versa.

Acknowledgements

Supported by US PHS grant NS-09914 and NIMH grant HD-03110

References

Al Satli M (1979) Données nouvelles sur les mécanismes sérotoninergiques
    de l'ovulation au cours du cycle chez la ratte.   com ren séan Soc
    Biol 173:132.
Crowley WR, O'Donohue TL, George JM, Jacobowitz DM (1978) Changes in
    pituitary oxytocin and vasopressin during the estrous cycle and after
    ovarian hormones: Evidence for mediation by norepinephrine.   Life
    Sciences 23:2579-2586.
Day TA, Blessing W, Willoughby TO (1980) Noradrenergic and dopaminergic
    projections to the medial preoptic area of the rat.   A combined
    horseradish peroxidase/catecholamine fluorescence study.   Brain Res
    193:543-548.
Dupont A, Barden N, Cusan L, Mérand Y, Labrie F, Vaudry H (1980)
    β-endorphins and Met-enkephalins: their distribution, modulation by
    estrogens and haloperidol, and role in neuroendocrine control.   Fed
    Proc 39:2544-2550.
Earley CJ, Leonard BE (1978) GABA and gonadal hormones.   Brain Res
    155:27-34.
Finley JCW, Maderdrut JL, Roger LJ, Petrusz P (1981) The immunohisto-
    chemical localization of somatostatin-containing cells in the rat
    central nervous system.   Neuroscience in press.
Grant LD, Stumpf WE (1975) Hormone uptake sites in relation to CNS
    biogenic amine system.   In: Stumpf WE, Grant LD (eds) Anatomical
    Neuroendocrinology.   Karger, Basel, pp.445-464.
Hancke JL, Wuttke W (1979) Effects of chemical lesion of the ventral
    noradrenergic bundle or of the medial preoptic area on preovulatory
    LH release in rats.   Exp Brain Res 35:127-134.
Heritage AS, Grant LD, Stumpf WE (1977) ^{3}H estradiol in catecholamine
    neurons of rat brain stem: Combined localization by autoradiography
    and formaldehyde-induced fluorescence. J Comp Neurol 176:607-630.
Heritage AS, Stumpf WE, Sar M, Grant LD (1980) Brainstem catecholamine
    neurons are target sites for sex steroid hormones.   Science 207:1377-
    1379.
Honma K, Wuttke W (1980) Norepinephrine and dopamine turnover rates in
    the medial preoptic area and the mediobasal hypothalamus of the rat
    brain after various endocrinological manipulations.   Endocrinology
    106:1848-1853.
Kahn D, Abrams GM, Zimmerman EA, Carraway R, Leeman SE (1980) Neurotensin
    neurons in the rat hypothalamus: An immunocytochemical study.   Endo-
    crinology 107:47-54.
Keefer DA, Stumpf WE, Petrusz P (1976) Quantitative autoradiographic
    assessment of ^{3}H estradiol uptake in immunocytochemically characteriz-
    ed pituitary cells.   Cell Tiss Res 166:25-35.

Kim YS, Stumpf WE, Sar M, Martinze-Vargas MC (1978) Estrogen and androgen target cells in the brain of fishes, reptiles and birds: Phylogeny and ontogeny. Am Zool 18:425–433.

Martinze-Vargas MC, Gibson DB, Sar M, Stumpf WE (1975) Estrogen target sites in brain of the chick embryo. Science 190:1307–1308.

Ondo JG (1974) Gamma-aminobutyric acid effects on pituitary gonadotropin secretion. Science 186:738–739.

Parker VD, Soliman KFA, Walker CA (1979) The involvement of serotonin in induced ovulation in the immature rat. Experientia 35:692–693.

Ricardo JA, Koh ET (1978) Anatomical evidence of direct projections from the nucleus of the solitary tract to the hypothalamus, amygdala and other forebrain structures in the rat. Brain Res 153:1–26.

Sar M, Stumpf WE (1972) Cellular localization of androgen in the brain and pituitary after the injection of tritiated testosterone. Experientia 28:1364–1366.

Sar M, Stumpf WE (1973) Neurons of the hypothalamus concentrate ^{3}H-progesterone or metabolites of it. Science 182:1266–1268.

Sar M, Stumpf WE (1979) Simultaneous localization of steroid and peptide hormones in rat pituitary by combined thaw-mount autoradiography and immunohistochemistry: Localization of dihydrotestosterone in gonadotropes, thyrotropes and pituicytes. Cell Tiss Res 203:1–7.

Sar M, Stumpf WE (1980) Simultaneous localization of ^{3}H estradiol and neurophysin I or arginine vasopressin in hypothalamic neurons demonstrated by a combined technique of dry-mount autoradiography and immunohistochemistry. Neuroscience Letters 17:179–184.

Sar M, Stumpf WE (1981) Combined autoradiography and immunohistochemistry for simultaneous localization of radioactively labeled steroid hormones and antibodies in the brain. J Histochem Cytochem in press.

Sar M, Stumpf WE, DeLuca HF (1980) Thyrotropes in the pituitary are target cells for 1,25 (OH)$_2$ vitamin D$_3$. Cell Tiss Res 309:161–166.

Sar M, Stumpf WE, Miller RJ, Chang K-J, Cuatrecasas P (1978) Immunohistochemical localization on enkephalin in rat brain and spinal cord. J Comp Neurol 182:17–38.

Sheridan PF, Sar M, Stumpf WE (1974) Autoradiographic localization of ^{3}H estradiol or its metabolites in the central nervous system of the developing rat. Endocrinology 94:1386–1390.

Stumpf WE (1968) Estradiol concentrating neurons: Topography in the hypothalamus by dry-mount autoradiography. Science 162:1001–1003.

Stumpf WE (1970) Estrogen-neurons and estrogen-neuron systems in the periventricular brain. Am J Anat 129:207–218.

Stumpf WE (1975) The Brain: An endocrine gland and hormone target, an introduction. In: Stumpf WE, Grant LD (eds) Anatomical Neuroendocrinology. Karger, Basel, pp.2–8.

Stumpf WE, Roth LJ (1966) High resolution autoradiography with dry-mounted, freeze-dried, frozen sections. Comparative study of six methods using two diffusible compounds, ^{3}H-estradiol and ^{3}H-mesobilirubinogen. J Histochem Cytochem 14:274–287.

Stumpf WE, Sar M (1973) Hormonal inputs to releasing factor cells, feedback sites. In: Gispen WH, Zimmerman E, Marks BH, de Wied D (eds) Progress in Brain Research 39, Elsevier, Amsterdam, pp.53–71.

Stumpf WE, Sar M (1975a) Autoradiographic techniques for localizing steroid hormones. In: O'Malley BW, Hardman JG (eds) Methods in Enzymology, Vol. XXXVI, Hormone Action, Part A. Steroid Hormones. Academic Press, New York, pp.135–156.

Stumpf WE, Sar M (1975b) Anatomical distribution of corticosterone concentrating neurons in rat brain. In: Stumpf WE, Grant LD (eds) Anatomical Neuroendocrinology. Karger, Basel, pp.82–103.

Stumpf WE, Sar M (1976) Autoradiographic localization of estrogen, androgen, progestin and glucocorticosteroid in "target tissues" and "non-target tissues". In: Pasqualini J (ed) Receptors and Mechanism of Action of Steroid Hormones, Modern Pharmacology-Toxicology, Vol. 8. Marcel Dekker, New York, pp.41-84.

Stumpf WE, Sar M (1977) Steroid hormone target cells in the periventricular brain: Relationship to peptide hormone-producing cells. Fed Proc 36:1973-1977.

Stumpf WE, Sar M (1978a) Anatomical distribution of estrogen, androgen, progestin, corticosteroid and thyroid hormone target sites in the brain of mammals: Phylogeny and ontogeny. Am Zool 18:435-445.

Stumpf WE, Sar M (1978b) Estrogen target cells in fetal brain. In: Dörner G, Kawakami M (eds) Hormones and Brain Development. Elsevier/North-Holland, Amsterdam, pp.27-33.

Stumpf WE, Sar M (1979) Clucocorticosteroid and mineral corticosteroid hormone target sites in the brain: Autoradiographic studies with corticosterone, aldosterone and dexamethasone. In: Jones MT, Dallman MF, Gillham B, Chattopadhyay S (eds) Interactions within the Brain-Pituitary Adrenocortical System. Academic Press, New York, pp.137-147.

Stumpf WE, Sar M, Reid FA, Tanaka Y, DeLuca HF (1979) Target cells for 1,25-dihydroxy-vitamin D_3 in intestinal tract, stomach, kidney, skin, pituitary and parathyroid. Science 206:1188-1190.

Uhl G, Goodman RR, Snyder S (1979) Neurotensin-containing cell bodies, fibers, and nerve terminals in the brainstem of the rat: immunohistochemical mapping. Brain Res 167:77-91.

Vandesande F, Dierickx K (1975) Identification of the vasopressin producing and of the oxytocin producing neurons in the hypothalamic magnocellular neurosecretory system of the rat. Cell Tiss Res 164:153-162.

Yukitake Y (1978) Possible relations between the secretory cycle of the neurosecretory cells in the rat paraventricular nucleus and the estrous cycle. Arch histol jap 41:471-482.

Estradiol Concentration in Dopamine-β-hydroxylase Containing Neurons of Lower Brain Stem Demonstrated by Combined Autoradiography and Immunohistochemistry

M. Sar and W.E. Stumpf, Chapel Hill

Central catecholamines play an important role in the regulation of hormone secretion from the pituitary gland (Kalra et al., 1972; Kalra and McCann, 1973; McCann and Moss, 1975). Norepinephrine has been shown to stimulate the release of luteinizing hormone probably by influencing the secretion of LH–RH (Simpkins and Kalra, 1979; Honma and Wuttke, 1980). The medial preoptic and hypothalamic areas, including the median eminence, contain noradrenaline terminals which originate from discrete noradrenaline cell groups in the lower brain stem (Dahlström and Fuxe, 1964). These cell groups are immunohistochemically identified with antiserum to dopamine-β-hydroxylase (DBH), the enzyme which converts dopamine to noradrenaline (Swanson and Hartmann, 1975). Steroid hormones have been shown to influence catecholamine metabolism in the central nervous system (Beattie et al., 1972; Crowley et al., 1978; Krieger and Wuttke, 1980; Stefano and Donoso, 1965). Estradiol concentrating neurons are localized by thaw–mount autoradiography in many areas of the lower brain stem where catecholamine neurons exist. Using a combined technique of autoradiography and immunohistochemistry developed in our laboratory (Sar and Stumpf, 1979, 1980a) we have demonstrated that certain DBH containing neurons in rat lower brain stem concentrate estradiol in their nuclei (Sar and Stumpf, 1980b), thus exhibiting direct morphological interrelationships between steroid hormone sites of action and noradrenaline producing neurons.

1. Materials and Methods

Adult female Holtzman Sprague–Dawley rats (n=6) castrated for 72 hours were injected intravenously with $0.5\,\mu\,g/100\,g$ b.w. of 2, 4, 6, 7-^{3}H estradiol -17β (specific activity 95 Ci/mM). After one hour, rats were decapitated, the lower brain stem was dissected, frozen in liquified propane ($-180^{\circ}C$) and processed for thaw-mount autoradiography (Stumpf and Sar, 1975). After a wash with PBS the autoradiographic slides were stained by the immunoperoxidase method described earlier (Sar et al., 1978; Sar and Stumpf, 1979) with antiserum to dopamine-β-hydroxylase at an optimal dilution of 1:500. For control, autoradiograms were incubated with normal rabbit serum at the same dilution.

2. Results

Autoradiograms of rat lower brain stem after ^{3}H-estradiol injection, when stained immunohistochemically with DBH antiserum, showed DBH positive cells in certain regions of the pons and medulla oblongata (Figs. 1-4). The strongest DBH positive staining was observed in cells of the locus ceruleus (Group A5). Approximately 30 to 40% of these cells showed nuclear concentration of radioactivity (Figs. 1,3). Similarly, about 30% of the DBH-stained cells which belong to the subceruleus group (Group A6) were labeled with ^{3}H-estradiol. These cells were located in the ventrolateral part of the pons around the lateral and dorsal aspect of the superior olivary nucleus and near the lateral lemniscus in the lateral tegmental area (Fig. 3).

In the medulla oblongata two groups of DBH positive cells were observed; a ventrolateral (A1) and a dorsomedial group (A2). The cells of the ventrolateral group were found around the lateral reticular nucleus. About 50% of these cells showed nuclear concentration of radioactivity (Fig. 4). The cells of the dorsomedial group were located within the nucleus of the solitary tract and about 70-80% of these cells were labeled with ^{3}H-estradiol (Fig. 2,4). In addition, some DBH positive cells of the area postrema showed nuclear concentration of ^{3}H-estradiol.

3. Discussion

The results of our combined autoradiography and immunohisto-

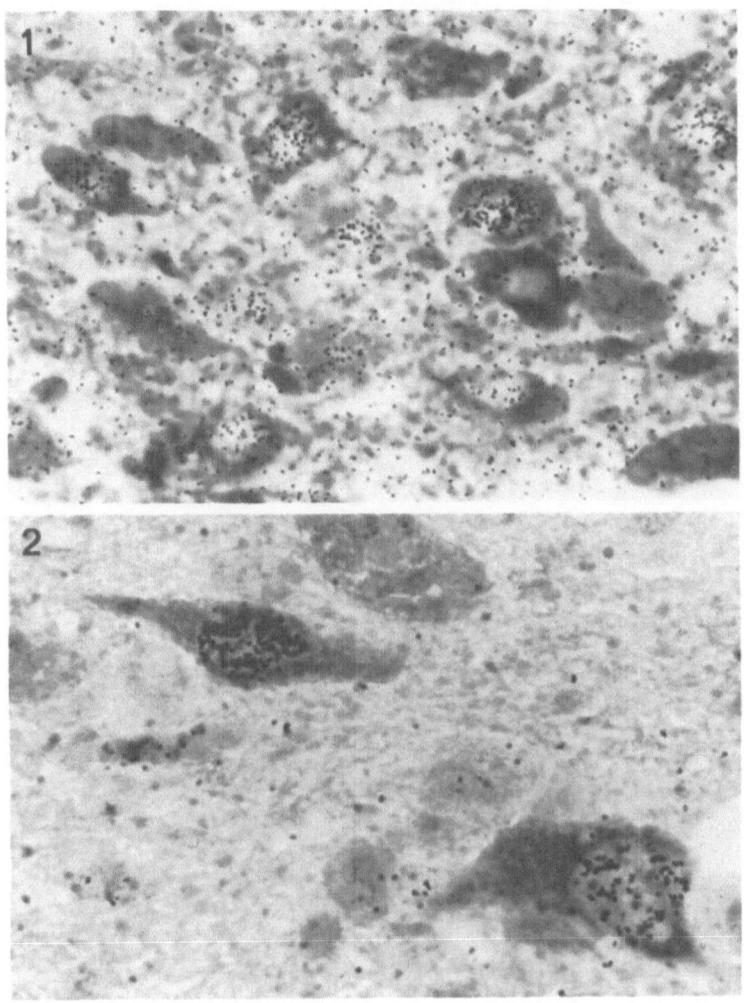

Figures 1-2:   Thaw-mount autoradiograms of rat lower brain stem prepared
one hour after injection of ^{3}H estradiol and stained by immunoperoxidase
method with DBH antiserum (1:500). Note the nuclear concentration of
radioactivity in DBH positive cells of the locus ceruleus (Fig. 4 x 1120)
and nucleus tractus solitarii (Fig. 5 x 1400)

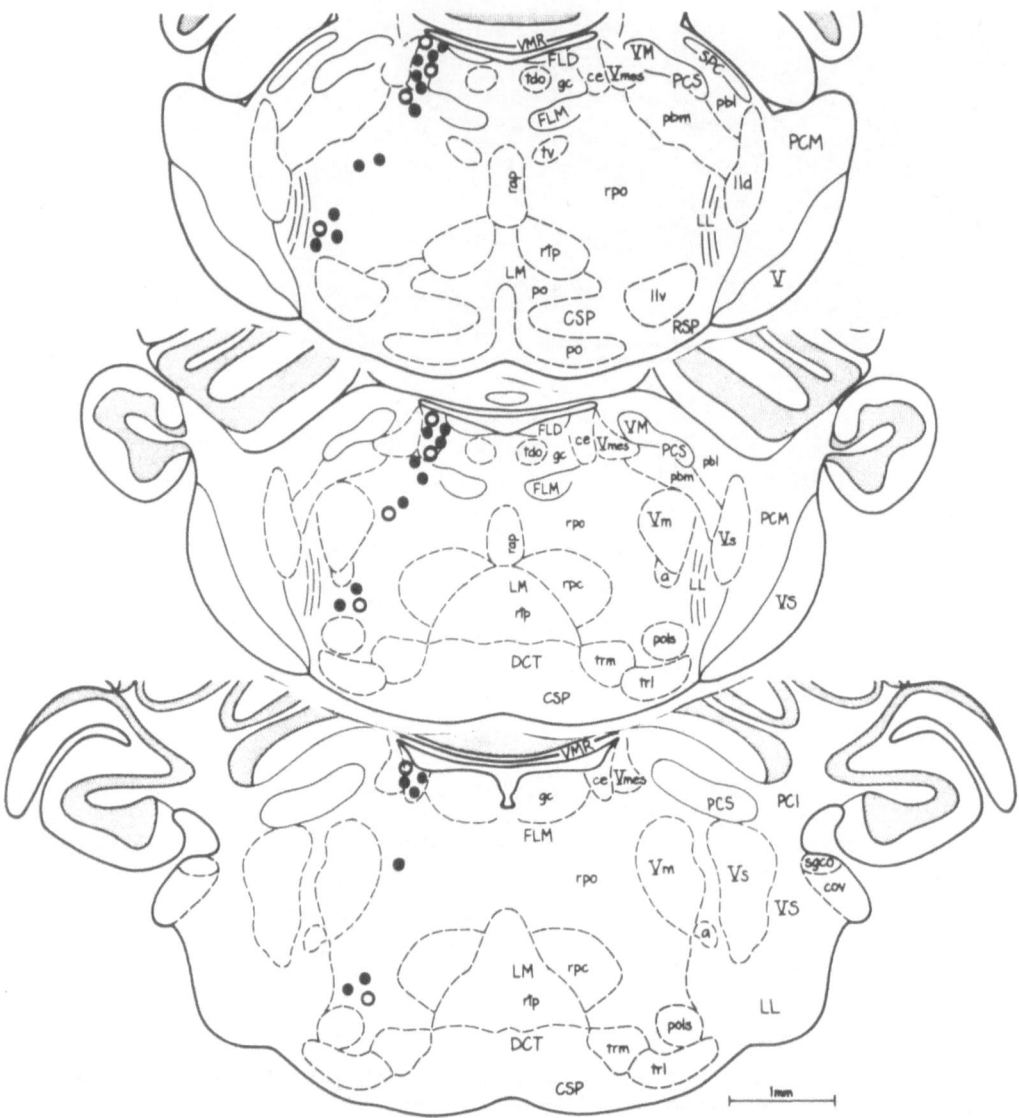

Figure 3: Legend see Figure 4 (next page)

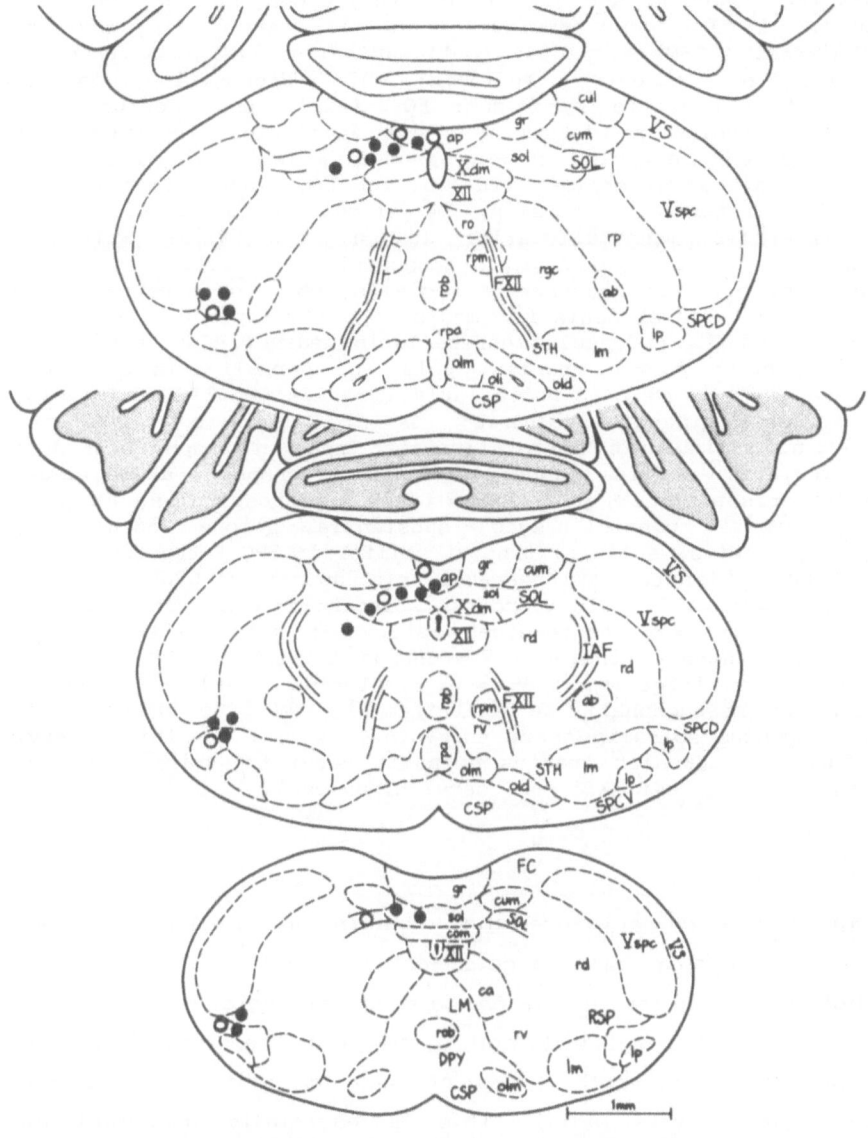

Figures 3-4: Schematic drawings (Frontal plane) show DBH containing neurons which concentrate estradiol (•) in pons (Fig. 3) and medulla oblongata (Fig. 4) at three different levels. Some DBH containing neurons (O) do not show nuclear concentration of radioactivity. (Abbreviations, see next page)

Abbreviations for Figures 3 and 4:   nucleus (n.) alpha; ab = n. ambiguus; ap = area postrema; ce = locus ceruleus; com = n. commissuralis; cov = n. cochlearis ventralis; CSP = tractus corticospinalis; culs = n. cuneatus lateralis;   cum = n.   cuneatus   medialis;   DCT = decussatio   corporis trapezoidei; DPY = decussatio pyramidum; FC = fasciculus cuneatus; FLD = fasciculus longitudinalis dorsalis; FLM = fasciculus longitudinalis medialis; gc = griseum centrale; gr = n. gracilis; IAF = fibrae arcuatae internae; LL = lemniscus lateralis; lld = n. lemnisci lateralis dorsalis; llv = n. lemnisci lateralis ventralis; LM = lemniscus medialis; lm = n. reticularis lateralis magnocellularis; lp = n. reticularis lateralis parvocellularis;   old = n.   olivarios   accessorius   dorsalis;   oli = n. olivaris; olm = n. olivaris accessorius medialis; pbl = n. parabrachialis lateralis;   pbm = n.   parabrachialis medialis; PCI = pedunculus cere-bellaris inferior; PCM = pedunculus cerebellaris medius; PCS = pedunculus cerebellaris superior; po = n. pontis; pols = n. paraolivaris superior; rap = n. raphes pontis; rd = n. reticularis dorsalis medullae oblongata; rgc = n. reticularis giagantocellularis; ro = n. Roller; rob = n. raphe obscurus; rp = n. reticularis parvocellularis; rpa = n. raphe pallidus; rpc = n. reticularis pontis caudalis; rpm = n. raphe paramedianus; rpo = n. reticularis pontis oralis; RSP = tractus rubrospinalis; rtp = n. reticularis   tegmenti   pontis;   sgco = substantia   gliosa   cochlearis; SOL = tractus solitarius; sol = n. tractus solitarii; SPC = tractus spino-cerebellaris; SPCD = tractus spinocerebellaris dorsalis; SPCV = tractus spinocerebellaris ventralis; STH = tractus spinothalamicus; tdo = n. teg-mentalis dorsalis; trl = n. trapezoides lateralis; trm = n. trapezoides medialis; tv = n. ventralis thalami; V = nervus trigeminus; VM = tractus mesencephalicus nervitrigemini; Vm = n.   motorius   nervi   trigemini; Vmes = n. tractus mesencephali nervi trigemini; VMR = velum medullare rostrale; VS = tractus spinalis nervi trigemini; Vs = n. sensibilis nervi trigemini; Vspc = n. caudalis tractus spinalis nervi trigemini; Xdm = n. dorsalis motorius nervi vagi; XII = n. nervi hypoglossi.

chemistry study provide evidence that certain DBH positive neurons in the lower brain stem are targets for estradiol.   This suggests that estradiol has a direct action on catecholaminergic neurons.   Our study with DBH antiserum did not distinguish noradrenaline and adrenaline neurons since both types of neurons contain the trans-mitter–synthesizing enzyme DBH.   This is especially important for catecholamine neurons in the region of nucleus tractus solitarii and nucleus reticularis lateralis where the existence of both noradrena-line and adrenaline neurons has been reported (Hökfelt et al., 1974).

Catecholamines in the medial preoptic area have been implicated in the control of thermoregulation (Day et al., 1979), cardiovascular functions (Struyker et al., 1975), and pituitary secretion (Kalra and McCann, 1973; McCann and Moss, 1975).   The NA turnover rate in the medial preoptic area has been well correlated with serum LH levels suggesting a stimulatory action of NE on LH–RH release (Honma and

Wuttke, 1980). Employing the combined localization of retrogradely transported HRP and CA - fluorescence, Day et al. (1980) demonstrated that the noradrenaline innervation of the medial preoptic area is derived from the nucleus tractus solitarii and nucleus reticularis lateralis of the medulla. In the medial preopic area DBH activity is reduced but norepinephrine turnover rate is increased (Krieger and Wuttke, 1980) following ovariectomy. The effect of estradiol on gonadotropin secretion may involve an activation of NA system through a genomic action of estradiol on catecholamine neurons in the lower brain stem. Thus NA terminals in the medial preoptic area which are derived from these neurons may directly stimulate LH–RH neurons to release LH–RH.

Acknowledgements

We thank Dr. T.H. Joh, Department of Neurology, Cornell Medical College, New York, for kindly supplying rabbit antiserum to rat DBH. Supported by PHS Grant NS-09914.

References

Beattie CW, Rodgers CH, Soyka LF (1972) Influence of ovariectomy and ovarian steroids on hypothalamic tyrosine hydroxylase activity in the rat. Endocrinology 91:226–279.

Crowley WR, O'Donohue JL, Wachslicht H, Jacobowitz DM (1978) Effects of estrogen and progesterone on plasma gonadotropins and on catecholamine levels and turnover in discrete brain regions of ovariectomized rat. Brain Res 154:345–357.

Dahlström A, Fuxe K (1964) Evidence for the existence of monoamine containing neurons in the central nervous system. Demonstration of monoamines in the cell bodies of brain stem neurons. Act Physiol Scand 62(Suppl 232):1–55.

Day TA, Blessing W, Willoughby JO (1980) Noradrenergic and dopaminergic projections to the medial preoptic area of the rat. A combined horseradish peroxidase/catecholamine fluorescence study. Brain Res 193:543–548.

Day TA, Willoughby JO, Geften LB (1979) Thermoregulatory effects of preoptic area injection of noradrenaline in restrained and unrestrained rats. Brain Res. 174:175–179.

Hökfelt J, Fuxe K, Goldstein M, Johnson O (1974) Immunohistochemical evidence for the existence of adrenaline neurons in the brain. Brain Res. 66:235–272.

Honma K, Wuttke W (1980) Norepinephrine and dopamine turnover rates in the medial preoptic area and the medial basal hypothalamus in the rat brain after various endocrinological manipulations. Endocrinology 106:1848–1853.

Kalra PS, Kalra SP, Krulich L, Fawcett CP, McCann SM (1972) Involvement of norepinephrine in transmission of the stimulatory influence of

35

progesterone on gonadotropin release. Endocrinology 90:1168–1176.

Kalra P, McCann SM (1973) Involvement of catecholamines in feedback mechanisms. Progr Brain Res 39:185–198.

Krieger A, Wuttke W (1980) Effects of ovariectomy and hyperprolactinemia on tyrosine hydroxylase and dopamine-β-hydroxylase activity in various limbic and hypothalamic structures. Brain Res 193:178–180.

McCann SM, Moss RL (1975) Putative neurotransmitters involved in discharging gonadotropin releasing neurohormones and the action of LH releasing hormone on the CNS. Life Sci 16:833–852.

Sar M, Stumpf WE (1979) Simultaneous localization of steroid and peptide hormones in rat pituitary by combined thaw-mount autoradiography and immunohistochemistry: Localization of dihydrotestosterone, in gonadotropes, and pituicytes. Cell Tiss Res 203:1.

Sar M, Stumpf WE (1980a) Combined autoradiography and immunohistochemistry for simultaneous localization of radioactively labeled steroid hormones and antibodies in the brain. J Histochem Cytochem, in press.

Sar M, Stumpf WE (1980b) Localization of ^{3}H estradiol in dopamine-β-hydroxylase containing neurons of lower brain stem. Science, submitted.

Sar M, Stumpf WE, Miller RJ, Chang K-J, Cuatrecasas P (1978) Immunohistochemical localization of Enkephalin in the rat brain and spinal cord. J Comp Neurol 182:17–38.

Simpkins JW, Kalra SP (1979) Blockade of progesterone-induced increase in hypothalamic luteinizing hormone-releasing hormone levels and serum gonadotropins by intrahypothalamic implantation of 6-hydroxydopamine. Brain Res 170:475–483.

Stefano FJE, Donoso AE (1965) Norepinephrine levels in the rat hypothalamus and during the estrous cycle. Endocrinology 81:1405–1411.

Struyker BH, Smeats G, Brouwer G, Van Rossum JM (1975) Central Nervous System α-adrenergic mechanisms and cardiovascular regulation in rats. Arch Int Pharmacodyn 213:285–293.

Stumpf WE, Sar M (1975) Autoradiographic techniques in localizing steroid hormones. In: O'Malley BW, Hardman JG (eds) Methods in Enzymology XXXVI, Hormone Action, Pa A. Steroid hormones, Academic Press, New York, pp.135–156.

Stumpf WE, Sar M (1975) Hormone architecture of mouse brain with ^{3}H estradiol. In: Stumpf WE, Grant LD (eds) Anatomical Neuroendocrinology, Karger, Basel, pp.104–119.

Swanson LW, Hartman BK (1975) The central adrenergic system: An immunofluorescence study of the location of cell bodies and their afferent connections in the rat utilizing dopamine-β-hydroxylase as a marker. J Comp Neurol 163:467–487.

Intracellular Actions of Gonadal Steroids

P.W. Jungblut, J. Gaues, L. Görlich, A. Hughes, E. Kallweit, J. Kielhorn, M. Little, I. Maschler, S. McCann, F. Parl, G.C. Rosenfeld, W. Sierralta, G. Stone, P.I. Szendro, C. Teran, A.J. Truitt and R.K. Wagner, Hannover

The experiments discussed in this lecture have been performed with steroid-sensitive uterine cells. The question then immediately arises, whether steroid-sensitive cells of the brain display the same basic molecular mechanisms in reacting to hormonal stimuli. Although backed only by circumstantial evidence, the answer is soundly affirmative: gonadal steroids – and all other steroid hormones – act intracellularly by interacting with specific proteins called "receptor". The complexes formed are non-covalent, but surprisingly stable. Equilibrium constants of association are in the $10^9 M^{-1}$ range; receptors bind "their" steroid with high specificity. These properties are shown by all receptors, independent of their tissuelar origin. Furthermore, the accumulation of steroid-receptor complexes in the nucleus, the site of action, is common to all target cells.

It is understandable, that in the past emphasis has been placed on the steroid as the active component, while a merely supportive role was assigned to the receptor. The non-covalent attachment, which is reversible in vitro, also suggested repeated usage of the intracellular steroid-"carrier", hence a slow turnover rate of the protein and a steady concentration level. Neither of these assumptions was correct. The essential element is the receptor, not the steroid, which "activates" the protein by inducing favorable conformational changes. Receptors do not shuttle between cytoplasm and nucleus; they are degraded after acting. Their action consists in an enhancement of transcription, the extent of which is not only receptor- but also cell-specific, meaning, that the scale of messages transcribed with the aid of an individual receptor depends on cell differentiation. At least one receptor governs the transcription of its

37

own message, the estradiol-receptive, transcription-regulating protein. The study of its turnover under controlled physiological conditions, therefore, is a promising approach for unveiling the unknown.

1. Subcellular Origins and Properties of Uterine Estradiol Receptors

Estradiol receptors have been found in three homogenate fractions of uterus: the soluble phase ("cytosol"), the nuclei and the microsomal particles. Of these, only one can be appropriately defined. Nuclei can be isolated to a high degree of purity and, after removing the outer layer of the nuclear envelope, allow for a quantitative assessment of their receptor content. The particle-free supernatant of homogenates is of course not identical with the cytosol, but rather represents a mixture of extra- and intracellular fluids, part of the latter possibly arising from cytoplasmic containements, ruptured during homogenization. Microsomes are fragments of rough and smooth endoplasmic reticulum and other membraneous structures of the cell and cannot be quantitatively recovered from homogenates. This hampers distribution studies, which, for the "cytosol" and the "microsomes", have to rely on reference markers. Fortunately, some physico-chemical differences between the receptors originating from the three subcellular sites are helpful discriminators.

The differences do not concern the steroid-binding site. Judging from their indistinguishably high affinity and steroid-binding specificity, it must be identical for the cytosol-, the nuclear- and the microsomal-estradiol receptor. They are rather due to the absence or presence of structural features adjacent to a common core and resulting in characteristic sedimentation velocities and electrophoretic mobilities.

(It ought to be mentioned here, that the early observed difference between the 9 S cytosol- and the 5 S nuclear receptor is likely a puzzling, still poorly understood artefact. The former can be produced by homogenizing tissue with low ionic strength buffer, the latter is extracted from nuclei by salt. Subsequent addition of salt to freshly prepared low ionic strength cytosols disperses the 9 S or larger receptor aggregates to a 4 S subunit.)

38

Since the sedimentation velocity of the microsomal receptor is lowest of all and also its electrophoretic mobility at pH 8.2 is markedly reduced as compared to that of the cytosol- and the nuclear receptor, it could be the common protein core awaiting some unknown posttranslational finishing. This "primordial" receptor is not only capable of steroid-binding, but already contains the structures required for a phenomenon interpreted as receptor "activation".

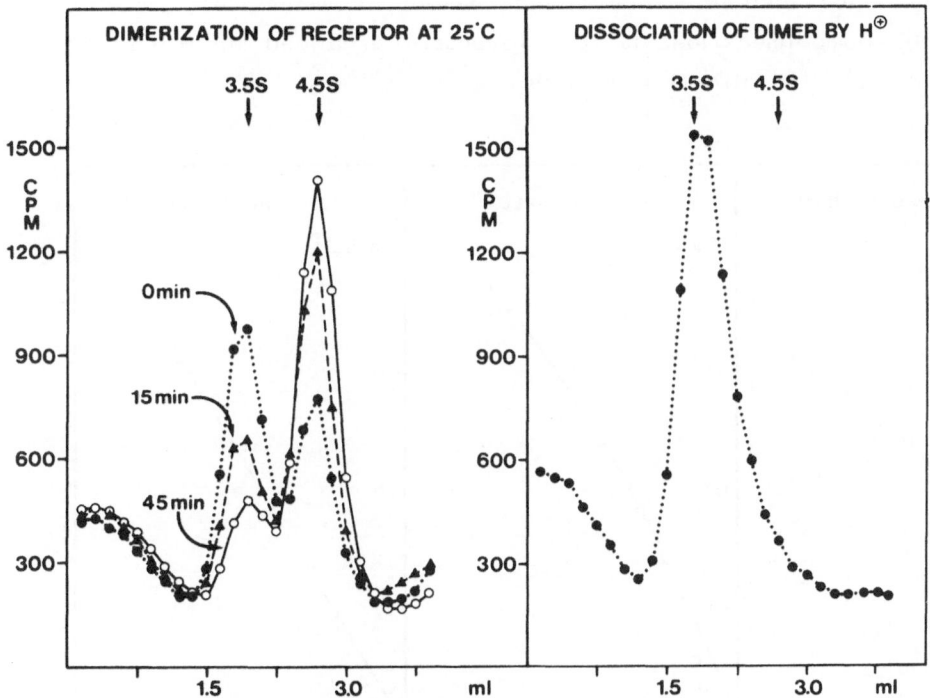

Figure 1:   Estradiol-facilitated conversion of microsomal 3.5 S ⇌ 4.5 S receptor (Little et al., 1973)

When estradiol-containing microsomal extracts are warmed, the macromolecular-bound labeled steroid is gradually shifted from the 3.5 S to the 4.5 S position in density gradient analyses (left hand panel Figure 1). The transition follows second order kinetics for dimerization (Figure 2). Stability studies (Figure 3) indicate the participation of histidyl- and tyrosyl residues, provided their "microscopic" pK's in the polypeptide are close to those of the free amino acids. While the decrease of 4.5 S receptor concentration above pH 10 is not matched by an increase of the 3.5 S complex (progressing denaturation), the dimer can be reversibly dissociated between pH 7.0 and 6.5 (right hand panel Figure 1). The back to back/head to toe model of the receptor dimer (Figure 4) is fictitious. Its actual shape might be more elongated, should the polar groups exist in closer vicinity, and the arrangement could be front to front/head to toe instead. For steric reasons, however, all possible forms of the homodimer must feature inversely arranged surface areas of its constituent (identical) monomers.

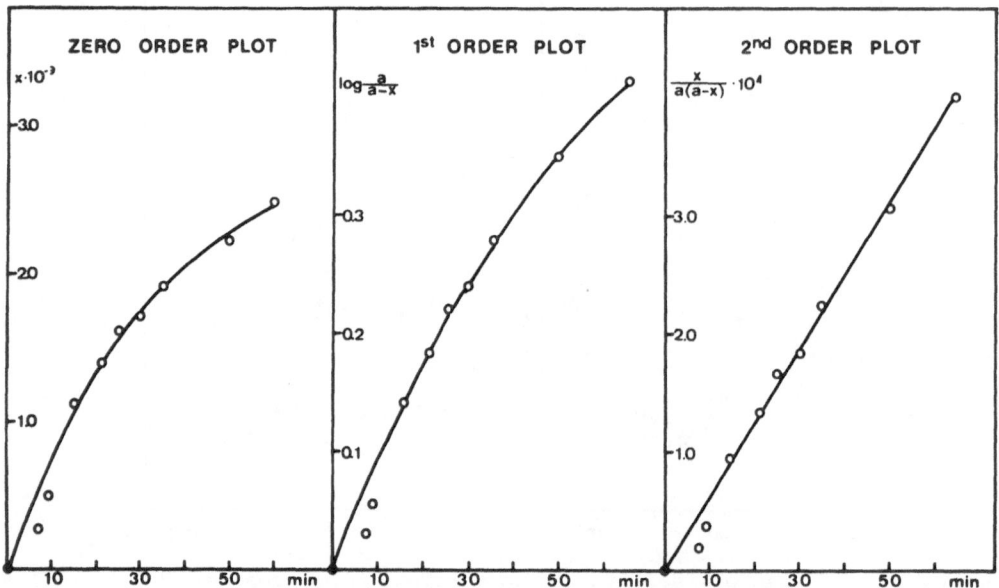

Figure 2: Kinetics of estradiol-facilitated conversion of microsomal 3.5 S → 4.5 S receptor (Little et al., 1973)

With some more difficulty than with the microsomal receptor, which lacks the tendency of forming uncontrollable homo- and hetero-aggregates, the same dimerization/dissociation processes are demonstrable for the cytosol receptor (Figure 5). Receptor extracted from highly purified nuclei after in vivo administration of estradiol

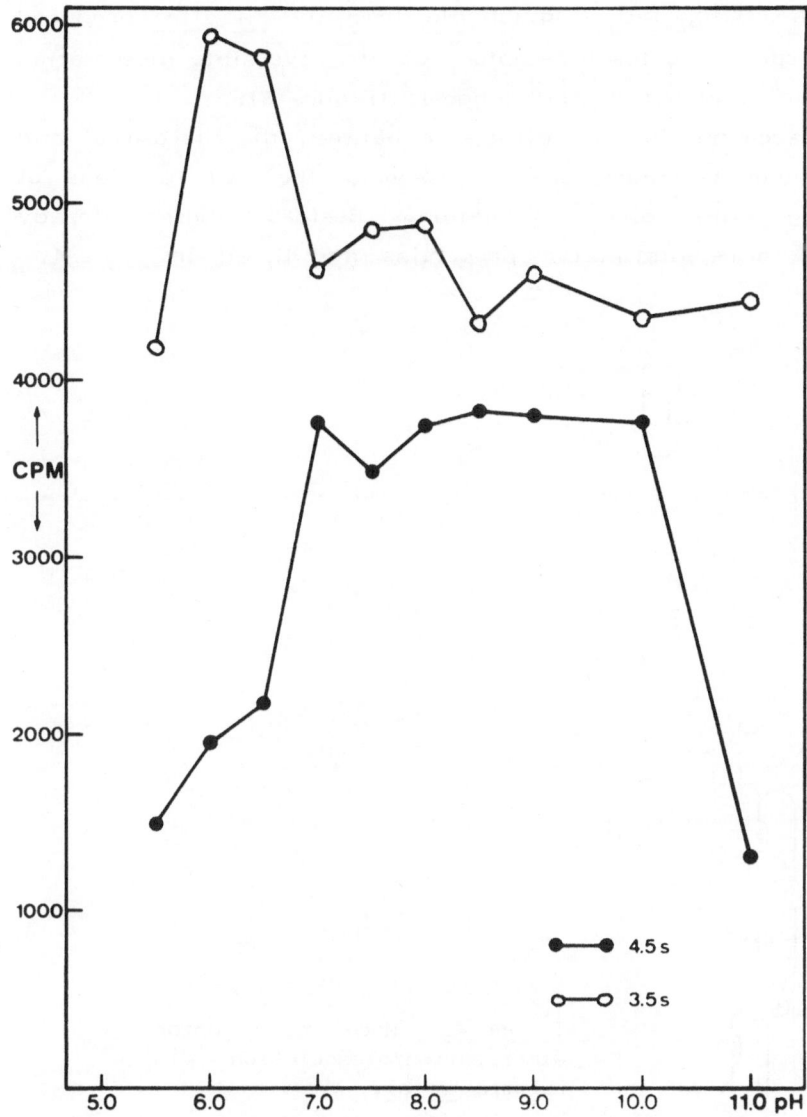

Figure 3:   Stability of 3.5 S and 4.5 S microsomal estradiol receptor complexes (Little et al., 1973)

is apparently a dimer, indistinguishable from the _in vitro_ produced dimer of the dispersed cytosol receptor, as its reversible dissociation by proton addition and withdrawal suggests (Figure 6).

Whatever accounts for the difference between the microsomal and the cytosol/nuclear receptors then is beyond the two functions of steroid binding and dimer formation. Besides those already mentioned, some more distinctive properties are listed in Table 1.

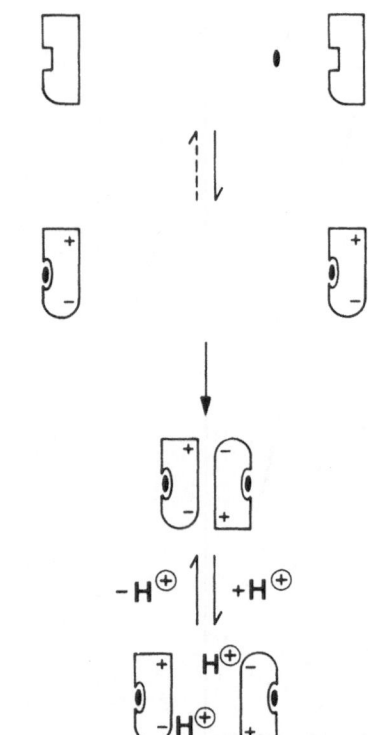

Figure 4:   Model of receptor dimerization/dissociation (Little _et al._, 1973)

They further add to the apparent identity of the cytosol and the nuclear receptor and, considering the total absence of microsomal-type receptor in purified nuclei (Figure 7), allow for a tentative functional assignment to the "finishing" entity: a participation in either nuclear uptake or retention or in both.

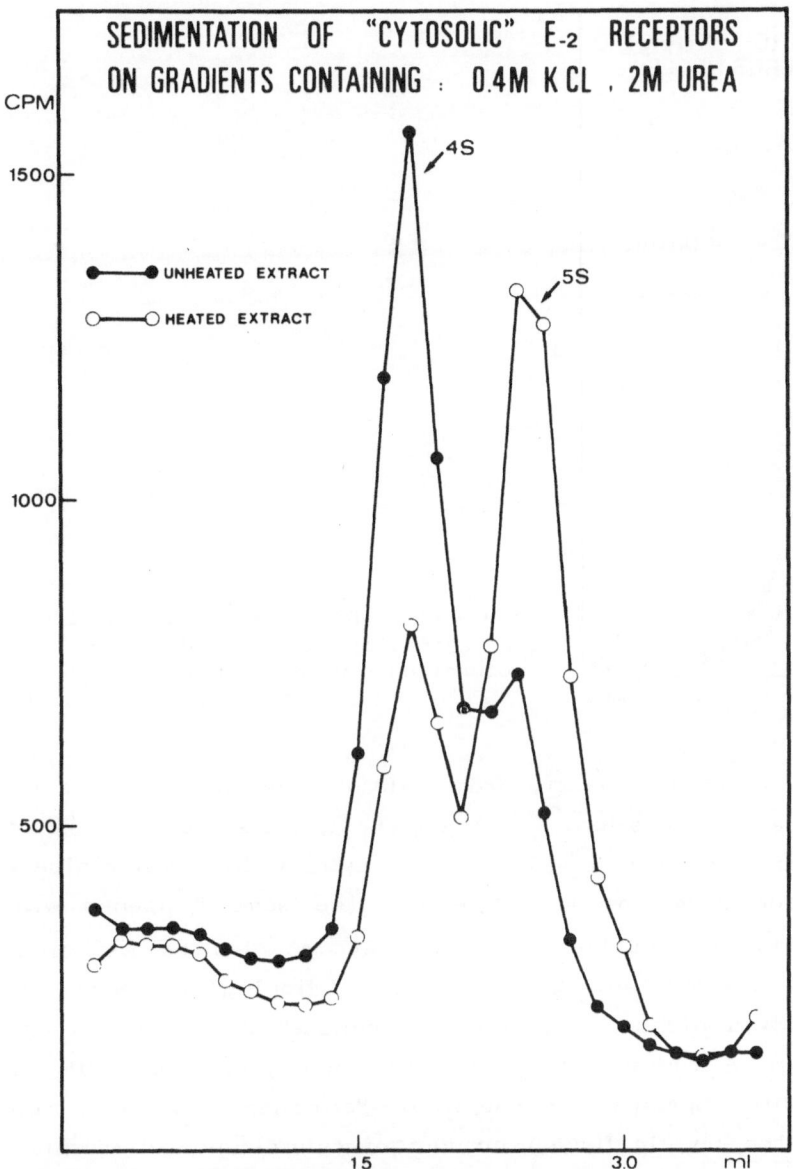

Figure 5: Estradiol-facilitated dimerization of cytosol $4\,S \rightarrow 5\,S$ receptor (Little et al., 1975).

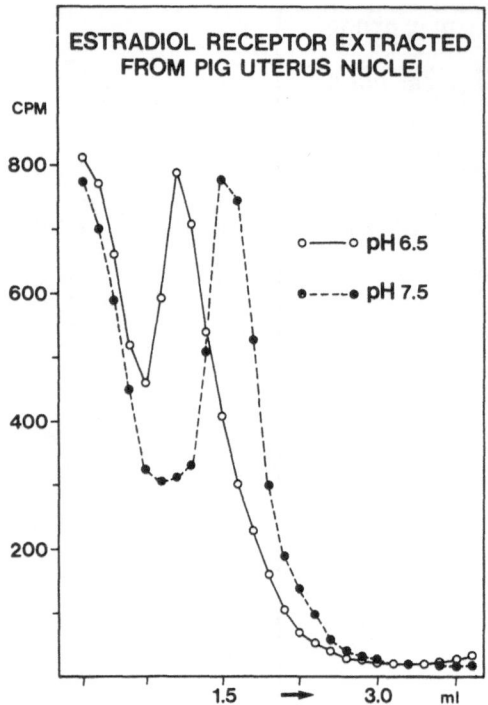

ESTRADIOL RECEPTOR EXTRACTED
FROM PIG UTERUS NUCLEI

o———o pH 6.5

●----● pH 7.5

Figure 6: Dissociation of nuclear 5 S estradiol receptor dimer by protonation (Jungblut et al., 1976)

The removal of this entity from cytosol- and nuclear receptor was a chance observation. Attempts to disperse suspected glycosamino-glycan-receptor aggregates in cytosol by hyaluronidase treatment, produced "microsomal" receptor. The same happened with receptor from purified nuclei (Figure 8), accompanied by 3-5 times higher receptor yields (Table 2). Since the "clipping" proceeds with both testes hyaluronidase and with "eliminase" from Streptomyces hyaluronolyticus, a contamination of both endoglycosidases with an identical, highly specific endopeptidase-"clippase" is a remote explanation. The tryptic fission product of cytosol/nuclear receptor, moreover, differs from that of hyaluronidase action. Whether "finished" receptor is indeed a hitherto unknown intracellular proteoglycan travelling along unfamiliar routes remains to be proven. The data available on this peculiar macromolecule are interpreted in Figure 9.

Table 1

PROPERTIES OF ESTROGEN RECEPTORS

Site of Extraction	"Microsomes"	"Cytosol"	Nucleus
K_A Estradiol	$\sim 5 \times 10^9 \ M^{-1}$	$\sim 5 \times 10^9 \ M^{-1}$	$\sim 5 \times 10^9 \ M^{-1}$
Velocity (S)	$3.5 \rightleftharpoons 4.5$ (low salt)	$4 \rightleftharpoons 5$ (high salt)	$5 \rightleftharpoons 4$ (high salt)
Mobility (pH 8.2)	$\ominus$	$\oplus$	$\oplus$
Heparin-Sepharose	not adsorbed	adsorbed	adsorbed
Protamine Chloride	not precipitated	precipitated	precipitated

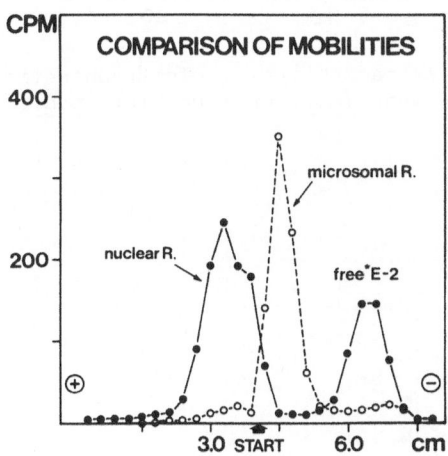

Figure 7:   Absence of microsomal–type receptor in purified and stripped uterine nuclei (Jungblut et al., 1978)

45

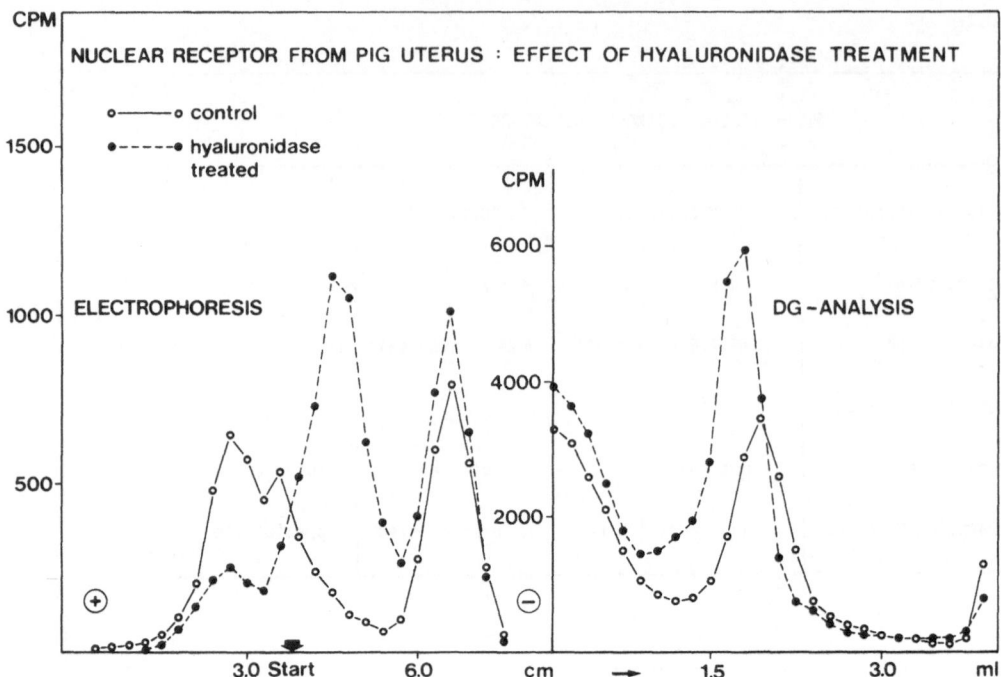

Figure 8: Effect of hyaluronidase extractability, electrophoretic mobility and sedimentation velocity of nuclear receptor (Jungblut et al., 1980)

Table 2

IMPROVEMENT OF RECEPTOR YIELDS FROM PIG UTERUS NUCLEI BY HYALURONIDASE

Ablative Treatment	Number of Binding Sites/Nucleus Extracted by	
	Salt only	Salt + Hyaluronidase
Ovariectomy	2,690	12,630
"	3,010	8,420
"	2,910	9,220
"	2,170	11,100
"	2,230	8,500
Ovariectomy and Adrenalectomy	2,230	4,760

ANATOMY OF ESTROGEN RECEPTOR

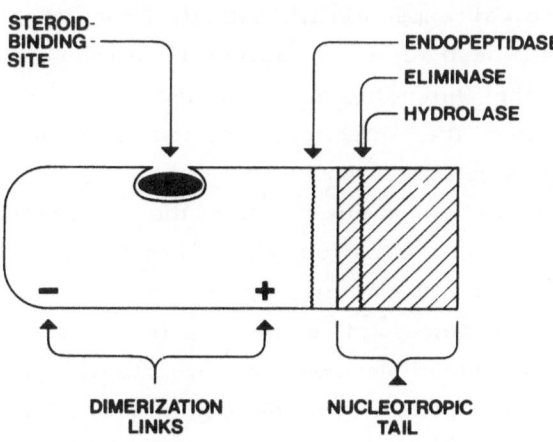

Figure 9: Model of "finished" estradiol receptor monomer (Jungblut et al., 1980)

2. Reaction of Uterine Cells to Pulse-administered Estradiol

The discovery of the small and less acidic microsomal estradiol receptor prompted the development of an experimental design for delineating its physiological role. We use German Landrace pigs for two reasons: 1. for securing sufficiently large quantities of tissue and 2. because the necessary manipulations can be carried out on wake, trained animals, which minimizes the complicating interference of adrenal-derived estradiol. In brief: 3 months old (premature) animals are ovariectomized and the left horn is detached from the corpus uteri. A silastic tubing containing a suspension of crystralline estradiol is subcutaneously implanted 4-6 days prior to the operation and left in situ until 8-10 days before the experiment, 2 months later. The treatment facilitates the operation, reduces the formation of adhesions and helps to standardize the size of the uterus. The chronically castrated pigs are then trained for tolerating a simulated insemination, which naturally proceeds in the sow via transcervical filling of the uterus with some 200 ml of ejaculate by the boar. In a typical experiment, instead, 20 ml of a 1×10^{-6}M solution of (unlabeled) estradiol in buffered saline are injected into the open horn, the animals are stunned and ex-sanguinated at various times after the injection, treated and un-treated horns are excised, chilled and processed.

The macroscopic effect seen at 90 minutes after the estradiol injection is shown in Figure 10. This so-called water imbibition of the treated horn, still missing at 60 minutes p.i., is a late phenomenon as compared to the swiftness of other events. It is preceeded by a rapid uptake of estradiol from the injectant, the steroid concentration of which drops within minutes below the $1^{\circ}/_{\circ\circ}$ level. Most of the estradiol passes through the uterine wall into the systemic circulation and is metabolized before reaching the "blind" control horn. We have thus the benefit of a pulse-exposure of target cells to a hormonal stimulus under optimal physiological conditions, to be compared with untreated cells of the same "walking incubator".

Although we have been improving the physiological technique over the past seven years to almost perfection, the originally intended purpose still suffers from biochemical shortcomings. As

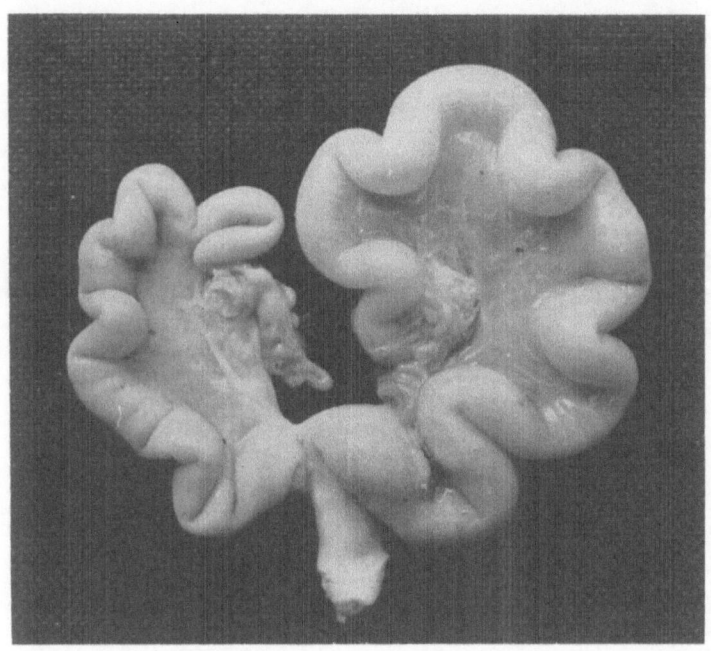

Figure 10:   Uterus of chronically castrated pig 90 minutes after injection of 20 ml of 1 x 10^{-6} M E-2 into open horn (right side of picture)

already mentioned, microsomes cannot be quantitatively harvested from homogenates, nor can we safely extract all microsomal receptor from the obtained particulate fraction.   If, however, receptor extracted by standardized procedures and referred to protein concentration and marker enzyme activity should be representative, the "basic" microsomal 3.5 S estradiol receptor qualifies as the precursor of the cytosol/nuclear receptor.   Its "specific" concentration rises within 30-60 minutes after an estradiol pulse to over fourfold.

Compared to this problem, the pursuit of estradiol- and receptor uptake by the nucleus is an easy task, provided, the nuclei analyzed have been carefully purified and stripped off the outer layer of the nuclear envelope, which is rough ER and contains microsomal receptor.   (We contend that experiments with crude, 600 x g nuclear sediments are hazardous.   The sediments trap up to 60% of the microsomal fraction of uterine homogenates and exchange experiments – "cold" for "hot" estradiol with concomitant receptor extraction – are unavoidably confused by the admixture of extranuclear receptors.) We split the nuclei isolated at various times after estradiol injection for parallel receptor and estradiol assays. The extracted receptor is labeled by exchange with tritiated estradiol at elevated temperature and quantitated by density gradient centrifugation or electrophoresis; the accumulated ("cold") estradiol is measured in the other aliquot by radioimmunoassay. Both values are expressed per nucleus.

The time course (Figure 11) shows a sudden and equimolar increase of estradiol and receptor content in the nucleus proper, albeit arising from different starting levels. This is followed by a slow and parallel decline of both concentrations until some 8 hours after the pulse, whereafter estradiol continues fading away from the nucleus, while the receptor content levels off to the starting concentration in the vicinity of 10,000/nucleus. The increase in nuclear

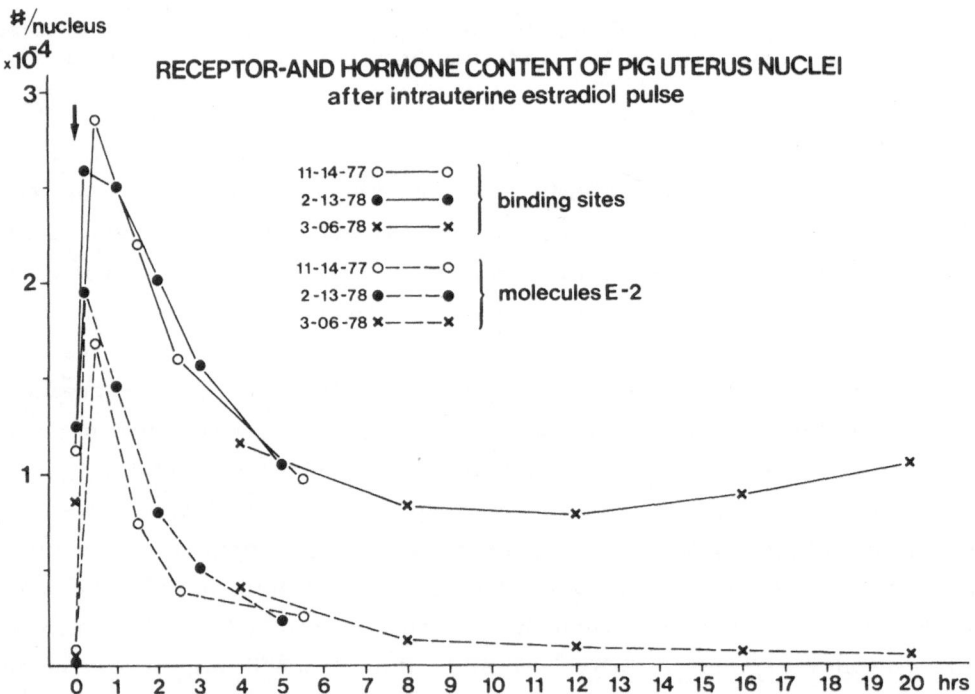

Figure 11: Comparison of nuclear estradiol and receptor contents (Jungblut et al., 1979b)

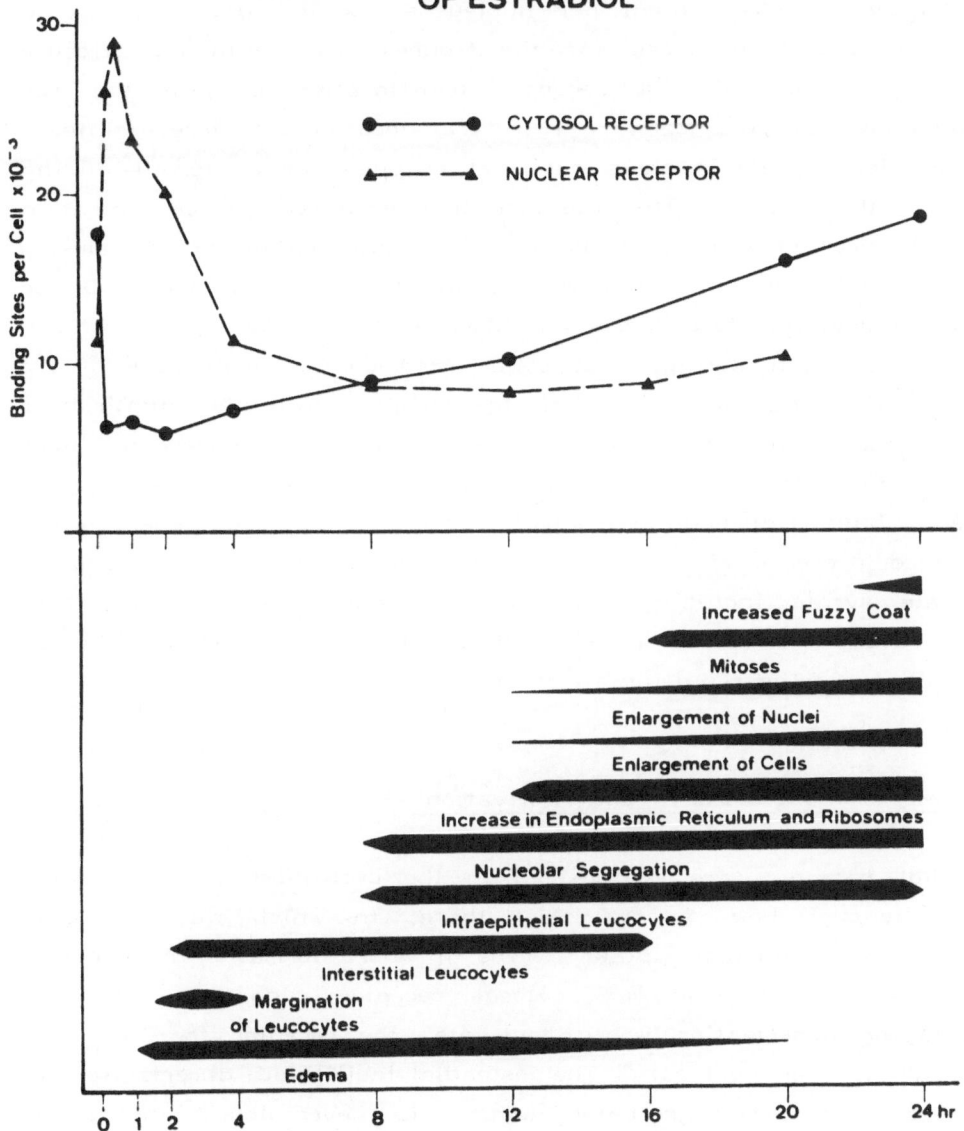

Figure 12: Correlation of biochemical and morphological events after estradiol pulse (Jungblut et al., 1979b).

51

receptor content coincides with the disappearance of receptor from the cytosol (upper panel Figure 12). (The cytosol receptor concentration per cell is calculated from the DNA concentration of the homogenate divided by the DNA content per nucleus = 7×10^{-12}g). The timing of the shift and the close absolute figures are convincing evidence for an estradiol-mediated receptor translocation between the two compartments of the cell. This translocation is irreversible. Receptor leaving the nucleus does not reappear as a steroid-binding entity in the cytosol. The late rise in cytosol receptor concentration which is preceeded by that of its presumable microsomal precursor, can be inhibited by (locally administered) actinomycin D or puromycin and therefore depends on de-novo synthesis.

It is worth noting, that major morphological responses of the stimulated endometrial epithelium are missing until the eighth hour after estradiol injection and are then sequentially patterned (lower panel figure 12). At this time, nuclear estradiol- and receptor contents have returned to control levels. The requirement of a prolonged presence of active steroid-receptor-complexes for promoting the late events including cell division cannot be concluded from these data. It rather appears that the hormone-receptor complex merely has a trigger-pulling function.

3. Receptor "Nucleotropy" and "Activation"

Estradiol receptors are synthesized in the cytoplasm and act inside the nucleus. How do they get there, in which way are they conditioned for nuclear uptake? The in vitro formation of nuclear-type 5 S receptor from 4 S cytosol receptor suggested, that the underlaying dimerization would "activate" the receptor for its "pas-de-deux" to the nucleus. The estradiol-facilitated dimerization of the 3.5 A microsomal receptor (which is never found inside the nucleus) did cast some doubt on this notion, although logistical restraint might be the physiological cause. There was however one observation at hand for testing the issue: estrone, in contrast to estradiol, does not facilitate the formation of receptor dimers; estriol is somewhat less effective than estradiol. The relative potencies of the three estrogens are equally demonstrable for the microsomal

52

receptor (Figure 13) and – with adapted experimental conditions – for the cytosol receptor. If then only receptor twins should be allowed into the nucleus, estrone would be an uneffective usher. It is by no means! Estrone, like estradiol, promotes a rapid translocation of receptor from the cytosol into the nucleus (upper panel Figure 14). But, the estrone-mediated translocation does not last; it is quickly followed by a receptor reshuttle. We must thus conclude, that monomeric receptor can enter the nucleus and that the enhancement of its "nucleotrophy" is a process different from dimerization. The nuclear retention of receptor, however, appears to be related to the

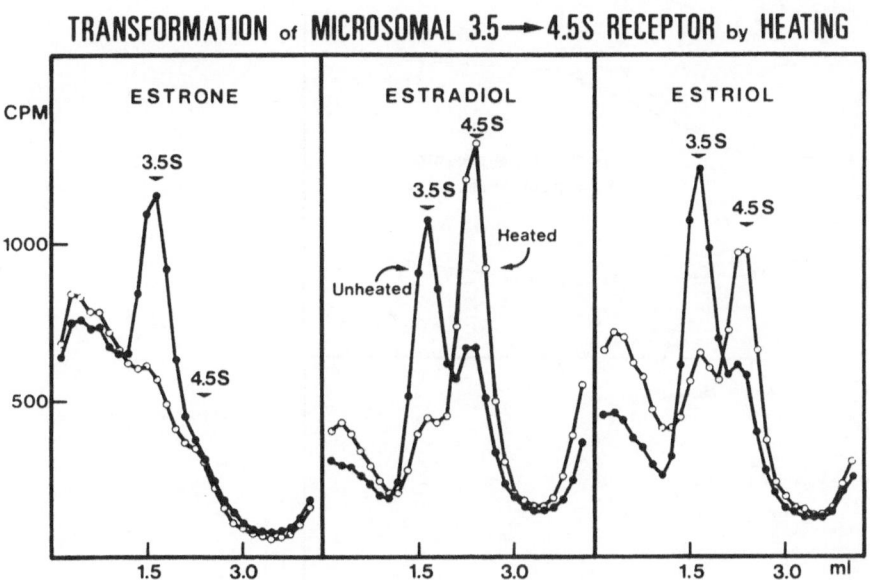

Figure 13: Relative potencies of estrone, estradiol and estriol in facilitating receptor dimerization (Little et al., 1973)

estrogen involved. It is longest with estradiol, shorter if estriol is administered (not shown) and missing after estrone. This order is the same as that for facilitating receptor dimerization and, provided retention time correlates to activity, receptor dimers should then be the active element in the nucleus.

Two aspects of the estrone experiments remain to be discussed: first, does estrone – and all other estrogens – enhance receptor "nucleotropy" by unfolding a "sticky tail", like that portion of the cytosol (and nuclear) receptor, which can be removed by hyaluronidase (converting it to microsomal–type receptor)? The thought is intriguing, because all but 100 seconds would be needed for a reverse "fly–catch" mechanism of total receptor depletion in the cytosol in favour of the nucleus, by postulating an unhindered diffusion in the cytoplasm and a size–average diffusion constant of the receptor. In essence, a model resembling the interactions of

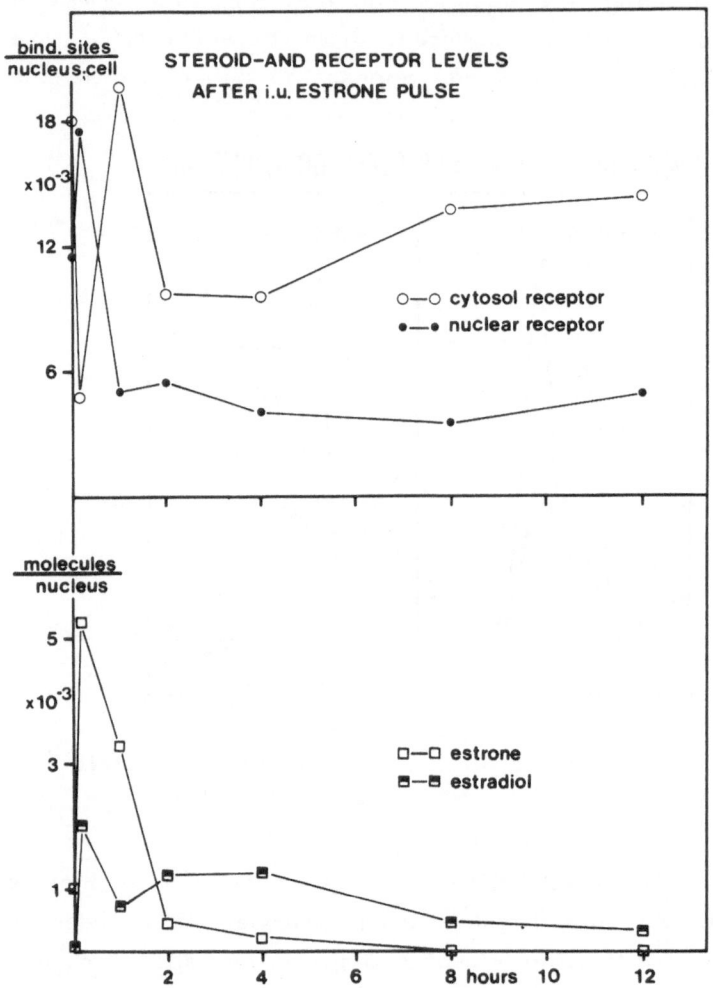

Figure 14: Reshuttle of receptor after estrone–facilitated translocation (Jungblut et al., 1979b)

54

hormones and antigens with plasma membrane receptors! Occuring within the confinement of the cytoplasm, it could practically achieve a unidirectional flux.

The second aspect concerns the fate of receptor, which is quickly "replenished" into the cytosol after estrone-facilitated translocation into the nucleus, but then vanishes before the onset of receptor synthesis, brought about by the complicating action of estradiol 17β-ol-oxidoreductase (lower panel Figure 14). The disappearance of the nucleus-released receptor might well be considered the second limb of a unidirectional migration, ending in receptor degradation. The site at which the degradation takes place is as yet unknown. Some observations indicate an involvement of lysosomes, which in porcine endometrial cells also contain a highly active estradiol 17β-ol-dehydrogenase. Unless the fate of receptor translocated with estrone-support is exceptional, the nucleus itself does not "process" the receptor to non-steroid-binding fragments. Whether it "conditions" the receptor for extra-nuclear degradation remains to be elucidated.

4.   Ovarian- and Steroid-independent Fluctuations of Uterine Estradiol Receptor Levels

We and others have been plagued by seasonal variations of receptor levels in immature animals and postmenopausal women. These can be attributed to a changing influence of the adrenal cortex, which in summertime and in stress releases increased quantities of estrogen precursors. A not too pronounced circadian rhythm of rat uterine estradiol receptor concentrations should have the same reason. But this explanation fails for the 7-12 day up and down periods of cytosol receptor concentration in the uteri of ovariectomized/hypophysectomized rats. We suspected a slow turnover of the receptor in the absence of steroid, likely without the implication of a nuclear passage. It was not until the pulse-administration experiments with pigs had arrived at the pure nuclei perfection, that we reconsidered. Like everybody else, we clung to the idea, that possibly the steroid, but not the receptor, could independently enter the nucleus. Considering the lability of the receptor and the excellent extractability of the stable, non-covalently bound steroid, each analysis of nuclei should then have shown an apparent excess of steroid. The failure in meeting this expectation has already been stated. In retrospect, the later on discovered difference between receptor "nucleo-tropy" and the formation of active dimers might have appealed as a handy explanation. "Finished" cytosol receptor could have a somewhat less effective "sticky tail" without the steroid and gradually enter the nucleus. It would remain there for some time as "unfilled site", in the inactive, monomeric form.

This retrospective hypothesis is only in part a true reflection. Uterine nuclei of ovariectomized and successfully adrenalectomized pigs are completely devoid of estradiol. They do contain some monomeric receptor, but, as late as 33 days after removing the second adrenal, the majority of receptor present is in its dimeric form (Figure 15). Both processes, nuclear entrance and dimerization, are therefore essentially steroid-independent. It still could be disputed, if this is sufficient evidence for a steroid-independent

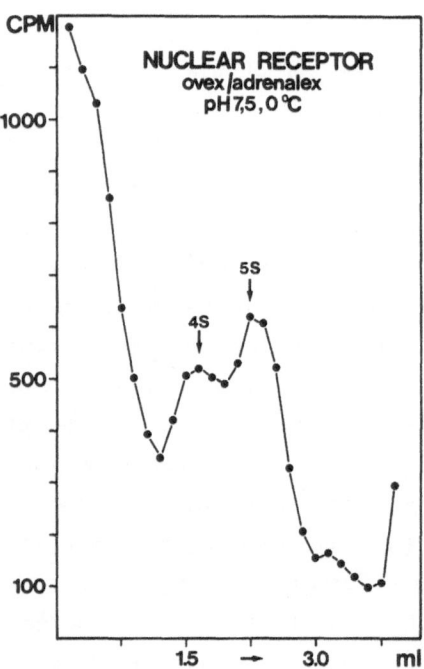

Figure 15: Presence of monomer and dimer estradiol receptor in uterine nuclei from ovariectomized/adrenal-ectomized pigs (Jungblut et al., 1978)

action of the receptor. But, since the estradiol receptor is good only for one nuclear passage and part of its action is the provision of its own message for resynthesis, admittedly proven only with steroidal support, an entirely different mechanism in the absence of estradiol can hardly be envisaged. A quantitative difference in receptor turnover, and all related processes, rather than a qualitative one in the presence or absence of steroid is the more reasonable alternative.

5. The Basic Mechanism of Estradiol Receptor Action

Recognizing the receptor protein as the essential element does not curtail the importance of the steroid. Called for only is substituting the "all or nothing" theorem by the less absolute "very much or very little" in explaining the physiological reality. (This might impress as a hair-splitting exercise, but there is at least one situation possible, in which the steroid-independent turnover of the estradiol, and other steroid receptors, could exceed the leisurely basal rate of cellular activity: the cancerous growth of "derailed" target cells. Should they retain receptor-dependency as an essential mechanism, withdrawal of the steroidal conformation catalysts might not suffice for a total blockade, which would require an effective "poisoning" of the transcription-regulating proteins, called receptor.)

Our present view of estradiol/receptor action is outlined in Figure 16. The diagram emphasizes the unidirectional voyage of the receptor, many stations of which are still in a haze. The sites of core-protein synthesis and receptor-"finishing" remain to be pin-pointed, as is the site of receptor degradation. The structure of the "nucleotropic tail" must be identified before the penetration of the nuclear envelope can be understood. Where exactly in the nucleus the receptor lodges for action is unknown. The dimer-structure of the receptor, however, allows for a reasonable assumption. Its toppled Janus-head features can only align to stretches of double-stranded DNA with fitting nucleotide sequences or to other inversely arranged macromolecular twin structures, hitherto unknown. Although our old hypothesis, that the receptor dimer would act as an unwinding protein for transcription retains its appeal, direct proof

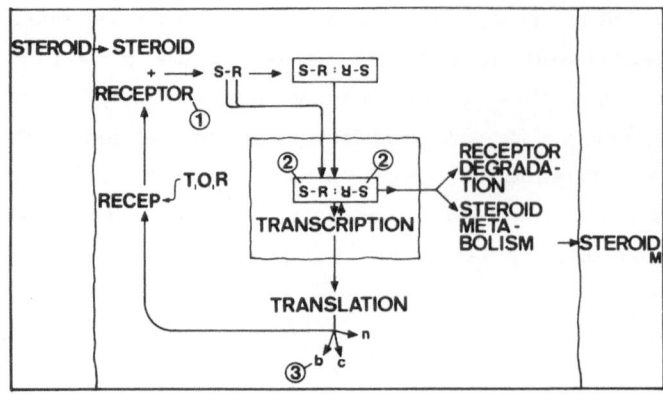

Figure 16: Basic mechanism of estradiol/receptor action

is hard to come by. The "sticky" nucleotropic tail complicates experiments with isolated systems, which cannot copy the intricate arrangement of macromolecules in the intact nucleus whereby un-specific adsorptions are obviously avoided, as the shedding of (monomeric) estrone receptor complex shows.

There are many indications, that the estrogen receptor's mode of action exemplifies those of all other steroid hormone receptors. Understandably, their sites of interaction and hence the products are different. At least one of them, the progestagen receptor, does not enhance the transcription of its own message, which is taken care of by the estrogen receptor. This is indicated by 3 in the diagram; 1 = cytosol estradiol receptor and 2 = estradiol in the cell nucleus are additional parameters which we recommend to analyze as criteria of persisting hormone-responsiveness in mammary cancer biopsies. (Wave-functions cannot be described by a single point!)

6. How to Succeed in Mapping the Steroid-sensitive Areas of the Brain?

The very last remarks connect to the plight of the neurophysiologist, which is twofold: the scarcity of steroid-responsive neural cells and their variable states of response. .The collection of sufficient amounts of topically well-defined cells already is a painstaking exercise, lest the various biochemical microanalyses necessary for monitoring the response situation,

What is the alternative? Recalling that the receptor, but not its specific steroid-"catalyst" can enter the cell nucleus independent-ly, Walter Stumpf's technique of injecting labeled hormone and tracking it by radioautography is of convincing safety. Whether the silver grains mirror the injected steroid or some active metabolite can with some certainty be checked on other, more abundant target cells, for as long as hypothetical cell-specific steroid receptors do not materialize. Proper timing for optimal accumulation must be taken care of by time course experiments.

The Stumpf technique, however, can only identify "resting" target cells, containing high concentrations of cytoplasmic receptor, which swiftly takes the marker steroid along into the nucleus. It "blacks-out" those cells, which have recently been exposed to endogeneous steroid and are in a state of "saturation" or "recovery". Italo NENCI's immunohistochemcial procedure for locally arresting steroids after their release from denatured receptor could fill the gap left by "occupied" nuclei.

Used in combination under well-defined physiological conditions, the two methods certainly will add to our knowledge. They are not only first choice for exploring the topography of steroid-responsive perikarya, but also could reveal, whether all cells of the organism containing identical steroid-receptor systems are "in phase" or not.

Note to the Reader

The manuscript has been written post festum. It follows closely the outline of the lecture given, framed by the order of slides. Naturally, none of the experimental data are original. All have been previously published or are in press. The references necessary for their critical evaluation are listed below. They also give credit to the many other groups active in steroid receptor research. Since foot-notes are carreer-neutral, my colleagues are named as co-lecturers. The last chapter was not presented at the symposium. It is an epilogue, prompted by re-flections and after-hours-discussions which might be the true benefit of meetings, although they usually have not printed record.

P.W.J.

References

Entenmann AH, Sierralta W, Jungblut PW (1980) Studies on the involvement of lysosomes in estrogen action. III. The dehydrogenation of estradiol to estrone by porcine endometrial lysosomes. Hoppe-Seyler's Z Physiol Chem 361:959-968.
Hughes A, Jacobson HI, Wagner RK, Jungblut PW (1976) Ovarian-independent

fluctuations of estradiol receptor levels in mammalian tissues; Mol Cell Endocrinol 5:379–388.

Hughes A, Szendro PI, Teran C, Kielhorn J, Sierralta W, Stone G, Little M, Jungblut PW (1977) Biosynthesis of steroid-hormone receptors. In: Vermeulen A et al. (eds) Research on steroids VII, North Holland, pp.149–167.

Jungblut PW, McCann S, Görlich L, Rosenfeld GC, Wagner RK (1970) Binding of steroids by tissue proteins. Steroid hormone "receptors". In: Finkelstein M, Klopper A, Conti C, Cassano C (eds) Research on steroids IV. Pergamon Press, pp.213–232.

Jungblut PW, Gaues J, Hughes A, Kallweit E, Sierralta W, Szendro PI, Wagner RK (1976) Activation of transcription-regulating proteins by steroids. J Steroid Biochem 7:1109–1116.

Jungblut PW, Hughes A, Sierralta W, Wagner RK (1977) A proposal for assessment of hormone sensitivity and consequent endocrine therapy of breast cancer. Europ J Cancer 13:1201–1202.

Jungblut PW, Kallweit E, Sierralta W, Truitt AJ, Wagner RK (1978) The occurrence of steroid-free, "activated" estrogen receptor in target cell nuclei. Hoppe-Seyler's Z Physiol Chem 359:1259–1268.

Jungblut PW, Hughes A, Gaues J, Kallweit E, Szendro PI, Truitt AJ, Wagner RK (1979a) Functional activities of estradiol receptor in the presence and in the absence of steroid. In: Proceedings of the International Symposium: Neuroendocrine regulatory mechanisms, Scientific Assemblies Vol. VI, Department of Sciences No. 2, Serbian Academy of Sciences and Art, Belgrade.

Jungblut PW, Hughes A, Gaues J, Kallweit E, Maschler I, Parl F, Sierralta W, Szendro PI, Wagner RK (1979b) Mechanisms involved in the regulation of steroid receptor levels. J Steroid Biochem 11:273–278.

Jungblut PW, Meyer HHD, Wagner RK (1980) The interrelationship of estrogen receptors extracted from various subcellular compartments. In: Bresciani F (ed) Perspective in steroid receptor research. Raven Press, in press.

Little M, Rosenfeld GC, Jungblut PW (1972) Cytoplasmic estradiol "receptor" associated with the "microsomal" fraction of pig uterus. Hoppe-Seyler's Z Physiol Chem 353:231–242.

Little M, Szendro PI, Jungblut PW (1973) Hormone-mediated dimerization of microsomal estradiol receptor. Hoppe-Seyler's Z Physiol Chem 354:1599–1610.

Little M, Szendro PI, Teran C, Hughes A, Jungblut PW (1975) Biosynthesis and transformation of microsomal and cytosol estradiol receptor. J Steroid Biochem 6:493–500.

Neural Estrogen Receptors in the Life Cycle of the Albino Rat

B.S. McEwen, New York

Steroid hormones are among the most selective and specific of the chemical signals reaching the brain from the blood. Among the effects of these hormones are the activation of behavior and regulation of neuroendocrine function in adult animals and the organization of behavioral and neuroendocrine systems in the course of neural development.

It is generally believed that steroid hormone action involves intracellular receptor sites which translocate with the hormone from the cytoplasm to the nucleus. Many of the original studies which identified and characterized steroid receptors and established their nuclear translocation dealt with estrogen receptors. Estrogen receptors have also occupied a central position in the study of neural responses to steroid hormones, for they were the first to be studied in the brain and they are perhaps the most versatile in terms of their physiological involvements. The present article will amplify this statement by describing estrogen receptors and then discussing the various facts of estrogen action and estrogen receptor function in neural tissue throughout the life history of the albino rat.

1. Identification and Properties of Estrogen Receptors

Reproductive tract: The chemical synthesis of high specific activity tritiated estrogens (Jensen, 1960; Glascock and Pope, 1960) enabled several laboratories to demonstrate the uptake and retention of these hormones by reproductive tract tissues (Glascock and Hoekstra, 1959; Jensen and Jacobson, 1962). The inference from this work that an intracellular receptor mechanism was responsible for estrogen action

(Jensen and Jacobson, 1962) was elucidated by the demonstration of cell nuclear retention of radioactive estradiol in uterine tissue and

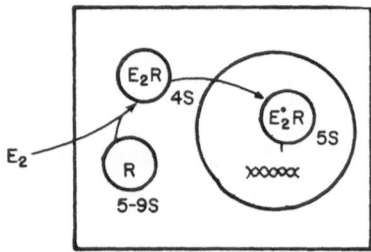

Figure 1: Model of estradiol (E_2) interaction with target cells. Diffusion of E_2 passively across cell membrane. Formation of E_2-receptor complex (E_2R) and translocation to cell nucleus. Activation of E_2R (E_2R) and 4S→ 5S transformation

by the characterization of soluble estrogen binding proteins in uterus (see Gorski et al., 1970; Jensen and DeSombre, 1973 for reviews). The presence of both soluble and cell nuclear estrogen binding sites was codified into a model of estrogen action involving a two-step transfer of estradiol first to the soluble (and presumably cyto-plasmic) receptor and then to the cell nucleus in combination with the soluble receptor (Jensen et al., 1968). Entry of estradiol into uterine cells is believed to be due to passive diffusion (Müller and Wotiz, 1979). This scheme is summarized in Fig. 1. The uterine cytosol estrogen receptor exists as a complex of a number of estrogen binding subunits with sedimentation (S) coefficients in sucrose densit-y gradients of 5-9S (Puca et al., 1972). When estrogens enter the target cells, the first stept in the nuclear translocation process may be the transformation of the native 5-9S receptor to a stable $\simeq$ 4S form by a Ca^{++}-dependent receptor transforming factor (Puca et al., 1972). The next step involves activation of the 4S estrogen-receptor complex, defined as increased binding to DNA or to isolated nuclei (eg., Yamamoto and Alberts, 1974), and transformation of the receptor to a 5S form (see Jensen and DeSombre, 1973). The 5S receptor appears to be a heterodimer consisting of an estrogen binding 4S monomer and a $\simeq$ 50,000 molecular weight protein (Notides and Nielsen, 1974). One view has been that the 4→5S transformation is synonymous with the activation process (eg., Notides and Nielsen, 1974; Yamamoto and Alberts, 1974; Weichman and Notides, 1979). The other, more recent, view is that the activation process, which appears to be a first order reaction and may be due to a conformational change, is independent of the 4→5S transformation, which is a second order reaction (Bailly et al., 1980). In any event, the activated state of the estrogen receptor is distinguished by having a slower dissociation rate for estradiol than the non-activated receptor; and the lesser estrogenic potency of estriol (E_3) and estrone (E_1) compared to estradiol is reflected in relatively greater dissociation rates of E_3 and E_1 from the activated receptors, rather than in differences in rates of receptor activation (Weichman and Notides, 1980).

The interaction of activated receptors with DNA and chromosomal proteins is believed to have considerable bearing upon the hormone-induced alterations in genomic activity, especially transcription of RNA (Buller and O'Malley, 1977; Spelsburg et al., 1975). The interactions in vitro of estrogen-receptor complexes with nuclei (Chamness et al., 1974) and with DNA (Yamamoto and Alberts, 1974; Andre and Rochefort, 1975) are described as largely nonsaturable, and it has been suggested that only a small proportion of the interactions of activated receptors with DNA is of significance for gene activation and that these may represent a saturable binding (Yamamoto and Alberts, 1974). Supporting such notions are indications of specificity in estrogen-receptor interactions with nucleic acids: preference for DNA over RNA; for double-stranded DNA over single-stranded DNA; for pyrimidine-rich over purine-rich polydeoxy-ribonucleotides (Kallos and Hollander, 1978; Thanki et al., 1978).

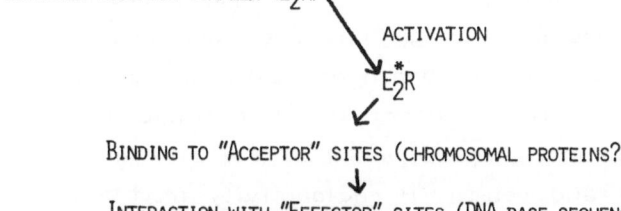

ESTROGEN-RECEPTOR COMPLEX (E_2R)

ACTIVATION

E_2^*R

BINDING TO "ACCEPTOR" SITES (CHROMOSOMAL PROTEINS?)

INTERACTION WITH "EFFECTOR" SITES (DNA BASE SEQUENCES?) TO PROMOTE TRANSCRIPTION

Figure 2: Model of E_2R interaction with postulated acceptor and effector sites (see text)

The notion of limited numbers of loci for receptor action on gene transcription has been codified into a model (Fig. 2) involving two kinds of interaction sites: acceptor sites and effector sites (Buller and O'Malley, 1977). This model is most apt for the progestin receptors of the chick oviduct which have been found to have a subunit which binds to chromosomal protein (proposed as acceptor sites) and a subunit which binds to DNA (proposed as effector sites) (see Buller and O'Malley, 1977). A similar situation is not thus far known to exist for estrogen receptors. However, two other features of the model summarized in Fig. 2 make it worth considering for the estrogen receptor system. One way of regarding the acceptor and effector sites is in terms of a receptor translocation model (Palmiter et al., 1976) in which the receptors move from initial unproductive (acceptor) sites to productive (ie., effector) sites. This is postulated to be a rate-limiting process and to explain the delayed appearance of ovalbumin m-RNA in the oviduct after estrogen treatment (Palmiter et al., 1976). Another aspect pertaining to the hypothetical effector sites is that they may differ in number and/or affinity for activated receptor even within the same target cells – this explanation has been proposed to explain different dose-response characteristics of estrogen action upon ovalbumin and conalbumin m-RNA production (Mulvihill and Palmiter, 1977).

Having summarized some of the basic facts and issues pertaining to estrogen receptors in non-neural target tissues, where much of our knowledge of their molecular biology has been obtained, let us now consider estrogen receptors in the brain and pituitary gland.

Brain and pituitary: The availability of tritiated estrogens enabled various investigators to demonstrate that the pituitary gland and hypothalamus take up and retain ^{3}H radioactivity from pulses of ^{3}H estradiol much as does the uterus (Eisenfeld and Axelrod, 1965; Kato and Villee, 1967; McEwen and Pfaff, 1970). The technique of steroid autoradiography permitted the localization of the neural uptake of ^{3}H estradiol to neurons of the hypothalmus, preoptic area and amygdala (Attramadal, 1965; Michael, 1965; Pfaff, 1968a,b; Stumpf, 1968, Anderson and Greenwood, 1969; Warembourg, 1970a,b; Pfaff and Keiner, 1973). Cell fractionation studies of brain and pituitary tissue patterned on the model of the studies of uterus, resulted in the demonstration of both soluble (for reference see McEwen, 1978) and cell nuclear (Zigmond and McEwen, 1970; Chader and Villee, 1970) forms of the estrogen receptors. As in uterus, cell nuclear translocation of estrogen receptor is accompanied by depletion of cytosol estrogen receptors (MacLusky et al., 1976), although this depletion appears to be less pronounced in brain than in pituitary or uterine tissue (Lieberburg et al., 1980). Repletion of cytosol estrogen receptors appears to involve a step which is dependent on protein synthesis (Cidlowski and Muldoon, 1974), as is also the case for the uterus (Scarff and Gorski, 1972).

The 4S→5S transformation has been demonstrated to occur in neural tissue (Linkie, 1977; Fox, 1977). The in vivo transformation of 4S to 5S occurs more slowly in hypothalamus compared to pituitary and uterus (Linkie, 1977). The in vitro transformation of 4S to 5S form in hypothalamic cytosol requires the presence of DNA-cellulose as well as 37° temperature and appears therefore to be a slower process than that occurring in the uterus (Fox, 1977). The proportion of activated estrogen receptor complexes in untreated brain cytosol capable of binding to DNA also appears to be lower than that in uterine cytosol (Fox and Johnstone, 1974).

In view of both similarities and differences between uterus and brain estrogen receptors, what is the evidence regarding their identity or non-identity? The physicochemical data and specificity of neural estrogen receptors (eg., see McEwen and Luine, 1978) reveals them to be very similar to uterine receptors. Moreover, the 5S receptor of hypothalamus, like that of the uterus, forms a complex with an unusual immunoglobulin-like protein present in many hyper-immune sera (Fox, 1977). In this connection, it should be noted that antisera prepared against calf uterine estrogen receptors (estro-philin) have been obtained which cross-react (Table 1) with estro-philin from other species and other tissues including pituitary and breast tumor cells, but not with receptors of other steroid hormones (Greene et al., 1979). Thus we have no reason at this stage to suspect that estrogen receptors of brain and pituitary are in fact different proteins from those in the uterus. Rather, certain aspects of cellular receptor processing may differ. For example, the slower 4→5S transformation in hypothalamus might be due to a limitation of the amount of the non-estrogen binding subunit (see above). Another

Table 1: Cross-reactivity of Estrogen Receptor (E_2R) from Various Tissues and Species with Rabbit IG-I

---

1. Rabbit IG-I reacts with rabbit, calf, rat, sheep, guinea pig, monkey and human E_2R.
2. Rabbit IG-I reacts with pituitary, uterine, mammary E_2R.
3. Rabbit IG-I does not react with androgen or progestin receptors or with alpha fetoprotein.

According to Greene, Closs, DeSombre and Jensen, 1979

factor which differentiates neural from non-neural targets is that neural estrogen receptors are present in excess over the amount which is required for nuclear translocation (Lieberburg et al., 1980).

2. Ontogeny of Neural Estrogen Receptors

The beginning of the life history of neural estrogen receptors concerns their elaboration in late fetal stages of the rat and mouse (Vito et al., 1979; MacLusky et al., 1979a). Though detectable in late fetal life in the rat, their level undergoes a marked increase in the two days preceding birth (MacLusky et al., 1979a). This is illustrated in Fig. 3, which also shows that there are no major sex differences in receptor levels or developmental time course. Neural progestin receptors, which are not detected on the day of birth, are elaborated early in the neonatal period (Fig. 4) in limbic structures and in cerebral cortex (MacLusky and McEwen, 1980). It should be noted in Fig. 3 that estrogen receptors are also laid down in the developing cerebral cortex of the male and female rat as well as in hypothalamus, preoptic area, and amygdala (referred to in Figure 3 as limbic structures). The cortical estrogen receptors, which have been visualized by autoradiography (McEwen, 1978; Sheridan, 1979), decline to the low levels found in the adult cortex during the third

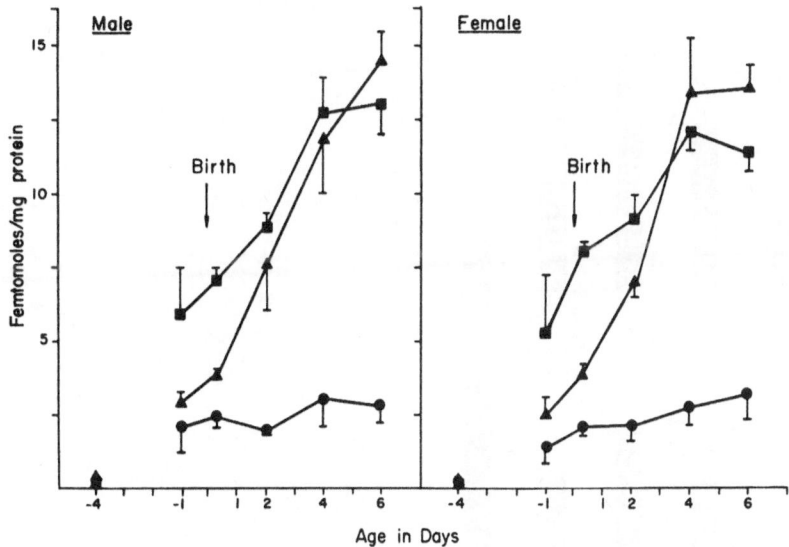

Figure 3: Perinatal ontogeny of soluble cytoplasmic estrogen receptor sites in the brains of male and female rats. Cytosols were prepared from either midbrain and brain stem (●), cerebral cortex (▲) or pooled hypothalamus, preoptic area and amygdala (■) and were labeled in vitro with 2 nM (^{3}H)moxestrol. Receptor-bound radioactivity was measured by Sephadex LH-20 gel filtration. Each data point represents the mean (±S.E.M.) of 4 determinations at each age. Reprinted from MacLusky et al., 1979 by permission

postnatal week of life (MacLusky et al., 1979b). Cortical progestin receptors remain elevated into adulthood and at no stage of development can they be elevated by estrogen treatment, even though the diencephalic progestin receptors can be elevated by estradiol priming starting in the second postnatal week of life (Fig. 4).

We are presently investigating the factors which influence the elaboration of estrogen and progestin receptors in the fetal hypothalamus by transplanting hypothalamic tissue on day 17 or 18 of fetal life into adult female hosts. We have established by autoradiography that estrogen receptors are elaborated outside of the fetal environment together with other hypothalamic charcteristics when the grafts are made into intact cycling female hosts (Stenevi et

67

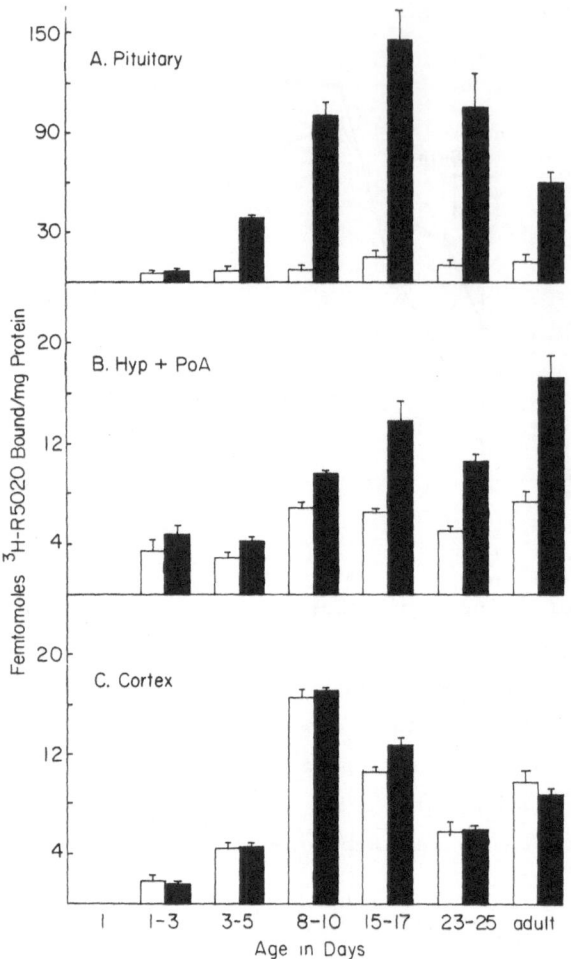

Figure 4: Ontogeny of cytosol high-affinity (^{3}H)R5020 binding sites. Animals were injected subcutaneously 44h before sacrifice with either R2858 (250 g/kg; solid bars) in 50μl oil, or the oil vehicle alone (open bars). Where an age range is given, the first figure represents the age at R5828 or vehicle injection. Adult rats were ovariectomized 7 days before use. All others were used intact. Cytosols were incubated for 4h at 2-4°C with 0.4 nM (^{3}H)R5020, in the presence and absence of 20 nM R5020. Bound (^{3}H)R5020 in the incubates was measured using Sephadex LH-20 gel filtration. Saturable (^{3}H)R5020 binding, defined as the difference between the results in the presence and absence of unlabeled R5020, is expressed per mg cytosol protein. Results represent the means (±S.E.M.) of either 4 (adults) or 3 (rest) observations. Total pituitary saturable (^{3}H)R5020 binding, expressed as femtomoles/pituitary, was as follows: days 1-3:Oil, 0.11 0.07; R2858, 0.17 0.01; days 3-5: Oil, 0.16 0.03: R2858, 0.98 0.07; days 8-10; Oil, 0.44 0.03; R2858, 5.04 0.18; days 15-17: Oil, 0.70 0.19; R2858, 7.44 1.08; days 23-25: Oil, 1.54 0.42; R2858, 18.0 2.2. Adult: Oil, 16.5 4.1; R2858, 97.6 10.3. Reprinted from MacLusky and McEwen, 1980 by permission.

al., 1980). It remains to be seen whether endocrine ablation such as adrenalectomy and ovariectomy will influence the course of receptor development.

3. Involvement of Estrogen and Estrogen Receptors in Brain Sexual Differentiation and in Neural Growth Processes

The perinatal increase of neural estrogen receptors coincides with the onset of the critical period during which testosterone suppresses the development of the potential for feminine sexual behavior and ovulation in rats (for review see Plapinger and McEwen, 1978). This action of testosterone is mediated by the conversion of testosterone to estradiol (McEwen et al., 1977; Vreeburg et al., 1977). Enzymes for this conversion are present in the perinatal rat brain (Reiddy et al., 1974; Weisz and Gibbs, 1974; Lieberburg et al., 1977) and result in substantial occupation of estrogen receptor sites in the perinatal male rat limbic brain (Lieberburg et al., 1979). Not all estrophilic cells are capable of aromatization – eg., those in the cerebral cortex and about half of those in the limbic brain (Lieberburg et al., 1979; Krey et al., 1980a). In those estrophilic cells of the limbic brain which aromatize, the normal levels of circulating testosterone in the neonatal male rat result in an occupation of 50% of their estrogen receptor capacity, a figure which is in agreement with the operating range of other steroid receptor systems (Krey et al., 1980a). Progestin receptors, which are elaborated at the start of the critical period (Fig. 4), may participate in an antagonistic action of progestins, leading to an attenuation of the effects of testosterone on rat brain sexual differentiation (McEwen et al., 1979). The cellular basis for this antagonism is unclear, but it may be another example of the kind of progesterone inhibition seen on the growth response of the uterus to estradiol (Bronson and Hamilton, 1972).

A principal action of estradiol during the neonatal critical period is to promote outgrowth of neuronal processes and to promote the formation of synaptic connections. This has been inferred from electron microscopic examination of synaptic density as a function of estrogen treatment within the hypothalamic arcuate nucleus (Arai et al., 1978; cf. also Raisman and Field, 1973) and from observations on neurite outgrowth from explants of hypothalamic tissue of newborn mice in response to estradiol and testosterone treatment (Toran-Allerand, 1976; 1978; 1980). In such explants, neurite outgrowth emanates from regions of the explant which contain estrophilic neurons (Toran-Allerand et al., 1979). Thus the estrogen action on growth appears to be a primary effect of the hormone rather than a secondary effect mediated by other cell types.

Although the principal developmental effects of estrogens on sexual differentiation occur within the first week of postnatal life in the rat, there are indications that estrogens may exert other, more subtle, long-term effects later in life. For example, the presence of the ovaries in female rats given low doses of testosterone attenuates the developmental effects of testosterone on sexual behavior and exploratory behaviors (Blizzard and Denef, 1973; Hendricks and Duffy, 1974; Hendricks and Weltin, 1976). A possible explanation for this from morphological studies is that estrogens given after the critical period continue to promote the formation of axodendritic synapses in the hypothalamic arcuate nucleus (Arai et al., 1978).

Estrogens also promote the enhancement of feminine sexual behavior in male rats after septal lesions (Nance et al., 1975; 1977). The authors of these studies suggest that estrogens modify the recovery process and reorganization of neural connections which follows brain damage. Related to this is the morphological observation in adult rats that estrogen treatment promotes collateral sprouting and reinvervation of synaptic sites vacated by degeneration in the arcuate nucleus following surgical lesions (Arai et al., 1978).

The ability of PMSG to promote precocious puberty in female rats is accompanied by a marked increase in the synaptic density within the arcuate nucleus; this action of PMSG requires the presence of the ovaries, a finding which once again implicates estrogens (Matsumoto and Arai, 1977).

Estrogen receptors in the perinatal rat cerebral cortex (Fig. 3) do not participate in the effects of testosterone because the cortex does not have aromatizing enzymes (Lieberburg et al., 1979). Yet they may be involved in certain aspects of cerebral cortical development resulting in sex differences in the thickness of the cerebral cortex (Diamond, M., personal communication).

4. The Transition From Organization to Activational Effects of Estrogens

Organizational effects are those permanent effects of estrogens which pertain to neural development (eg., sexual differentiation), whereas activational effects are those reversible actions of estradiol such as the priming of sexual behavior or ovulation. There is a transition period during the second postnatal week of life when organizational effects are waning (though not entirely absent – see above) and when activational effects begin to emerge. For example, at normal ambient temperatures, female rats begin around postnatal day 15 to show receptive and proceptive responses to manual stimulation after exogenous estradiol and progesterone (Södersten, 1975). Moreover, progesterone treatment of estrogen-primed rats at elevated body temperature will accentuate sexual responses in rats as young as 8-10 days of age (Williams, 1979). Fig. 4 shows that around 8-10 days of age one can first see signs of the estrogen induction of progestin receptors which become adult-like in magnitude by day 15. It seems likely that the emergence of progestin receptor inducibility by estradiol after the end of the critical period for brain sexual differentiation is a sign that the target cells are changing in their predominant mode of response to the estrogen-receptor complexes from one involving growth and other organizational effects to a mode emphasizing the reversible modification of chemical features of the estrophilic cells which are referred to under the heading of "activation" (MacLusky and McEwen, 1980).

5. Activational Effects of Estrogens and the Diversity of Cell Functions Associated with Estrophilic Neurons

The principal actions of estradiol in the adult female rat brain are to activate sexual behavior and ovulation. Progesterone synergizes with estradiol in enhancing these effects. Estrogens also play a role in male rats. In the male brain, estrogens derived from testosterone by aromatization participate in the activation of masculine sexual behavior. (For review see McEwen et al., 1979; MCcEwen, 1980). In this connection, it is interesting to note that the system of estrophilic cells in the brain (see Pfaff and Keiner, 1973) contain neurons capable of progestin receptor induction (Moguilewsky and Raynaud, 1977; Kato and Onouchi, 1977; MacLusky and McEwen, 1978; Warembourg, 1978) as well as neurons which convert testosterone to estradiol (Lieberburg and McEwen, 1977). Not all estrophilic neurons aromatize – eg., only about half of the limbic brain estrogen receptor capacity is present in such cells (Krey et al., 1980a). And not all estrophilic neurons show progestin receptor induction – eg., those of the amygdala clearly do not (MacLusky and McEwen, 1980; Moguilewsky and Raynaud, 1979). Some neurons of the hypothalamus and preoptic area contain both capabilities, as judged from the observation that testosterone treatment induces progestin receptors and activates sexual behavior and ovulation in OVX female rats by a process which is inhibited by a competitive inhibition of aromatization, ATD (Krey et al., 1980b).

Other demonstrated effects of estrogens in the limbic brain include the induction of choline acetyltransferase (Luine et al., 1980) and of muscarinic cholinergic receptors (Rainbow et al., 1980); the down regulation of type A monoamine oxidase (Luine and McEwen, 1977), of glutamic acid decarboxylase (Wallis and Luttge, 1980), and of tyrosine hydroxylase (Luine et al., 1977); and the induction of β-adrenergic receptors (Vacas and Cardineli, 1980). In short, the effects of estrogens on target cells in the adult rat brain may be as diverse as the target cells themselves rather than involving a property or properties common to all cells. The examples cited above indicate that estrogen effects on neurons involve the modulation of cellular constituents which are involved in synaptic transmission of electrical signals. A fuller discussion of the relevancy of estrogen action to synaptic function may be found in two recent reviews (McEwen, 1980a,b).

6. Neural Estrogen Receptors and Aging

Aging in female rats is associated first with the cessation of estrous cycles (Aschheim, 1976) and later with a decline in sexual receptivity (Peng et al., 1977). Since it is believed that the brain may be the primary site of the aging process in relation to the endocrine system (Finch, 1975; 1976), the study of estrogen feedback in the brain of aging animals is an appropriate way of approaching this problem. The aspect of estrogen feedback dealing with neural estrogen receptors has received only limited attention. However, there is agreement among three published studies that ^{3}H estradiol uptake by hypothalamus and ^{3}H estradiol binding to neural cytosol estrogen receptors are reduced in aging female rats (Kanungo et al., 1975; Peng et al., 1971; Haji et al., 1980). Since neural estrogen receptor levels in adult ovariectomized female rats are not altered by recent estrogen priming (Parsons et al., 1980), a gradual decline in estrogen titers in the blood does not appear to be a likely explanation for the decline of receptors with age. Rather, a loss of estrophilic neurons or a decline of the capacity of estrophilic cells to produce estrogen receptors should be considered as possibilities.

7. Conclusion

The study of estrogen receptors as a starting point for investigations of brain function has revealed a wide spectrum of hormone-regulated cellular events, some of which may well be responsible for the organization of behavior and neuroendocrine function early in life and others of which may be involved in the activation of behavior and neuroendocrine events in adult life. It is likely, because of their strong similarities among tissues and across species, that the estrogen receptors, which enable the target cells to respond to hormonal signals at various stages in the animal's life, do not themselves change as the animal develops; rather, it is the cellular responses to estrogens which change as the target cells differentiate.

The cellular responses to estrogens are indicative of the ways in which brain cells adapt to their environment. One type of response is growth and this leads neurons to meet other neurons and form synaptic connections. Growth responses of neurons to chemical signals such as estrogens are one of the predominant modes of response of developing neurons.

They are not totally absent in prepubertal and even adult hyothalamic tissue, as the discussion above has indicated. As we have also seen, another type of cellular response to hormonal signals is the induction or down-regulation of specific gene products that appear to be associated with synaptic function and neurotransmission. It remains to be seen exactly when these reversible responses to hormones appear in the course of neural development and differentiation. For such studies, we have as the model the emergence of the estrogen induction of progestin receptors (Fig. 4). The fact of their regulation by estrogens suggest that particular gene products (eg., neurotransmitter receptors, biosynthetic and degradative enzymes) may be rate limiting for neurotransmission in particular neural pathways via the up or down regulation of such gene products. The existence of this type of regulatory control by steroids over neural activity adds another level of complexity to the picture of chemical communication between neurons which is emerging from the recognition that there are neurohormones and neuromodulators as well as classical neurotransmitters (see Dismukes et al., 1979).

Acknowledgments

Research in the author's laboratory is supported by USPHS Grant NS07080 and by an institutional grant RF70095 from the Rockefeller Foundation for research in reproductive biology. The editorial assistance of Mrs. Oksana Wengerchuk is gratefully acknowledged.

References

Anderson CH, Greenwald SS (1969) Autoradiographic analysis of estradiol uptake in the brain and pituitary of the female rat. Endocrinology 85:1160–1165.

Andre J, Rochefort H (1975) In vitro binding of the estrogen receptor to DNA: absence of saturation at equilibrium. FEBS Letters 50:319–323.

Arai Y, Matsumoto A, Nishizuka M (1978) Synaptogenic action of estrogen on the hypothalamic arcuate nucleus (ARCN) of the developing brain and of the deafferented adult brain in female rats. In: Dörner G, Kawakami M (eds) Hormones and Brain Development, Elsevier/ North-Holland, pp.43–48.

Ascheim P (1976) Aging in the hypothalamic-hypophyseal ovarian axis in the rat. In: Everitt AV, Burgers JA (eds) Hypothalamus pituitary and aging, Charles C. Thomas, Springfield, pp.376–418.

Attramadal A (1965) Distribution and site of action of oestradiol in the brain and pituitary gland of the rat following intramuscular administration. In: Proc 2nd Internat Congress of Endocrinology, Part 1, pp.612–616.

Bailly A, LeFevre B, Savouret J-F, Milgrom E (1980) Activation and changes in sedimentation properties of steroid receptors. J Biol Chem 255:2729-2734.

Blizard D, Denef C (1973) Neonatal androgen effects on open-field activity and sexual behavior in the female rat: the modifying influence of ovarian secretions during development. Physiol Behav 11:65-69.

Bronson FH, Hamilton TH (1972) A comparison of nuclei acid synthesis in the mouse oviduct and uterus: interactions between estradiol and progesterone. Biol Reprod 6:160-167.

Buller RE, O'Malley BW (1976) The biology and mechanism of steroid hormone receptor interaction with the eukaryotic nucleus. Biochem Pharmac 25:1-12.

Chader GJ, Villee CA (1970) Uptake of oestradiol by the rabbit hypothalamus. Biochem J 118:93-97.

Chamness GC, Jennings AW, McGuire WL (1974) Estrogen receptor binding to isolated nuclei. A nonsaturable process. Biochemistry 13:327-331.

Cidlowski JA, Muldon TG (1974) Estrogenic regulation of cytoplasmic receptor populations in estrogen-responsive tissues of the rat. Endocrinology 95:1621-1629.

Dismukes RK (1979) New concepts of molecular communication among neurons. Behav Brain Sci 2:409-448.

Eisenfeld AJ, Axelrod J (1965) Selectivity of estrogen distribution in tissues. J Pharmacol Exp Therap 150:469-475.

Finch CE (1975) Neuroendocrinology of aging: a view of an emerging area. Bioscience 25:645-650.

Finch CE (1976) The regulation of physiological changes during mammalian aging. Quarterly Rev Biol 51:49-83.

Fox TO (1977) Conversion of the hypothalamic estradiol receptor to the "nuclear" form. Brain Res 120:580-583.

Fox TO, Johnston C (1974) Estradiol receptors from mouse brain and uterus: binding to DNA. Brain Res 77:330-336.

Glascock RF, Hoekstra WG (1959) Selective accumulation of tritium-labeled hexoestrol by the reproductive organs of immature female goats and sheep. Biochem J 72:673-682.

Glascock RF, Pope GS (1960) The preparation and purification of tritium-labeled hexoestrol of very high specific activity on the 5 mg scale. Biochem J 75:328-335.

Gorski J, Shyamala G, Toft D (1970) The search for hormone receptors: studies on estrogen binding in the uterus. In: Danielli JF, Moran JF, Triggle DJ (eds) Fundamental concepts in drug-receptor interaction, Academic Press, pp.215-228.

Greene GL, Closs LE, DeSombre ER, Jensen V (1979) Antibodies to estrophilin: comparison between rabbit and goat antisera. J Steroid Biochem 11:333-341.

Gupta GN (1960) The fate of tritium-labeled estradiol 17β in rat tissues. Ph.D. Thesis, University of Chicago, Dissertation Abstracts Int 34, 1972.

Haji M, Kato K, Nawata H, Ibayashi H (1981) Age-related changes in the concentration of cytosol receptors for sex steroid hormones in the hypothalamus and pituitary gland of the rat. Brain Res (in press).

Hendricks SE, Duffy JA (1974) Ovarian influences on the development of sexual behavior in neonatally androgenized rats. Develop Psychobiol 7:297-298.

Hendricks SE, Weltin M (1976) Effect of estrogen given during various periods of prepubertal life on the sexual behavior of rats. Physiol. Psychol 4:105-110.

Jensen EV (1960) Studies of growth phenomena using tritium-labeled steroids. Proc 4th Internat'l Congress of Biochem, Vienna, 1958, Vol 15, Pergamon, Oxford, p.119.

Jensen EV, DeSombre ER (1973) Estrogen-receptor interaction. Science 182:126-134.

Jensen EV, Jacobson HI (1962) Basic guides to the mechanism of estrogen action. Rec Progr Horm Res 18:387-408.

Jensen EV, Suzuki T, Kawashima T, Stumpf WE, Jungblut PW, DeSombre ER (1968) A two-step mechanism for the interaction of estradiol with rat uterus. Proc Nat Acad Sci USA 59:632-638.

Kallos J, Hollander VP (1978) Assessment of specificity of oestrogen-receptor-DNA interaction by a competitive assay. Nature 272:177-179.

Kanungo MS, Patnaik SK, Koul O (1975) Decrease in 17β-oestradiol receptor in brain of aging rats. Nature 253:366-367.

Kato J, Onouchi T (1977) Specific progesterone receptors in the hypothalamus and anterior hypophysis of the rat. Endocrinology 101:920-928.

Kato J, Villee CA (1967) Preferential uptake of estradiol by the anterior hypothalamus of the rat. Endocrinology 80:567-575.

Krey LC, Kamel F, McEwen BS (1980a) Parameters of neuroendocrine aromatization and estrogen receptor occupation in the male rat. Brain Res (in press).

Krey LC, MacLusky NJ, Davis PG (1980b) Neuroendocrine mechanisms underlying testosterone priming for lordosis and cyclic LH release in the rat. Abstracts, The Endocrine Society 2nd Annual Mtg., Washington, DC, Abstract 106.

Lieberburg I, Krey LC, McEwen BS (1979) Sex differences in serum testosterone and in exchangeable brain cell estradiol during the neonatal period in rats. Brain Res 178:207-212.

Lieberburg I, MacLusky NJ, McEwen BS (1980) Cytoplasmic and nuclear estradiol-17β binding in male and female rat brain: regional distribution, temporal aspects and metabolism. Brain Res (in press).

Lieberburg I, McEwen BS (1977) Brain cell nuclear retention of testosterone metabolites, 5α dihydrotestosterone and estradiol 17β, in adult rats. Endocrinology 100:588-597.

Lieberburg I, Wallach G, McEwen BS (1977) The effects of an inhibitor of aromatization (1,4,6-androstatriene-3,17-dione) and an anti-estrogen (CI-628) on in vivo formed testosterone metabolites recovered from neonatal rat brain tissues and purified cell nuclei. Implications for sexual differentiation of the rat brain. Brain Res 128:176-181.

Linkie DM (1977) Estrogen receptors in different target tissues: similarities of form - dissimilarities of transformation. Endocrinology 101:1862-1870.

Luine VN, McEwen BS (1977) Effect of oestradiol on turnover of type A monoamine exidase in brain. J Neurochem 28:1221-1227.

Luine VN, Park D, Joh T, Reis D, McEwen BS (1980) Immunochemical demonstration of increased choline acetyltransferase concentration in rat preoptic area after estradiol administration. Brain Res 191:273-277.

MacLusky NJ, Chaptal C, Lieberburg I, McEwen BS (1976) Properties and subcellular inter-relationships of presumptive estrogen receptor macromolecules in the brains of neonatal and prepubertal female rats. Brain Res 114:158-165.

MacLusky NJ, Chaptal C, McEwen BS (1979b) The development of estrogen receptor systems in the rat brain and pituitary: postnatal development. Brain Res 178:143-160.

MacLusky NJ, Lieberburg I, McEwen BS (1979) The development of estrogen receptor systems in the rat brain: perinatal development. Brain Res 178:129–142.

MacLusky NJ, McEwen BS (1978) Oestrogen modulates progestin receptor concentrations in some rat brain regions but not in others. Nature 274:276–278.

MacLusky NJ, McEwen BS (1980) Progestin receptors in the developing rat brain and pituitary. Brain Res 189:262–268.

MacLusky NJ, McEwen BS (1980) Progestin receptors in rat brain: distribution and properties of cytoplasmic progestin binding sites. Endocrinology 106:192–202.

Matsumoto A, Arai Y (1977) Precocious puberty and synaptogenesis in the hypothalamic arcuate nucleus in pregnant mare serum gonadotropin (PMSG)-treated immature female rats. Brain Res 129:375–378.

McEwen BS (1978) Gonadal steroid receptors in neuroendocrine tissues. In: O'Malley B, Birnbaumer L (eds) Hormone Receptors, Vol I Steroid Hormones, Academic Press, N.Y., pp.353–400.

McEwen BS (1978) Sexual maturation and differentiation: the role of the gonadal steroids. Progr Brain Res 48:291–307.

McEwen BS (1980) Mechanisms of gonadal steroid action in the brain viewed as the end product of sexual differentiation. Science (in press).

McEwen BS, Davis PG, Parsons B, Pfaff DW (1979) The brain as a target for steroid hormone action. In: Cowan M (ed) Annual Review of Neuroscience, pp.65–112.

McEwen BS, Lieberburg I, Chaptal C, Davis PG, Krey LC, MacLusky NJ, Roy EJ (1980) Attenuating the defeminization of the neonatal rat brain: mechanisms of action of cyproterone acetate, 1,4,6-androstatriene-3,17-dione and a synthetic progestin, R5020. Horm Behav 13:269–281.

McEwen BS, Lieberburg I, Chaptal C, Krey LC (1977) Aromatization: important for sexual differentiation of the neonatal rat brain. Horm Behav 9:249–263.

McEwen BS, Luine VN (1978) Specificity, mechanisms and functional significance of steroid-receptor interactions in the brain and pituitary. In: Vincent J-D, Kordon C (eds) Biologie Cellulaire des Processus Neurosecretoires Hypothalamique, Colloques Internationaux du CNRS No. 280, Paris, pp.239–267.

McEwen BS, Pfaff DW (1970) Factors influencing sex hormone uptake by rat brain regions: I. Effects of neonatal treatment, hypophysectomy, and competing steroid on estradiol uptake. Brain Res 21:1–16.

Michael RP (1965) Oestrogens in the central nervous system. Brit Med Bull 21:87–90.

Moguilewsky M, Raynaud J-P (1977) Progestin binding sites in the rat hypothalamus, pituitary and uterus. Steroids 30:99–109.

Moguilewsky M, Raynaud JP (1979) Estrogen-sensitive progestin-binding sites in the female rat brain and pituitary. Brain Res 164:165–179.

Müller RE, Wotiz HH (1979) Kinetics of estradiol entry into uterine cells. Endocrinology 105:1107–1114.

Mulvihill ER, Palmiter RD (1977) Relationship of nuclear estrogen receptor levels to induction of ovalbumin and conalbumin mRNA in chick oviduct. J Biol Chem 252:2060–2068.

Nance DM, Phelps C, Shryne JE, Gorski RA (1977) Alterations by estrogen and hypothyroidism in the effects of septal lesions on lordosis behavior of male rats. Brain Res Bull 2:49–53.

Nance DM, Shryne J, Gorski RA (1975) Facilitation of female sexual behavior in male rats by septal lesions: an interaction with estrogen. Horm Behav 6:289–299.

Notides AC, Nielsen S (1974) The molecular mechanism of the in vitro 4S to 5S transformation of the uterine estrogen receptor. J Biol Chem 249:1866–1873.

Palmiter RD, Moore PB, Mulvihill ER (1976) A significant lag in the induction of ovalbumin messenger RNA by steroid hormones: a receptor translocation hypothesis. Cell 8:557–572.

Parsons B, MacLusky NJ, Krieger MS, Pfaff DW, McEwen BS (1980) The effects of long-term exposure on the induction of sexual behavior and on brain estrogen and progestin receptors in the female rat. Horm Behav 13:301–313.

Peng TM, Chuong CF, Peng YM (1977) Lordosis response of senile female rats. Neuroendocrinology 24:317–324.

Peng MT, Peng YM (1973) Changes in the uptake of tritiated estradiol in the hypothalamus and adenohypophysis of old female rats. Fertil Steril 24:534–539.

Pfaff DW (1968a) Uptake of estradiol-17 $-^3$H in the female rat brain: an autoradiographic study. Endocrinology 82:1149–1155.

Pfaff DW (1968b) Autoradiographic localization of radioactivity in rat brain after injection of tritiated sex hormones. Science 161:1355–1356.

Pfaff DW, Keiner M (1973) Atlas of estradiol-concentrating cells in the central nervous system of the female rat. J Comp Neurol 151:121–158.

Plapinger L, McEwen BS (1978) Gonadal steroid-brain interactions in sexual differentiation. In: Hutchinson JB (ed) Biological Determinants of Sexual Behavior, Wiley, N.Y., pp.153–218.

Puca GA, Nola E, Sica V, Bresciani F (1972) Estrogen-binding proteins of calf uterus. Interrelationship between various forms and identification of a receptor-transforming factor. Biochemistry 11:4157–4165.

Rainbow TC, DeGroff V, Luine VN, McEwen BS (1980) Estradiol 17β increases the number of muscarinic receptors in hypothalamic nuclei. Brain Res (in press).

Raisman G, Field PM (1973) Sexual dimorphism in the neuropil of the preoptic area of the rat and its dependence on neonatal androgen. Brain Res 54:1–29.

Reddy VVR, Naftolin F, Ryan KJ (1974) Conversion of androstenedione to estrone by neural tissues from fetal and neonatal rats. Endocrinology 94:117–121.

Sarff M, Gorski J (1971) Control of estrogen binding protein concentration under basal conditions and after estrogen administration. Biochem 10:2557–2563.

Sheridan PJ (1979) Estrogen binding in the neonatal cortex. Brain Res 178:201–206.

Södersten PC (1975) Receptive behavior in developing female rats. Horm Behav 6:307–317.

Spelsburg TC, Webster R, Pikler GM (1975) Multiple binding sites for progesterone in the hen oviduct nucleus: evidence that acidic proteis represent the acceptors. In: Chromosomal Proteins and their Role in the Regulation of Gene Expression, Academic Press, N.Y., pp.153–186.

Stenevi U, Björklund A, Kromer LF, Paden CM, Gerlach JL, McEwen BS, Silverman AJ (1980) Differentiation of embryonic hypothalamic transplants cultured on the choroidal pia in brains of adult rats. Cell Tiss Res 209:217–228.

Stumpf WE (1968) Estradiol-concentrating neurons: topography in the hypothalamus by dry mount autoradiography. Science 162:1001–1003.

Thanki KH, Beach TA, Dickerman HW (1978) Selective binding of mouse estradiol-receptor complexes to oligo(dT)-cellulose. J Biol Chem 253:7744–7750.

Toran-Allerand CD (1976) Sex steroids and the development of the newborn mouse hypothalamus and preoptic area in vitro: implications for sexual differentiation. Brain Res 106:407-412.

Toran-Allerand CD (1978) Gonadal hormones and brain development: cellular aspects of sexual differentiation. Amer Zool 18:553-565.

Toran-Allerand CD (1980) Sex steroids and the development of the newborn mouse hypothalamus and preoptic area in vitro. II. Morphological correlates and hormonal specificity. Brain Res. 189:413-427.

Toran-Allerand CD, Gerlach JL, McEwen BS (1980) Autoradiographic localization of ^{3}H estradiol related to steroid responsiveness in cultures of the newborn mouse hypothalamus and preoptic area. Brain Res 184:517-522.

Vacas MI, Cardineli DP (1980) Effect of estradiol on α-and β-adrenoceptor density in medial basal hypothalamus, cerebral cortex and pineal gland of ovariectomized rats. Neurosci Letters 17:73-77.

Vito CC, Fox TO (1979) Embryonic rodent brain contains estrogen receptors. Science 204:517-519.

Vreeburg JTM, van der Vaart PDM, van der Schoot P (1977) Prevention of central defeminization but not masculinization in male rats by inhibition neonatally of oestrogen biosynthesis. J Endocrinol 74:375-382.

Wallis CJ, Luttge WG (1980) Influence of estrogen and progesterone on glutamic acid decarboxylase activity in discrete regions of rat brain. J Neurochem 34(3):609-613.

Warembourg M (1970a) Fixation de l'oestradiol ^{3}H dans le telecephale et le diencephale chez la souris femelle. Comptes Rendus Soc Biol 164:126-129.

Warembourg M (1970b) Fixation de l'oestradiol ^{3}H au niveau des noyaux amygdaliens, septaux et du systeme hypothalamo-hypophysaire chez la souris femelle. C R Acad Sci Paris 270:152-154.

Warembourg M (1978) Radioautographic study of the rat brain, uterus and vagina after (^{3}H)R-5020 injection. Mol Cell Endocr 12:67-79.

Weichman BM, Notides AC (1979) Analysis of estrogen receptor activation by its ^{3}H estradiol dissociation kinetics. Biochemistry 18:220-225.

Weichman BM, Notides AC (1980) Estrogen receptor activation and the dissociation kinetics of estradiol, estriol, and estrone. Endocrinology 106:434-439.

Weisz J, Gibbs C (1974) Metabolites of testosterone in the brain of the newborn female rat after an injection of tritiated testosterone. Neuroendocrinology 14:72-86.

Williams CL (1979) Steroids induce lordosis and ear wiggling in infant rats. Abstracts, Eastern Conference on Reproductive Behavior, New Orleans, June 8-9, 1979.

Yamamoto KR, Alberts B (1974) On the specificity of the binding of the estradiol receptor protein to deoxyribonucleic acid. J Biol Chem 249:7076-7086.

Zigmond RE, McEwen BS (1970) Selective retention of oestradiol by cell nuclei in specific brain regions of the ovariectomized rat. J Neurochem 17:889-899.

Effects of Sex Hormone Metabolites on the Secretion of Gonadotropins

M. Motta, F. Celotti, R. Massa, M. Zanisi and L. Martini, Milano

The anterior pituitary, the hypothalamus and other brain structures, known to be a target for androgens and progestagens with respect to the regulation of gonadotropin secretion, are able to convert testosterone and progesterone into their respective 5α-reduced metabolites. It has been shown that, in these central tissues of male mammals, as in the peripheral androgen sensitive structures, testosterone may be transformed into 5α-androstan-17β-ol-3-one (5α-dihydrotestosterone, DHT) and 5α-androstan-3α,17β-diol (3α-diol) (for references see Martini, 1976 and Celotti et al., 1979b). Minute amounts of 5α-androstan-3β,17β-diol(3β-diol) are also formed in the neuroendocrine structures (Van Doorn et al., 1975; Kao et al., 1977). These conversions occur under the influence of a 5α-reductase-3-hydroxysteroid dehydrogenase system.

Similar enzymatic activities have been found in the anterior pituitary and in the hypothalamus of female mammals, where progesterone is probably the physiological substrate. Several studies have demonstrated that, in these structures, progesterone is converted into 5α-pregnan-3,20-dione (dihydroprogesterone, DHP) and 5α-pregnan-3α-ol-20-one (3α-ol) (Massa et al., 1972; Karavolas and Nuti, 1976; Stupnicka et al., 1977).

It seems reasonable to postulate that the conversion of testosterone and progesterone taking place in these tissues might be an important component of the mechanisms whereby testosterone and progesterone exert their effects on gonadotropin secretion and on other neural processes (e.g. control of sexual behavior, etc.)

This paper summarizes findings of our laboratory aimed at clarifying: (a) the factors that modulate the activity of the 5α-reductase-3-hydroxysteroid dehydrogenase system in the anterior pituitary and in the hypothalamus of rats of both sexes; and (b) the mechanisms through which the 5α-reduced metabolites of testosterone and of progesterone may influence gonadotropin secretion, respectively in the male and in the female rat.

1. Endocrine Factors Which Control the 5α-Reductase Activity of the Anterior Pituitary and of the Hypothalamus

Effects of castration, androgens, and prolactin on the conversion of testosterone into its 5α-reduced metabolites. Little information is available on the endocrine factors which control the conversion of testosterone into its 5α-reduced metabolites. This study was performed in order to analyze whether endogenous or exogenous androgens might participate in such a control. The effect of castration was analyzed first. The enzymatic activities of the anterior pituitary and of the hypothalamus of male rats were evaluated in vitro using labeled testosterone as the substrate. The different metabolites have been identified using techniques previously described (Kniewald et al., 1971; Massa et al., 1977). Orchidectomy induces in 20 days a significant increase in the amounts of DHT and of the diols formed in the anterior pituitary. There are no significant effects of castration on testosterone metabolism at the hypothalamic level (Celotti et al., 1980). The effect of orchidectomy at the anterior pituitary level might be interpreted either as a direct one on the enzymatic activities involved, or, as an indirect one linked to the changes in the composition of pituitary cell population which occurr following the operation. It is known that castration increases the number and the size of the gonadotrophs in which the 5α-reductase-3-hydroxysteroid dehydrogenases are predominantly located, as indicated by in vitro and in vivo evidence the different tissues in the presence of labeled progesterone and by identifying, at the end of the incubation period, the different metabolites formed. A technique similar to that used for the studies on testosterone metabolism has been adopted (Kniewald et al., 1971;

Massa et al., 1977). Ovariectomy induces in 20 days a significant increase in the amounts of the 5α-derivatives formed by the anterior pituitary. On the contrary, the operation does not exert any relevant effect on the 5α-reductase and 3-hydroxysteroid dehydrogenase activities of the hypothalamus. The in vivo administration of estradiol to ovariectomized rats significantly decreases the 5α-reductase activity in the anterior pituitary of these animals. Estrogens do not exert any significant effect on the 5α-reductase activity of the hypothalamus (Stupnicka et al., 1977).

2. Effects of Testosterone and its 5 α –Reduced Metabolites on Gonadotropin Secretion

The observations mentioned in the preceeding sections of this paper, that the brain and the anterior pituitary convert testosterone into DHT, 3α-diol and 3β-diol, and the fact that these 5α-reduced metabolites are also present in the peripheral blood of male rats have led to the suggestion that these steroids might play a physiological role in the control of gonadotropin secretion.

Following the preliminary observations of Zanisi et al. (1973) several data in the literature have indicated that DHT and 3α-diol are more effective than testosterone in suppressing LH release (Swerdloff et al., 1973; Verjans and Eik-Nes, 1976, 1977; see also Celotti et al., 1979b for references). In a recent experiment, it has been confirmed once more that the administration of one single dose of either DHT or 3α-diol to adult castrated male rats is followed in 24 hr by a significant decrease of serum LH which is greater than that induced by a comparable dose of testosterone. Contrary to previous evidence in this experiment 3β-diol was found to be totally ineffective. It was thought that the ineffectiveness of 3β-diol might be due to the selection of an inappropriate sampling time. Consequently an experiment was run in which serum levels of LH have been obtained in this and other laboratories (Lloyd and Karavolas, 1975; Celotti et al., 1976; Denef, 1979).

The reverse experiment was then performed by administering, to castrated adult male rats, testosterone, DHT, 3α-diol and 3β-diol, i.e., the four androgens present physiologically in large amounts in the blood of the male rat (Gupta et al., 1975; Corpechot et al., 1977; Moger, 1977; Zamecnik et al., 1977). Treatment with all androgens decreased the formation of DHT and of the diols at the pituitary level. There was no effect of androgen administration at the hypothalamic level (Celotti et al., 1979a). These data underline once more that only the 5α-reductase 3-hydroxysteroid dehydrogenase system of the anterior pituitary is sensitive to androgens. However, it must be stressed that the results obtained after steroid treatment might be the reflection of the return of the gonadotrophs to normal size and number.

The effect of prolactin was studied next. The experiments were performed in adult castrated male rats in order to avoid any possible peripheral action of prolactin on testicular function (resulting in an increased production of testosterone) (Hafiez et al., 1972; McNatty et al., 1974). Subcutaneous injection of rat prolactin does not influence the formation of DHT and of the diols at the anterior pituitary level, but significantly decreases the formation of the 5α-reduced metabolites of testosterone in the hypothalamus (Martini et al., 1978). There is plenty of evidence (derived from electrophysiological, metabolic and feedback studies) which indicates that prolactin may act directly at hypothalamic level (Clemens et al., 1967; Clemens and Meites, 1968; Clemens et al., 1971; Yamada, 1975; Fuxe et al., 1977); the present data add new support to such a hypothesis. It is interesting to note that prolactin was active on the hypothalamus, i.e. on a structure in which androgens were not effective.

Effects of castration and estrogens on the conversion of progesterone into its 5α-reduced metabolites. The ability of the anterior pituitary and of the hypothalamus of female rats to convert progesterone into its 5α-reduced metabolites has been studied by incubating in vitro measured, by specific radioimmunoassay (Niswender et al., 1968), in adult castrated male rats 2, 5, and 8 hr following the administration of testosterone, DHT, 3α- and 3β-diol. It appears from Figure 1 that 3β-diol does inhibit LH release only at 2 hr and that its effects disappear after that time interval. Testosterone, DHT and 3α-diol exert a comparable LH-inhibiting effect at all time intervals consider-

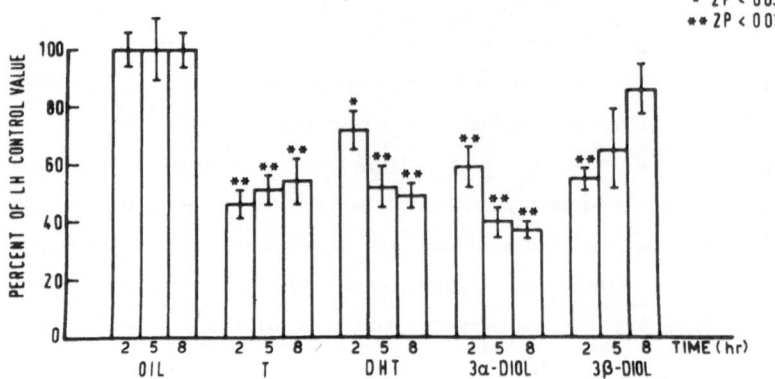

Figure 1: Effect of a single s.c. injection of 2 mg of various androgens on serum LH levels in long-term castrated male rats measured at different time intervals

ed.   The   negative   result   obtained   with   3β-iol   at   24 hr   might consequently   be   due   to   the   fact   that   this   steroid   loses   its   LH-inhibiting   activity   very   rapidly.   In   recent   studies,   it   has   been shown   that   3β-iol   is   further   converted   in   the   neuroendocrine structures   into   two   different   metabolites,   i.e.   5α-androstan-3β,6α,17β-triol   (6α-triol)   and   5α-androstan-3β,7α,17β-triol(7α-triol)   (Morfin   et al.,   1979;   Samperez   and   Jouan,   1979).   Nothing   is   known   in   the literature   on   the   feedback   activities   of   these   derivatives;   these   are at   present   under   investigation   in   our   laboratory.

A further   step   was   that   of   trying   to   identify   the   site   of   action (hypothalamus,   anterior   pituitary?)   of   testosterone   and   its   5α-reduced metabolites.   Several   approaches   have   been   utilized.   One   was   that of   directly   implanting   the   various   compounds   into   the   hypothalamus or   the   anterior   pituitary   (Motta   et   al.,   1980).   The   other   one   was that   of   studying   the   effect   of   the   various   androgens   on   the   hypo-thalamic   concentration   of   LHRH   as   measured   by   radioimmunoassay (Nett   et   al.,   1973).   It   is   known   that   (when   radioimmunoassays   are utilized)   castration   is   followed   by   a   significant   decrease   in   the concentrations   of   LHRH   at   the   hypothalamic   level   which   may   be brought   back   to   normal   by   the   administration   of   testosterone   (Shin and   Howitt,   1975,   1976).   Very   little   information   is   available   on   the effects   of   DHT   and   practically   nothing   on   those   of   3α-   and   3β-diol   on this   parameter.   In   our   experiments,   like   in   those   of   previous   authors (Shin   and   Howitt,   1975,   1976)   castration   is   followed   by   a   significant

84

decrease in hypothalamic stores of LHRH; the administration of testosterone is able to partially overcome this effect. On the contrary, DHT, 3α-diol and 3β-diol are not able to increase the hypothalamic stores of LHRH reduced by orchidectomy (Fig. 2).

This result seems to indicate that testosterone may operate in the feedback mechanisms controlling LH release acting also at hypothalamic level. The inefficacy of the 5α-reduced metabolites on the parameter considered opens the question whether the effect of testosterone on LHRH stores is brought about by the molecule as such, or following its conversion into estrogen through the well known aromatization process (see Celotti et al., 1979b, for references). The fact that DHT and the diols do not influence hypothalamic LHRH stores might be taken as evidence in favor of an intrapituitary mode of action of these steroids in the control of gonadotropin secretion. However, this interpretation is not supported by previous data from this laboratory which indicate that testosterone, DHT and 3α-diol reduce serum levels of LH in castrated animals following intrahypothalamic but not following intrapituitary placement (Motta et al., 1980). The answer will have to be derived

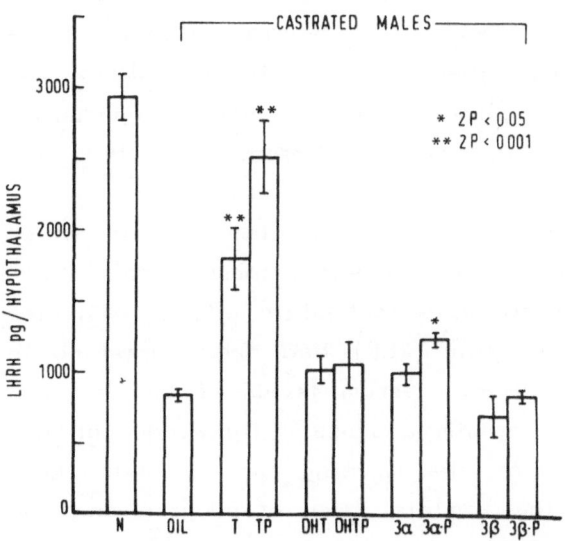

Figure 2: Effect of 6-day treatment with various androgens (2 mg rat/day) on hypothalamic stores of LHRH in long-term castrated adult male rats

from additional experiments, since the measurement of hypothalamic stores of LHRH does not provide any indication on how much LHRH is released into the pituitary vessels. It is known that stores may be changed either by modifications in the synthesis of a hormone or by a variation in its release and/or degradation.

3.   Effects of Progesterone and its 5 α -Reduced Metabolites on Gonadotropin Secretion

It is known that, depending on the circumstances, progesterone may exert either an inhibitory (negative feedback) or a stimulatory (positive feedback, or facilitatory) effect on gonadotropin secretion (Motta et al., 1970; Neill and Smith, 1974). The hypothesis that the 5α-reduced metabolites of progesterone might represent the mediators of the actions of the hormone on LH and FSH secretion has been consequently investigated. First of all, it has been shown that in ovariectomized, estrogen-primed rats, DHP and 3α-ol exert a stimulatory effect on the release of LH of a magnitude comparable to that of progesterone (Zanisi and Martini, 1975). DHP and 3α-ol are also able to induce the release of FSH in the same animals; the activity on this gonadotropin is similar for the two steroids but is, however, lower than that of progesterone (Zanisi and Martini, 1975). These results have been confirmed by others, using different doses and schedules of administration of estrogens and various progesterone derivatives (Brown-Grant, 1974; Fink and Henderson, 1977; Nuti and Karavolas, 1977).

To gain additional information on the mechanisms through which DHP and 3α-ol may modify gonadotropin secretion, these steroids have now been administered subcutaneously, dissolved in oil, to castrated female rats, in which ethinyl estradiol (EE) had been implanted in the median eminence 5 days earlier. Serum levels of LH and FSH have been measured by specific radioimmunoassays (Niswender et al., 1968; Daane and Parlow, 1971) on the morning of the sixth post-implantation day, 17 hr after the administration of progesterone and its 5α-reduced metabolites. The 3β-epimer of 3α-ol (5α-pregnan-3β-ol-20-one, 3β-ol) was included in this study even if this steroid is not a regular metabolite of progesterone in the brain or in the

86

anterior pituitary. However, it has been shown to be present in the general circulation of the female rat (Holzbauer, 1971, 1975) as the other 5α-reduced derivatives (Ichikawa et al., 1971, 1974).

The implantation of EE into the median eminence of castrated female rats is followed by a dramatic decrease in serum LH levels. The administration of either progesterone or DHP to EE-implanted animals brings about a significant increase of serum LH levels. The increase induced by DHP is significantly higher than that induced by progesterone. Neither 3α- nor 3β-ol is able to increase serum levels of LH in the EE-implanted animals (Fig. 3).

The implantation of EE also induces a significant decrease in serum levels of FSH. The subsequent administration of progesterone does not increase serum FSH. On the contrary, DHP, 3α- and 3β-ol are all able to enhance serum levels of FSH (Fig. 3).

The data confirm once more, using a more sophisticated technique, that progesterone and DHP may exert a stimulatory effect on LH release (Zanisi and Martini, 1975). Contrary to the data in which estrogens were given systemically (Brown-Grant, 1974; Fink and Henderson, 1977; Nuti and Karavolas, 1977; Zanisi and Martini, 1975), FSH is not affected by progesterone in animals bearing median

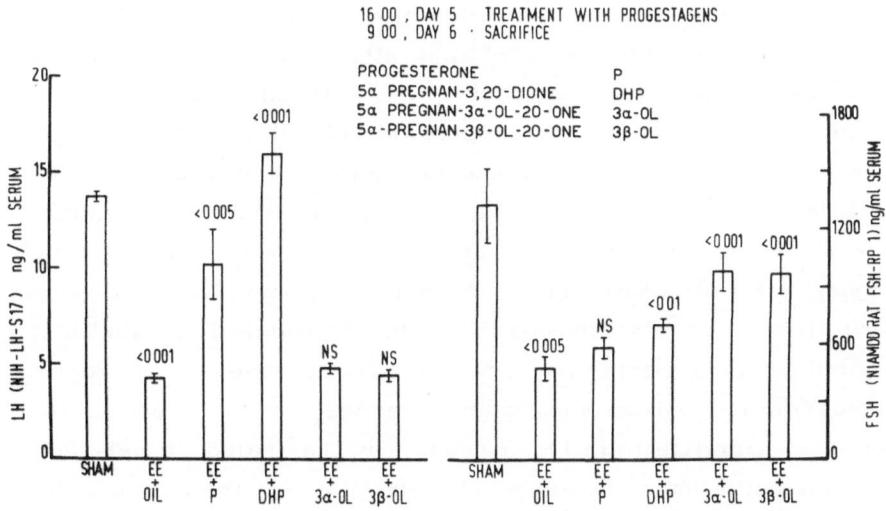

Figure 3: Effect of treatment with 100 µg/rat of progesterone and of its 5α-reduced metabolites on serum LH and FSH levels in long-term castrated female rats implanted in the median eminence with ethinyl estradiol (EE) 5 days earlier

eminence implants of EE. This discrepancy may be explained by two facts. First, a smaller dose of estrogens has been used in the present series of experiments when compared to the doses used systemically. Second, in the present study, the effects of progesterone were evaluated much later than previous experiments (17 versus 9 hr). It is consequently possible that in these experiments, the FSH peak has been missed. At variance with the earlier results in animals given estradiol systemically (Zanisi and Martini, 1975), in the present experiments 3α- and 3β-ol were found to be ineffective in increasing serum levels of LH. The reason for such a discrepancy may be found in the different time interval between treatment and sacrifice. The efficacy of DHP, 3α- and 3β-ol on the release of FSH following systemic administration in animals implanted with estrogens is in line with previous observations from this and other laboratories (Brown-Grant, 1974; Fink and Henderson, 1977; Nuti and Karavolas, 1977; Zanisi and Martini, 1975).

4. Summary and Conclusions

It emerges from the data that the metabolism of testosterone and of progesterone occurring in the neuroendocrine structures may play an important role for the expression of the effects of the two hormones on the secretion of pituitary gonadotropins. It appears first of all that DHT and 3α-diol are potent suppressors of LH secretion; 3β-diol shares this property, but with a shorter duration of action. Testosterone is able to restore LHRH intrahypothalamic stores in castrated male rats, while its 5α-reduced metabolites are ineffective; this fact might suggest a different site of action (hypothalamus versus anterior pituitary) for testosterone and the 5α-reduced metabolites. However, additional experiments are needed because of a conflict with previous data. Dihydroprogesterone appears more effective than progesterone in facilitating LH release in castrated female rats bearing intrahypothalamic implants of estrogen; in the same animal mode, the other 5α-reduced derivatives of progesterone appear ineffective on LH secretion, but strongly stimulate FSH release. This finding opens new possibilities: that the different metabolites of progesterone might be responsible for the differential feedback control of the secretion of the two gonadotropins. The fact that the enzymatic activities of the anterior pituitary might be modulated in opposite directions by the elimination of endogenous sex steroids and by the administration of exogenous androgens and estrogens also favors the view that the process of 5α-reduction may represent an important step in the mode of action of testosterone and progesterone.

Acknowledgements

The experiments described in this paper have been supported by grants from the Ford Foundation, New York; the Consiglio Nazionale delle Ricerche, Rome, through the Program Biology of Reproduction, to Dr. L. Martini; and by a grant from the Consiglio Nazionale delle Ricerche to Dr. M. Motta. All such support is gratefully acknowledged. Materials for LH and FSH radioimmunoassay have been kindly provided by the Rat Pituitary Hormone Distribution Program of the National Institutes of Arthritis, Metabolism and Digestive Diseases of the National Institutes of Health, Bethesda, Md. Thanks are also due to Mrs. Paola Assi Brunone and Mrs. Giovanna Miccichè Anzani for their skilfull technical assistance.

References

Brown-Grant K (1974) Steroid hormone administration and gonadotrophin secretion in the gonadectomized rat. J Endocrinol 62:319-332.

Celotti F, Farina J, Cresti L, Massa R, Martini L (1976) 5α-reductase activity (5 -R) in rat pituitary homografts under the kidney capsule. Program 5th Intern Congr Endocrinology, pp.44-45.

Celotti F, Farina JMS, Santaniello E, Martini L, Motta M (1979a) Effect of testosterone, its 5α-reduced metabolites and the corresponding propionates on testosterone metabolism. I. In the hypothalamus and in the anterior pituitary. J Steroid Biochem 11:215-219.

Celotti F, Massa R, Martini L (1979b) Metabolism of sex steroids in the central nervous system. In: De Groot LJ (ed) Endocrinology, Vol 1, Grune and Stratton, New York, pp.41-53.

Celotti F, Ferraboschi P, Negri-Cesi P, Martini L (1980) Control of the metabolism of testosterone in the prostate and in other androgen-dependent structures. In: Jacobelli S (ed) Hormones and Cancer, in press.

Clemens JA, Meites J (1968) Inhibition by hypothalamic prolactin implants of prolactin secretion, mammary growth and luteal function. Endocrinology 82:878-881.

Clemens JA, Gallo RV, Whitmoyer DI, Sawyer CH (1971) Prolactin responsive neurons in the rabbit hypothalamus. Brain Res 25:371-379.

Clemens JA, Sar M, Meites J (1967) Inhibition of lactation and luteal function in postpartum rats by hypothalamic implantation of prolactin. Endocrinology 84:868-872.

Corpechot C, Eychenne B, Robel P (1977) Simultaneous radioimmunoassay of testosterone, dihydrotestosterone, 5α-androstane-3α,17β-diol and 5α-androstane-3β,17β-diol in the plasma of adult male rats. Steroids 29:503–516.

Daane TA, Parlow AF (1971) Periovulatory patterns of rat serum follicle stimulating hormone during the normal estrous cycle: effect of pentobarbital. Endocrinology 88:653–663.

Denef C (1979) Evidence that pituitary 5α-dihydrotestosterone formation is regulated through changes in the proportional number and size of the gonadotrophic cells. Neuroendocrinology 29:132–139.

Fink G, Henderson SR (1977) Steroids and pituitary responsiveness in female, androgenized female and male rats. J Endocrinol 73:157–164.

Fuxe K, Hokfelt T, Eneroth P (1977) Prolactin-like immunoreactivity: localization in nerve terminalis of rat hypothalamus. Science 196:899–900.

Gupta D, Zarzycki J, Rager K (1975) Plasma testosterone and dihydrotestosterone in male rats during maturation and following orchidectomy and experimental bilateral cryptorchidism. Steroids 25:33–42.

Hafiez AA, Lloyd CW, Bartke A (1972) The role of prolactin in the regulation of testis function: the effects of prolactin and luteinizing hormone on the plasma levels of testosterone and adrostenedione in hypophysectomized rats. J Endocrinol 52:327–332.

Holzbauer M (1971) In vivo production of steroids with central depressant actions by the ovary of the rat. Br J Pharmacol 43:560–569.

Holzbauer M (1975) Physiological variations in the ovarian production of 5α-pregnane derivatives with sedative properties in the rat. J Steroid Biochem 6:1307–1310.

Ichikawa S, Morioka H, Sawada T (1971) Identification of the neutral steroids in the ovarian venous plasma of LH-stimulated rats. Endocrinology 88:372–383.

Ichikawa S, Sawada T, Nakamura Y, Morioka H (1974) Ovarian secretion of pregnane compounds during the estrous cycle and pregnancy in rats. Endocrinology 94:1615–1620.

Kao LWL, Lloret AP, Weisz J (1977) Metabolism in vitro of dihydrotestosterone, 5α-adrostane-3α,17β-diol and its 3β-epimer, three metabolites of testosterone, by three of its target tissues, the anterior pituitary, the medial basal hypothalamus and the seminiferous tubules. J Steroid Biochem 8:1109–1115.

Karavolas HJ, Nuti KM (1976) Progesterone metabolism by neuroendocrine tissues. In: Naftolin F, Ryan KJ, Davies IJ (eds) Subcellular Mechanisms in Reproductive Neuroendocrinology, Elsevier Amsterdam, pp.305–326.

Kniewald Z, Massa R, Martini L (1971) Conversion of testosterone into 5α-androstan-17β-ol-3-one at the anterior pituitary and hypothalamic level. In: James VHT, Martini L (eds) Hormonal Steroids, Excerpta Medica, Amsterdam, pp.784–791.

Lloyd RV, Karavolas HJ (1975) Uptake and conversion of progesterone and testosterone to 5α-reduced products by enriched gonadotropic and chromophobic rat anterior pituitary cell fractions. Endocrinology 97:517–526.

Martini L (1976) Androgen reduction by neuroendocrine tissues: physiological significance. IN: Naftolin F, Ryan KJ, Davies IJ (eds) Subcellular Mechanisms in Reproductive Neuroendocrinology Elsevier, Amsterdam, pp.327–345.

Martini L, Celotti F, Massa R, Motta M (1978) Studies on the mode of action of androgens in the neuroendocrine tissues. J Steroid Biochem 9:411–417.

Massa R, Cresti L, Martini L (1977) Metabolism of testosterone in the anterior pituitary gland and the central nervous system of the European starling (Sturnus vulgaris). J Endocrinol 75:347-354.

Massa R, Stupnicka E, Martini L (1972) Metabolism of progesterone in the anterior pituitary, the hypothalamus and the uterus of female rats. Excerpta Medica Intern Congress Series 256:118.

McNatty KP, Sawers RS, McNeilly AS (1974) A possible role for prolactin in the control of steroid secretion by the human Graafian follicle. Nature 250:653-655.

Moger WH (1977) Serum 5α-androstane-3α,17β-diol, androsterone and testosterone concentrations in the male rat. Influence of age and gonadotropin stimulation. Endocrinology 100:1027-1032.

Morfin R, Guiraud J-M, Ducouret B, Samperez S, Jouan P (1979) Mise en évidence du 5α-androstane-3β,6α,17β-triol et du 5α-androstane-3β,7α,7β-triol dans l'Hypophyse antérieure du rat male prépubère. C R Acad Sci 288:437-440.

Motta M, Massa R, Zanisi M, Martini L (1980) Mode of action of androgens and progestagens in neuroendocrine tissues. In: Genazzani E, di Carlo F, Mainwaring I (eds) Pharmacological Modulation of Steroid Action, Raven Press, New York, pp.187-204.

Motta M, Piva F, Martini L (1970) The hypothalamus as the center of endocrine feedback mechanisms. In: Martini L, Motta M, Fraschini F (eds) The Hypothalamus, Academic Press, New York, pp.463-489.

Neill JD, Smith MS (1974) Pituitary-ovarian interrelationships in the rat. In: James VHT, Martini L (eds) Current Topics in Experimental Endocrinology, Academic Press, New York, Vol. 2, pp.73-106.

Nett TM, Akbar AM, Niswender GD, Hedlund MT, White WF (1973) A radio-immunoassay for gonadotropin-releasing hormone (Gn-RH) in serum. J Clin Endocrinol Metab 36:880-885.

Niswender GD, Midgley AR Jr., Monroe SE, Reichert LE Jr. (1968) Radio-immunoassay for rat luteinizing hormone with antiovine LH serum and ovine LH-^{131}I. Proc Soc Exp Biol Med 128:807-811.

Nuti KM, Karavolas HJ (1977) Effect of progesterone and its 5α-reduced metabolites on gonadotropin levels in estrogen-primed ovariectomized rats. Endocrinology 100:777-781.

Samperez S, Jouan P (1979) Androgen metabolism, androgen and oestrogen receptors in the male rat anterior pituitary. J Steroid Biochem 11:819-831.

Shin SM, Howitt CJ (1975) Effect of castration on luteinizing hormone and luteinizing hormone releasing hormone in the male rat. J Endocrinol 65:447-448.

Shin SM, Howitt CJ (1976) Effect of testosterone on hypothalamic LH-RH content. Neuroendocrinology 21:165-174.

Stupnicka E, Massa R, Zanisi M, Martini L (1977) Role of anterior pituitary and hypothalamic metabolism of progesterone in the control of gonadotropin secretion. In: Hubinont PO, L'Hermite M, Robyn C (eds) Clinical Reproductive Neuroendocrinology, Karger, Basel, pp.88-95.

Swerdloff RS, Grover PK, Jacobs HS, Brain J (1973) Search for a substance which selectively inhibits FSH. Effect of steroids and prostaglandins on serum FSH and LH levels. Steroids 21:704-722.

Van Doorn EJ, Burns B, Wood D, Bird CE, Clark AF (1975) In vivo metabolism of ^{3}H-dihydrotestosterone and ^{3}H-androstene-diol in adult male rats. J Steroid Biochem 6:1549-1554.

Verjans HL, Eik-Nes KB (1976) Effects of androstenes, 5α-androstanes, 5β-androstanes, oestrenes and oestratienes on serum gonadotrophin levels and ventral prostate weights in gonadectomized, adult male rats. Acta Endocrinol 83:201-210.

Verjans HL, Eik-Nes KB (1977) Comparison of effects of C19 (androstene or androstane) steroid on serum gonadotrophin concentrations and on accessory reproductive organ weights in gonadectomized, adult male rats. Acta Endocrinol 84:829–841.

Yamada Y (1975) Effects of iontophoretically-applied prolactin on unit activity of the rat brain. Neuroendocrinology 18:263–271.

Zamecnik J, Barbe G, Moger WH, Armstrong DT (1977) Radioimmunoassays for androsterone, 5α-androstane-3α,17β-diol and 5α-androstane-3β, 17β-diol. Steroids 30: 679–689.

Zanisi M, Martini L (1975) Effects of progesterone metabolites on gonadotrophin secretion. J Steroid Biochem 6:1021–1023.

Zanisi M, Motta M, Martini L (1973) Inhibitory effect of 5α-reduced metabolites of testosterone on gonadotrophin secretion. J Endocrinol 56:315–316.

Estrogen Effects on LH-RH Degrading Brain and Pituitary Enzymes

K. Bauer, S. Beier, B. Horsthemke, H. Knisatschek and J. Sievers, Berlin

As we know from autoradiographic studies (see chapter by W. Stumpf, this volume) steroid hormones are discretely localized in certain brain areas and hypophyseal cells. Estrogen effects on neural and pituitary processes not only alter RNA and protein synthesis but also alter tissue specific products and functions. In the brain, altered gene expression apparently leads to changes in electrical activities of the neurons, which affects the metabolism and/or release of neurotransmitters and releasing hormones. In the pituitary we observe fluctuations of cellular functions during the estrous cycle and steroid hormones are known to affect strongly the sensitivity to hypothalamic hormones and the metabolism of gonadotropins (see reviews by McEwen and Knobil, this volume).

For the hypothalamic hypophysiotrophic hormones which act at higher centers of biological control cascades, any alteration in their concentrations, either at the site of synthesis and/or target interaction, might result in major changes within the hypothalamus–pituitary–target organ axis. The concentrations of these substances are of course a result of the rate of synthesis and/or release over the rate of destruction. Some authors therefore postulated that the enzymatic degradation of neuropeptides might be involved in the metabolic regulation of these peptides and thus in the regulation of the peptides' neuroendocrine or behavioral effects (Griffiths et al., 1975; Kuhl and Taubert, 1975; Fridkin et al., 1977; Griffiths and Kelly, 1979).

It would be easy to conceive such a regulatory function of neuropeptide degrading enzymes, provided:

A.   The degradation is catalyzed by a neuropeptide-specific enzyme, and

B.   the enzymes activity represents the limiting factor within the regulatory system.

If so, one should consequently expect,

a)   that these enzyme activities are controlled by feedback regulatory mechanisms, and

b)   that changes in enzyme activities correlate in time with changes in neuroendocrine or behavioral events.

The LH-RH degrading hypothalamic or hypophyseal tissue enzymes, for example, should be regulated by steroid hormones. Experimental manipulations such as gonadectomy and estradiol administration should cause significant changes in the activities of LH-RH degrading enzymes. This working hypothesis has been tested by several investigators. Using radioimmunological methods Griffiths et al. (1975) observed some changes in the rate of LH-RH degradation by hypothalamic tissue extracts of experimentally manipulated rats. Testing the LH-RH degrading enzyme activity from the pituitary Fridkin et al. (1977) reported that ovariectomy caused a 50% decrease, while estradiol replacement restored enzyme activity to pre-castration levels. With synthetic arylamides as presumptive substrates of the LH-RH degrading enzyme(s), fluctuation of enzyme activities after estradiol administration was also observed by Kuhl and Taubert (1975). Loudes et al. (1978), however, reported that castration neither alters the affinity of LH-RH degrading brain and pituitary enzymes nor the specific activities of the overall peptidasic activity which can be evaluated by radioimmunological methods.

To some extent these conflicting results might be due to differences in assay condition which had not been optimized for the enzymes to be tested. Furthermore, these results are difficult to interpret since the experimental conditions used do not permit one to differentiate between various LH-RH degrading enzymes present in brain and pituitary homogenates.

1. Degradation of LH-RH by Brain and Pituitary Enzymes

Recently we demonstrated (Bauer et al., 1979; Horsthemke and Bauer, 1980; Knisatschek and Bauer, 1979) that the inactivation of LH-RH is not catalyzed by a LH-RH specific enzymes, as suggested by Fridkin et al. (1977), but mainly by 3 enzymes: E_1, a pyroglutamate aminopeptidase hydrolyzing LH-RH at the < Glu–His bond, E_2, a non-chymotrypsin like endopeptidase cleaving preferentially the Tyr-Gly bond, and E_3, a post proline cleaving enzyme hydrolyzing LH-RH at the Pro-Gly bond (Figure 1).

These three enzymes, which account for about 95% of the total LH-RH degrading peptidasic activities, have been characterized as general proteolytic enzymes. By convential chromatographic methods (Horsthemke and Bauer, 1980) these enzymes have been separated from each other and also from various arylamidases. It could be shown that the cystinyl arylamidase acts as a typical aminopeptidase which may be involved in secondary cleavage of LH-RH fragments but not in the primary cleavage of LHRH itself.

Enzyme specific tests have been developed to determine selectivity of the enzyme activities (Horsthemke and Bauer, 1980;

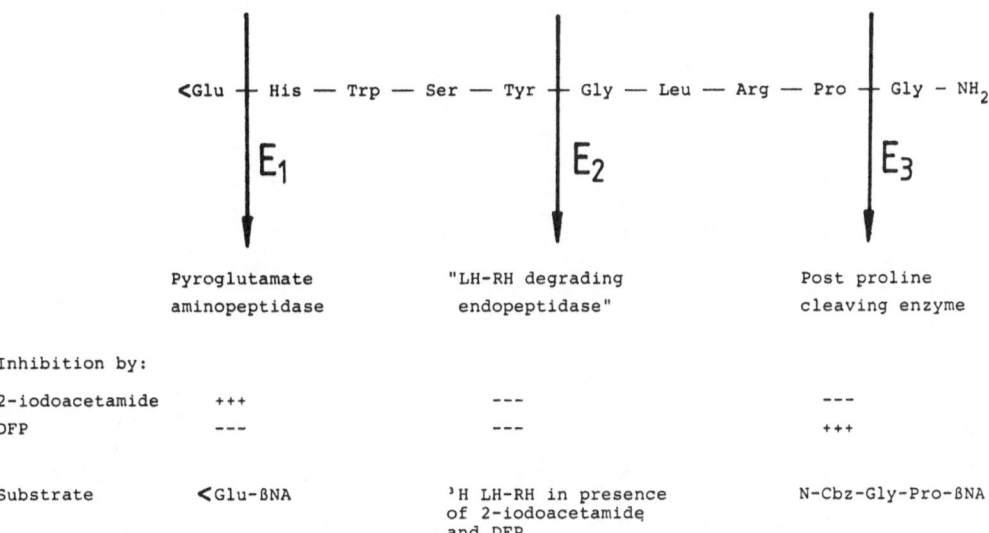

Inhibition by:			
2-iodoacetamide	+++	---	---
DFP	---	---	+++
Substrate	<Glu-βNA	³H LH-RH in presence of 2-iodoacetamide and DFP	N-Cbz-Gly-Pro-βNA

Figure 1: Fragmentation of LH-RH by brain and pituitary enzymes

Table 1: Assay conditions for enzymes

Enzyme	Substrate	Conc. mM	p_H of assay	Buffer	Addition	Temp.	Compound measured	Ref.
Total LH-RH degrading activity	³H LH-RH	0.002	7.4	A	2 mM DTE 2 mM EDTA	37°C	Residual ³H LH-RH	13
Pyroglutamate aminopeptidase	Glu-βNA	0.1	7.4	A	2 mM DTE 2 mM EDTA	37°C	β-NA	23
Post proline cleaving enzyme	N-Cbz-Gly-Pro-βNA	0.01	7.4	A	2 mM DTE 1 mM EDTA	37°C	β-NA	15
"LH-RH degrading endopeptidase	³H LH-RH	0.002	8.0	A	.2 mM DTE 1 mM JAc .3 mM DFP	37°C	Residual ³H LH-RH	23
Glutaryl-Gly-Gly-Phe-βNA hydrolyzing enzyme	Glutaryl-Gly-Gly-Phe-βNA	0.1	7.5	B	10 mM $CaCl_2$	37°C	β-NA	13
Aminopeptidases (Arylamidases)	Leu-βNA	0.1	7.4	A	1 mM DTE	37°C	β-NA	1
	Cys-βNA	0.01	7.4	A	1 mM DTE	37°C	β-NA	1
	Arg-βNA	0.1	7.4	A	1 mM DTE	37°C	β-NA	1
	Tyr-βNA	0.1	7.4	A	1 mM DTE	37°C	β-NA	1
Post proline dipeptidyl aminopeptidase (Dipeptidylamino-peptidase IV)	Gly-Pro-βNA	0.1	7.8	B	1 mM DTE	37°C	β-NA	1

Enzyme	Substrate		pH	Buffer	Additions	Temp.	Measurement	Ref.
Dipeptidylamino-peptidase III	Arg-Arg-βNA	0.04	9.0	B	1 mM DTE	37°C	β-NA	18
Dipeptidylamino-peptidase I	Ser-Tyr-βNA	0.1	4.0	C	5 mM NaCl 2 mM DTE	37°C	~β-NA	18
Acid phosphatase	p-Nitrophenyl-phosphate	5.0	5.0	D	1 mM DTE 1 mM EDTA	37°C	Nitro-phenol	19
5'Nucleotidase	2-^{3}H Adenosin 5-monophosphate	0.005	8.5	B	12 mM $MgCl_2$	37°C	5'Adenosin	24
Lactate dehydrogenase	Pyruvate NADH	0.31 0.20	7.4	A	--	20°C	E_{340}	5
Glucose-6-phosphate dehydrogenase	Glucose-6-phosphate NADP	0.67 0.50	7.8	B	--	20°C	E_{340}	5

Four groups each of 15 female rats (Wistar, 180–200 g b.w.) were used and maintained in standard conditions. Animals of group 1 (intact rats, controls) and group 2 (rats ovariectomized 25 days before) received 5 daily injections (s.c.) of 0.2 ml vehicle (benzyl benzoate/castor oil 1:9 v/v). Animals of group 3 (intact rats) and group 4 (rats ovariectomized 25 days before) received 5 daily injections of 20 μg estradiol benzoate dissolved in 0.2 ml vehicle. The animals were sacrificed by decapitation. The anterior pituitary and the hypothalamus were quickly removed and bulked together for homogenization in 25 volumes buffer (20 mM Tris·HCl, pH 7.4 and 2 mM DTE) using a motor driven teflon glass homogenizer (800 rpm). The homogenate was sonicated 3 times for 5 seconds using a Branson sonifier. Enzyme activities were assayed as indicated. Protein content was measured by the method of Lowry according to Peterson (1979). Buffers used: A: 100 mM potassium phosphate; B: 50 mM Tris·HCl; C: 70 mM sodium succinate; D: 50 mM sodium acetate. Abbreviations: DTE: dithioerythritol; JA: 2 iodoacetamide; DFP: Diisopropyl fluorophosphate; βNA: β-naphtylamine.

Szewczuk and Kwiatkowky, 1970; Knisatschek et al., 1980) in brain and pituitary homogenates of ovariectomized and estradiol benzoate treated rats. These changes in enzyme activities were compared with other enzymatic activities catalyzing cellular events (see Table 1).

2. Changes in Enzyme Activities After Experimental Manipulation

Enzyme activities are expressed in specific activities in order to account for considerable changes in pituitary weight and protein content as a consequence of the experimental conditions of the animals.

Confirmatory to the findings of Loudes et al. (1978) we observed no significant changes in total LH-RH degrading activities of hypothalamic homogenates from gonadectomized or estradiol benzoate treated rats. In addition, significant changes in specific activities of the individual LH-RH degrading enzymes could also not be observed (Table 2). However, the specific activities of the total peptidasic pool of hypophyseal LH-RH degrading enzymes increases after estradiol benzoate administration and slightly decreases after ovariectomy for 25 days (Fig. 2). The specific activity of the post proline cleaving enzyme follows the same pattern whereas the specific activity of the "LH-RH degrading endopeptidase" is slightly reduced after ovariectomy as well as after estradiol administration. These findings are in agreement with our kinetic studies which indicated that the rate of LH-RH degradation by pituitary enzymes is mainly determined by the activity of the post proline cleaving enzyme.

For comparison, other enzymes were also tested (Fig. 3). In agreement with earlier reports by Vanha Pertulla (1969) we observed that injections of estradiol benzoate into ovariectomized rats did not significantly alter the specific activities of various arylamidases (aminopeptidase). However, changes in specific enzyme activities comparable to those of the LH-RH degrading enzymes could be observed for other peptidases such as the dipeptidyl aminopeptidases I, III and IV and for a Glutaryl-Gly-Gly-Phe-β-naphthylamide hydrolyzing activity (Horsthemke and Bauer, 1980). As a consequence of estradiol administration, we, as others (McEwen and Luine, 1978),

98

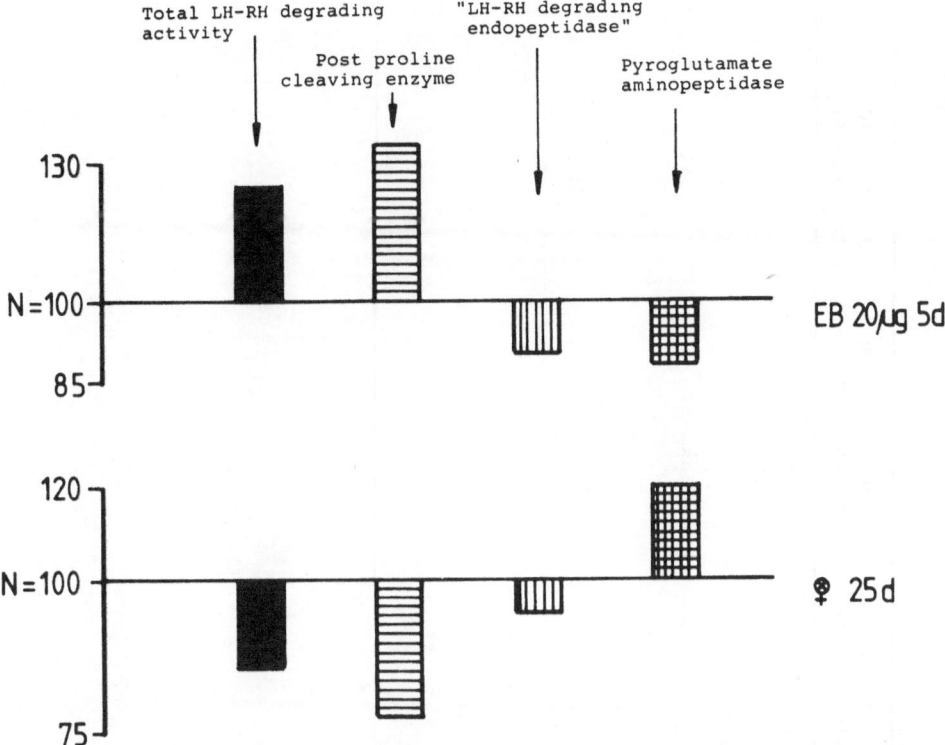

Figure 2: Specific activities of LH-RH degrading enzymes from ovariectomized (♀) or estradiol benzoate (EB)-treated rats compared to control animals taken as 100%

Table 2: Specific activities of hypothalamic enzymes from experimentally manipulated rats

Rats	E N Z Y M E S			
	Total LH-RH degrading activity	Post proline cleaving enzyme	"LH-RH degrading endopeptidase"	Pyroglutamate aminopeptidase
Normal controls	100	100	100	100
Normal, 20 µ g EB for 5 days	102	101	95	98
ovariectomized 25 days	101	96	104	103
ovariectomized for 25 days, 20 µ g EB for 5 days	96	102	93	106

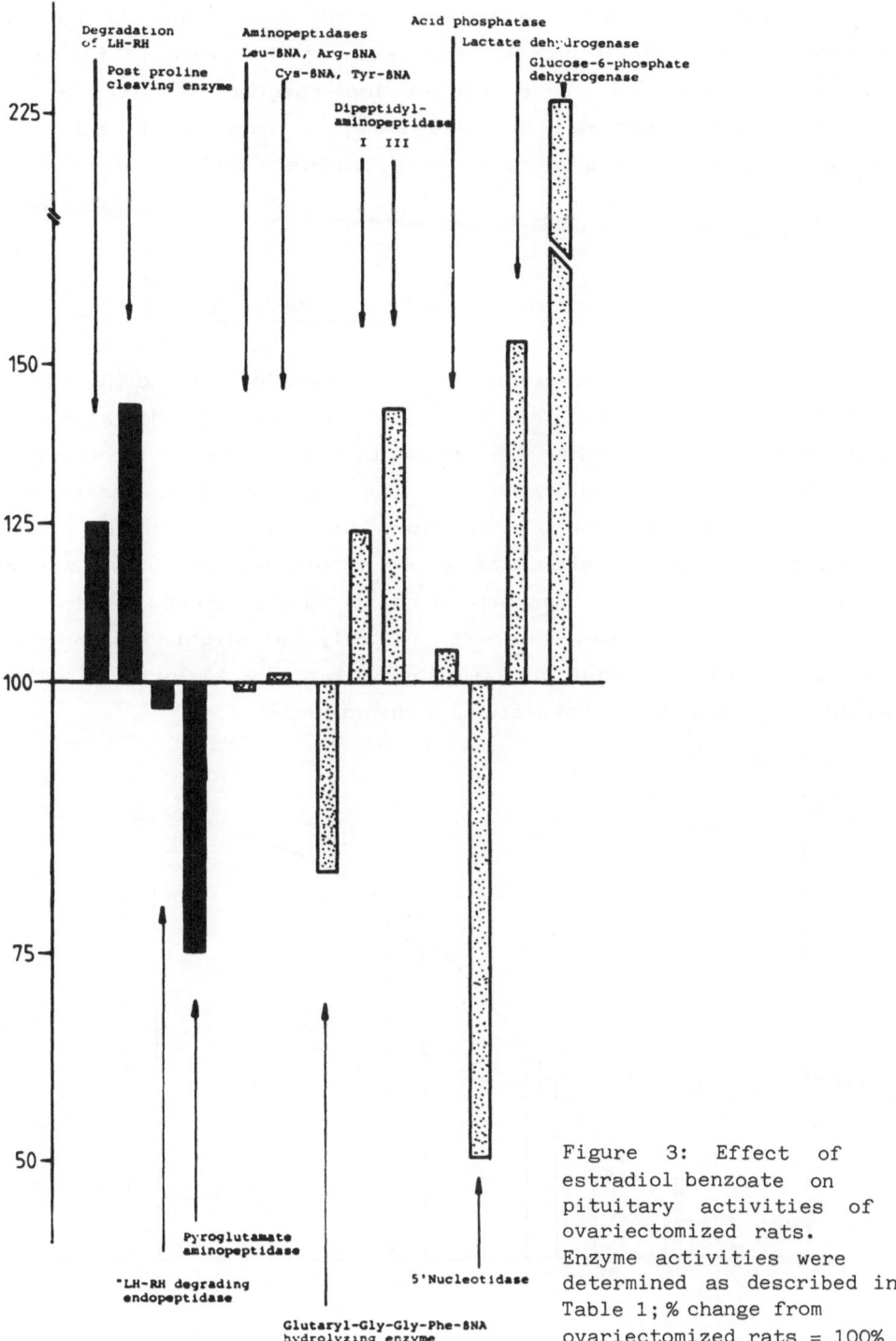

Figure 3: Effect of estradiol benzoate on pituitary activities of ovariectomized rats. Enzyme activities were determined as described in Table 1; % change from ovariectomized rats = 100%

observe significant changes in enzymes of glycolysis and the pentose phosphate pathway which provide energy for cell function. Estradiol administration significantly decreased the specific activity of the membrane marker enzyme 5'nucleotidase. The total pituitary activities of this membrane constituent enzyme remained unchanged, however.

3. Time Course of Estrogen Effects on Enzyme Activities

Based on the present analysis it is impossible to differentiate whether these changes in peptidase activities reflect alterations of enzyme activities in mechanisms regulating neuropeptide metabolism rather than in homeostatic adaption processes. As a necessary but not sufficient condition for a regulatory function, one should expect that changes in enzyme activities occur within the same time period in which neuroendocrine or behavioral changes occur. This is apparently not the case. There is only a slight increase in hypophyseal LH-RH degrading activities within the 24-36 hour period necessary for induction of ovulation or lordosis (Fig. 4).

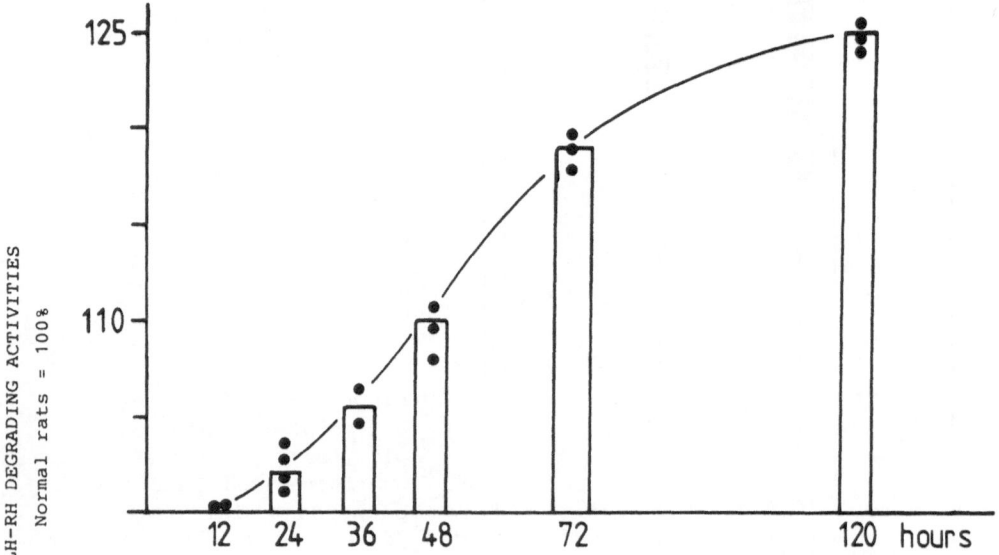

Figure 4: Time course of the effect of estradiol benzoate on the overall LH-RH degrading activity of pituitary enzymes.

4. Effect of Estrogen on GH-3 Cells

Since the LH-RH degrading enzymes are found ubiquitously distributed throughout all tissues and various cell lines, cell specific changes in enzyme activities might be obscured when enzyme activities are determined in whole tissue extracts. The gonadotrophic cells, for example, account only for a few percent of the total pituitary cell population. As a model for studying enzyme activities with a homogeneous population of target cells, the GH_3/B_6 cells were used. As known, secretion of prolactin by these cells is strongly affected by 17β-estradiol or thyroid hormones (Brunet et al., 1977) and stimulated by TRH (Tashjian et al., 1971). The specific activities of the TRH degrading enzymes, the pyroglutamate aminopeptidase and the post proline cleaving enzyme (Bauer and Kleinkauf, 1980), however, are not affected by the culture conditions, that is, when cells are grown in medium containing charcoal treated serum supplemented or not with 17β-estradiol and thyroid hormones (K. Bauer, D. Gourdji, A. Tixier-Vidal, unpublished).

At present, we cannot totally exclude the possibility that fluctuations in enzyme activities might occur within certain cellular compartments. This aspect warrants further investigations using more refined analytical methods.

5. Conclusions and Perspectives

For tissues as heterogeneous as the hypothalamus or the pituitary it is extremely difficult to interpret biochemical data in terms of physiological functions. This is especially true since the cellular localization of neuropeptide degrading enzymes, the mechanisms of neuropeptide biosynthesis as well as their mechanisms of action are poorly understood. So far, there is no experimental evidence supporting the hypothesis that neuropeptide degrading enzymes control neuropeptide metabolism. It has been shown that the LH-RH degrading enzymes are general cell constituent proteolytic enzymes. Therefore, these enzymes may provide a general and highly efficient degradation system for an unlimited number of neuropeptides (Bauer, 1980). The selectivity and specificity of the inactivating system

103

however, must be inherent to the mechanisms controlling the availability of the enzymes' substrates. These mechanisms but not the activities of the neuropeptide degrading enzymes represent most likely the limiting factors of neuropeptide degrading processes. The cellular compartmentalization of enzymes and substrates, the anatomical organization, and the mechanisms of intercellular communication may conceivably represent important elements of control. For example, neuropeptides might be removed by unknown uptake mechanisms or may be inactivated by enzymes present in intercellular fluid. In the substantia nigra, spontaneous as well as potassium stimulated release of acetycholinesterase has been described (Greenfield et al., 1980), and recently, de Cotte et al. (1980) reported that high concentrations of dopamine (10^{-4}M) stimulates the degradation of LH-RH by rat synaptosomes. This calcium dependent process requires the structural integrity of nerve endings and fluctuates with the reproductive state of the animal. It remains to be established whether these results reflect a physiological rather than a pharmacological effect and whether the release of LH-RH degrading enzymes is associated with changes in LH-RH transmission.

Based on studies concerning the metabolism of adenohypophyseal hormones, Farquhar (1971) and McDonald et al. (1971) proposed an interesting model for regulation of hormone turnover. Under conditions where hypophyseal hormone secretion is suppressed, excess secretion granules are taken up and disposed of by lysosomes, a process known as crinophagy. This model may also apply for neuropeptide synthesizing cells. In contrast to pituitary hormones which are degraded by lysosomal enzymes, TRH and LH-RH are most likely not degraded by lysosomal enzymes. We only observe degradation of TRH and LH-RH by enzymes acting in the pH range 6 to 9 with optimal activity between pH 7.2 and 8.2. However, after digestion of the granule membrane by lysosomal enzymes, these neuropeptides like other oligopeptides could diffuse through the lysosomal membrane into the cell sap, and then could be degraded into their constituent amino acids, which are then restored to the metabolic pool for reutilization within the cell (Fig. 5).

It is assumed that secretory granules are more or less continuously funneled into the lysosomal system according to the fluctuations in secretion activity. Since the concentration of mature

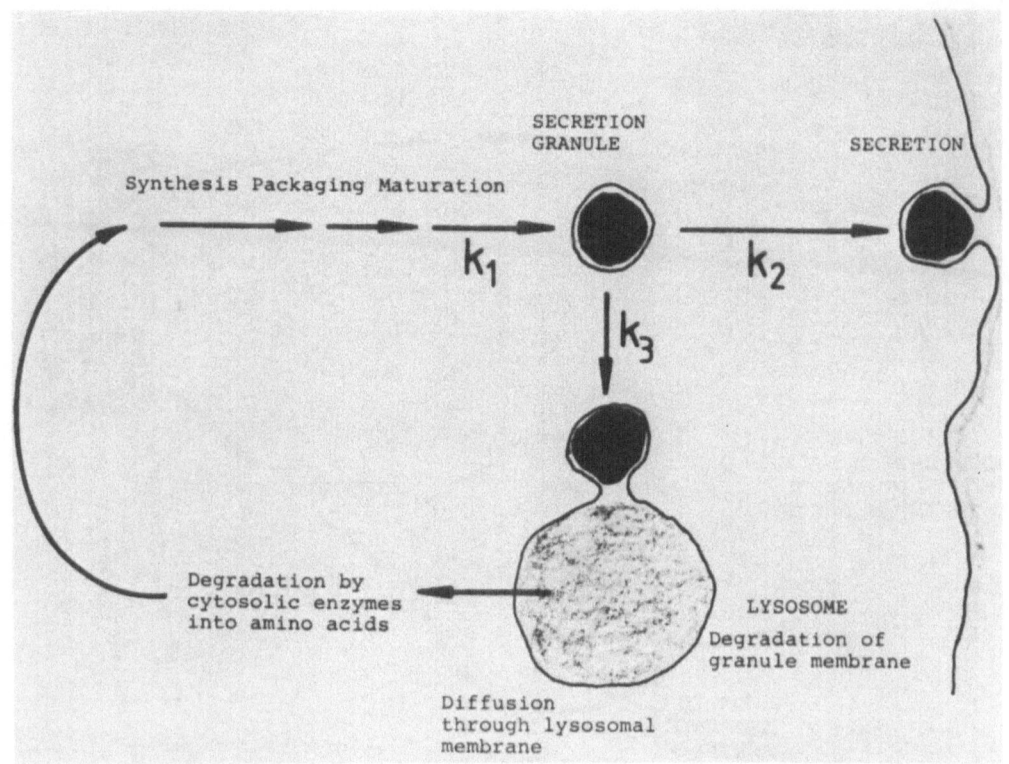

Figure 5: Hypothetical scheme of LH–RH metabolism by the LH–RH synthesizing cells

secretion granules is thereby determined by the rate constants K_1, K_2 and K_3, this control mechanism may not only act as a security device system but also as a buffer system whereby degradation itself would merely follow the principles of an unsaturated system: the more substrate available, the more degraded. For short term regulation neither synthesis nor degradation needs to be directly controlled and thus, overregulation could be easily avoided.

Principally, the same system may also operate at neuropeptide target sites (Fig. 6). After internalization, receptor–hormone complexes might be disposed of in lysosomes where degradation of receptors occurs. Again, the neuropeptide thus liberated could diffuse out of the lysosomes to be degraded by cytosolic enzymes.

Other control mechanisms could also be postulated. It is a common feature of such mechanisms, that degradation would not represent the limiting factor of regulation but would act as a

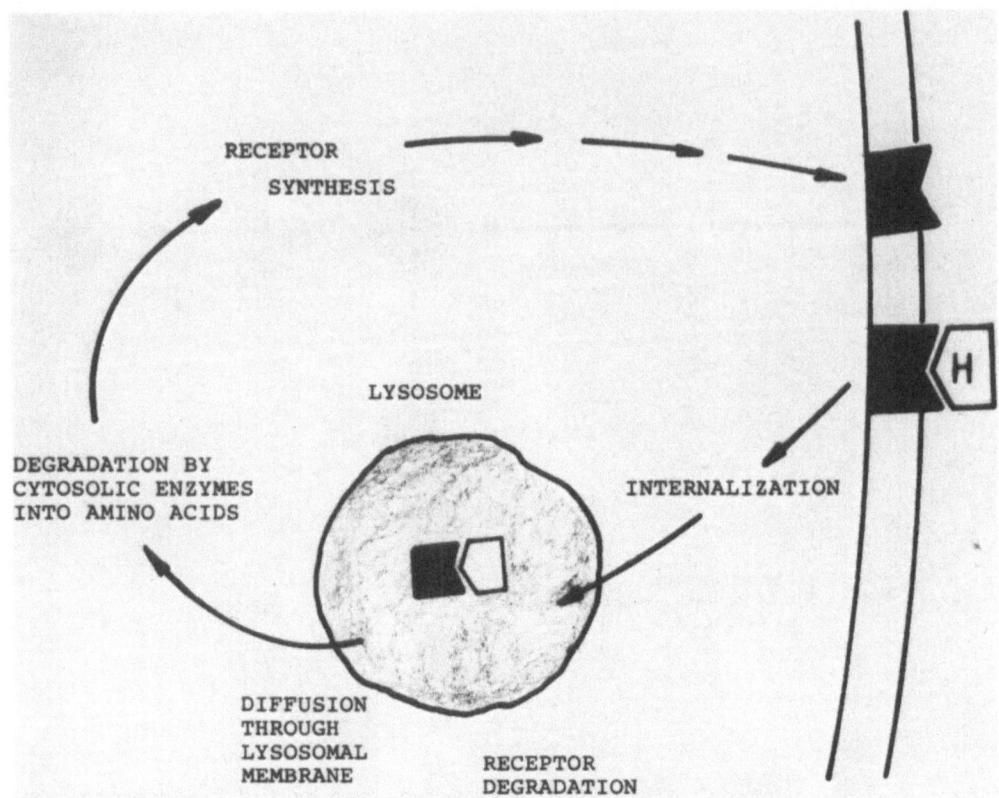

Figure 6: Hypothetical pathway of LH–RH degradation by LH–RH target cells

secondary control mechanism. It is obvious that under such conditions degradation would still represent a physiologically most
important event. The physiological role of neuropeptide degrading
enzymes, however, could not be easily evaluated by determining
enzyme activites under various physiological conditions. Under this
aspect some parallelism between the physiological role of neuropeptide
degrading enzymes and the monoamine metabolizing enzymes might be
seen. Therefore, it appears more adequate to determine enzyme
activities in certain cases of pathological disorders where enzyme
activity may represent the limiting factor. Alternatively, the
characterization of neuropeptide degrading enzymes should enable us
to synthesize enzyme specific inhibitors suitable for physiolgocial
and pharmacological studies. It is hoped that studies along such
lines might provide the tools for understanding the yet unkown
physiological function of neuropeptide degrading enzymes and finally
to elucidate the mechanisms controlling neuropeptide metabolism.

Acknowledgment

We thank Dr. H. Kleinkauf for continuous interest and support. We thank
Dr. D. Gourdji and Dr. A. Tixier-Vidal, Collège de France, Paris, for
stimulating discussions and for culturing the GH$_3$cells. The financial
support by the Deutsche Forschungsgemeinschaft is gratefully acknowledged.

References

1. Barrett AJ (1977) Barrett AJ (ed) Proteinases in mammalian cells and
    tissues North Holland Publishing Co., Amsterdam, pp.1-52.
2. Bauer K, Horsthemke B, Knisatschek H, Nowak P, Kleinkauf H (1979)
    Hoppe-Seyler's Z Physiol Chem 360:229.
3. Bauer K, Kleinkauf H (1980) Eur J Biochem 106:107-117.
4. Bauer K (1980) Wuttke W, Weindl A, Voigt KH, Dries RR (eds) Brain and
    Pituitary Peptides, S. Karger, Basel.
5. Bergmeyer HU (1970) Bergmeyer HU (ed) Methoden der enzymatischen
    Analyse, Verlag Chemie, Weinheim.
6. Brunet N, Gourdji D, Moreau MF, Grouselle D, Bournaud F, Tixier-Vidal
    A (1977) Ann Biol anim Biochem Biochys 17:413-424.
7. DeCotte DM, De Menzes CEL, Bennett GW, Edwardson JA (1980) Nature
    283:487-489.
8. Farquhar MG (1971) Mem Soc Endocrinol 19:79-122.
9. Fridkin M, Hazum E, Baram T, Lindner HR, Koch Y (1977) In: Goodman M,
    Meienhofer J (eds) Peptides, Proceedings of the Fifth American
    Peptide Symposium, Halsted Press, John Wiley & Sons, New York,
    pp.193-196.
10. Greenfield S, Cheramy A, Leviel V, Glowinski J (1980) Nature 284:355-
    357.
11. Griffiths EC, Hooper KC, Jeffcoate SL, Holland DT (1975) Brain
    Research 88:384-388.
12. Griffiths EC, Kelly JA (1979) Mol Cell Endocrinol 14:3-17.
13. Horsthemke B, Bauer K (1980) Biochemistry.
14. Knisatschek H, Bauer K (1979) J Biol Chem 254:10936-10943.
15. Knisatschek H, Kleinkauf H, Bauer K (1980) FEBS Letters 111:157-161.
16. Kuhl H, Taubert H-D (1975) Acta Endocrin 78:634-663.
17. Loudes C, Josepho-Bravo P, LeBlanc P, Kordon C (1978) Biochem Biophys
    Res Commun 83:921-926.
18. McDonald JK, Schwabe C (1977) In: Barrett AJ (ed) Proteinases in
    mammalian cells and tissues, pp.311-392.
19. McDonald JK, Reilly J, Zeitman BB, Ellis S (1968) J Biol Chem
    243:2028-2037.
20. McDonald JK, Callahan PX, Ellis S, Smith RE (1971) In: Barrett AJ,
    Dingle JT (eds) Tissues Proteinases, North-Holland, Amsterdam, pp.69-
    107.
21. McEwen BS, Luine VN (1978) In: Vincent JD, Kordon C (eds) Cell
    biology of hypothalamic neurosecretion, Edition du CNRS, Paris,
    pp.238-267.
22. Peterson GL (1979) Anal Biochem 100:201-220.
23. Szewczuk A, Kwiatkowsky J (1970) Eur J Biochem 15:92-96.
24. Sun AS, Poole B (1975) Anal Biochem 68:260-273.
25. Tashjian AH, Barowsky NJ, Jensen DK (1971) Biochem Biophys Res Commun
    43:516-523.
26. Vanha-Pertulla T (1969) Endocrinology 85:1062-1069.

Mediators of Feedback Message: Estrogens and/or Catecholestrogens?

R. Knuppen, Lübeck

Until now the mechanisms of action of the female sex hormone estradiol in the neuroendocrine systems are poorly understood. The understanding is complicated by the assumption of a biphasic nature of the action of estradiol itself in the regulation of pituitary hormone release initiating both positive and negative feedback effects. It is generally accepted and demonstrated by innumerable experiments that the negative feedback effect on gonadotrophin release can be attributed to estradiol itself, but the final proof as to whether estradiol itself or metabolic products of estradiol are responsible for the regulation of the positive feedback effect, is still missing.

In this connection, new concepts on the possible mechanism of action of estradiol have been experimentally tested in recent years, special interest being focused on the biological properties of a very important group of phenolic steroids, the so called catecholestrogens.

These catecholestrogens are naturally occurring steroids and those so far isolated from human urine are demonstrated in Fig. 1. From the quantitative point of view, 2-hydroxyestrone is the most important compound within this group (for details cf. Ball and Knuppen, 1980). Very recently 4-hydroxyestrone was also isolated from human urine (Emons, Hoppen, Ball and Knuppen: Steroids (1980), in press). The latter compound belongs to a very poorly characterized, but with regard to the biological properties, a highly interesting new class of catecholestrogens.

From the series of different methods developed in our laboratories the results obtained by RIA for both urinary excretion and

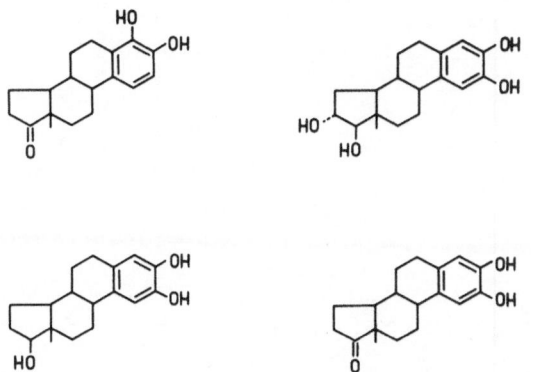

Figure 1:   Catecholestrogens isolated from human urine

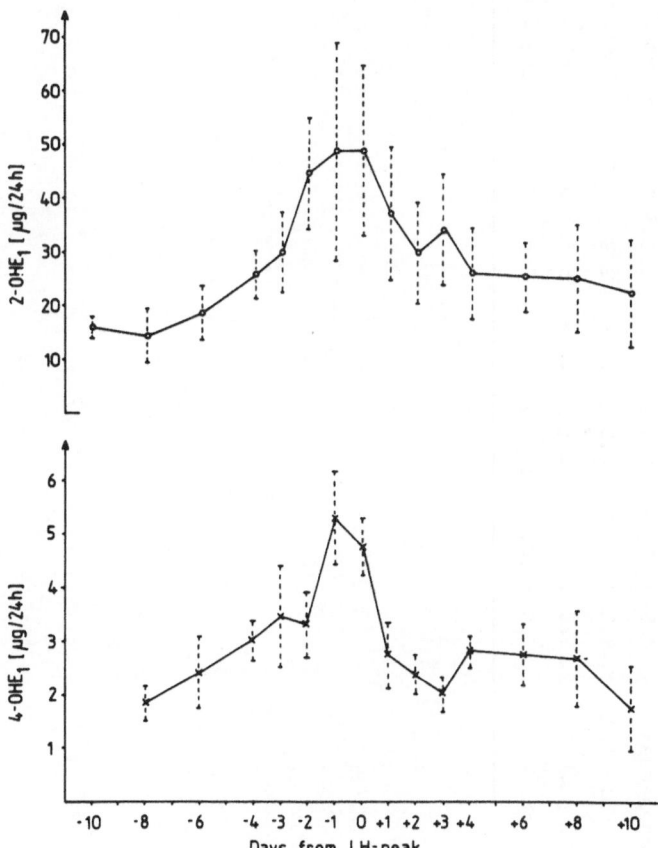

Figure 2: Excretion of 2-hydroxyestrone (o) and 4-hydroxyestrone (x) during the menstrual cycle

109

Table 1: Excretion of 2-substituted estrogens and 4-hydroxyestrone in human urine and plasma levels of 2- and 4-hydroxyestrone. For details cf. Ball et al., 1978b; Ball et al., 1979; Emons et al., 1979; Ball and Knuppen, 1980. ($2-OHE_1$ = 2-hydroxyestrone; $2-OHE_1$ 2-Me = 2-hydroxyestrone 2-methyl ether; $4-OHE_1$ = 4-hydroxyestrone).

Subject	$2-OHE_1$	Urine (μg/24h) $2-OHE_1$ 2-Me	$4-OHE_1$	Plasma (pg/ml) $2-OHE_1$	$2-OHE_1$ 2-Me
Children, female	1.1 ± 0.6	3.8 ± 1.6	0.4 ± 0.1	20 – 40	61 ± 16
Women, postmenopausal	4.6 ± 1.6	9.0 ± 3.5	1.5 ± 0.3	40 – 70	102 ± 26
Women, follic ph.	18.2 ± 12.2	14.2 ± 6.6	1.9 ± 0.5	50 – 70	96 ± 19
Women, periov. ph.	41.3 ± 17.0	22.6 ± 7.5	5.3 ± 0.8	65 – 95	181 ± 27
Women, luteal ph.	22.5 ± 10.0	16.4 ± 8.7	2.4 ± 0.3	55 – 85	152 ± 22

plasma levels of 2-hydroxy- and 4-hydroxyestrone are given in Table 1 (cf. Ball et al., 1978b; Ball et al., 1979a; Emons et al., 1979; Ball and Knuppen, 1980). Highest values were found in the reproductive phase of women, but it is also of interest that 2-hydroxyestrone is also excreted in relatively high amounts in the urine of postmenopausal women. As demonstrated in Fig. 2 the urinary amounts of 2- and 4-hydroxyestrone vary within the menstrual cycle with a proliferatory minimum, a sharp periovulatory peak and a broad maximum during the secretory phase (cf. Ball et al., 1979a; Emons et al., 1980).

In order to discuss whether estradiol and/or catecholestrogens are possibly involved in the regulation of gonadotrophin release a knowledge of the metabolism of estradiol and the formation of catecholestrogens in different tissues is necessary. It is well known that both the 2- and 4-hydroxyestrogens are formed from estradiol, mainly via estrone, in the liver of mammals including man (for details cf. Ball and Knuppen, 1980), 2-hydroxyestrogens being the main products. Of special interest was the finding of Fishman and coworkers (Fishman and Norton, 1975a,b; Fishman et al., 1976) that 2-hydroxylation of estradiol also occurred during incubation with hypothalamic, limbic, parietal cortex and pituitary tissue homogenates from humans and with hypothalamic tissues from rats. In comparative studies on the metabolism of $(6,7-{}^{3}H_2)$estradiol in the brain, the pituitary and the liver of rat and the human fetus, we isolated high amounts of 2-hydroxylated metabolites from the liver preparations but only low amounts after incubation with hypothalamic and pituitary tissue (Ball and Knuppen, 1978; Ball et al., 1978a). We were also able to identify and to quantitate 4-hydroxylated estrogens in the incubation media. It was demonstrated that relative low amounts of 4-hydroxyestradiol and 4-hydroxyestrone (when compared with 2-hydroxyestradiol and 2-hydroxyestrone) were found in the liver, whereas approx. equal amounts – when compared with 2-hydroxyestradiol and 2-hydroxyestrone – could be isolated from the pituitary and brain incubations. However, on the basis of wet weight the 2-hydroxylating capacity of the liver was about 50 times greater than that of the brain and the pituitary, while the 4-hydroxylating capacity was about the same in liver, brain and pituitary.

111

Studies carried out in rats have also shown that catechol-estrogens administered peripherally can cross the blood-brain barrier. Thus, i.v. or s.c. injected (^{14}C)hydroxyestrone resulted in a substantial incorporation of radioactivity in central tissues dissected 30 min after the injection (Fishman and Norton, 1977). We were able to demonstrate that radioactivity was present in central tissues up to 24 h after the i.v. injections of $(6,7-^3H_2)2-$ and 4-hydroxyestradiol in rats (Knuppen and Hiefner, unpublished results).

One prominent biotransformation that the catecholestrogens under-go is their catalytic methylation resulting in the formation of monomethyl ethers. Thereby the 2-hydroxyestrogens yield the iso-meric 2- and 3-monomethyl ethers, whereas 4-hydroxyestrone is almost exclusively methylated at the position 4 (for review, cf. Ball and Knuppen, 1980). The reactions are catalyzed by a catechol-0-methyl-transferase and it was shown that the catecholestrogen metabolizing enzyme is identical with that which methylates catecholamines (Ball et al., 1971; Ball et al., 1972a,b). In comparative kinetic studies with the catechol-0-methyltransferase from human liver it was demon-strated that the catecholamines showed a normal Michaelis-Menten kinetic, whereas the methylation of the catecholestrogens, especially of 2-hydroxyestrone and 2-hydroxyestradiol, showed a distinct maximum at 50 μM (Ball et al., 1972b). The latter finding indicated the bad methylation of high concentrations of catecholestrogens compared with catecholamines, and this point of view may be of physiological significance. Since the Michaelis constants for 2-hy-droxylated estrogens were approx. 10 times smaller than those for catecholamines, it can be assumed that the catecholestrogens have a higher affinity to the enzyme. These data were later confirmed by Breuer and Köster (1974) using the 150 000 × g supernatant from rat brain as enzyme source.

The catecholestrogens are in fact superior substrates for the catechol-0-methyltransferase and in a series of investigations we have demonstrated (for details cf. Ball and Knuppen, 1980) that the catecholestrogens are the strongest inhibitors of catecholamine degra-dation known so far. It should be added that in contrast to catecholestrogens the monophenolic precursors, i.e. estradiol or estrone, had little or no effect on catecholamine inactivation. More-

112

over, the effective competitive inhibition of catecholamine degradation by catecholestrogens was not only shown in experiments with purified enzymes, but also under in vivo conditions in rats and mice (for details cf. Ball and Knuppen, 1980).

The question arises: what is the possible physiological significance of these chemical, biochemical and analytical findings? One point of possible influence of catecholestrogens on gonadotrophin levels should be stressed. It has long been known that primary estrogens, such as estradiol, can induce negative and positive feedback effects on gonadotrophin secretion. It is also known that catecholamines play a primary role in the release of the hypo-thalamic hormones. However, the mechanism of interaction of primary estrogens with catecholamines remains to be established. On the basis of the above data it is conceivable that the catechol-estrogens may be the missing link connecting primary estrogens and catecholamines, thereby modifying or even regulating the hormonal effects of primary estrogens and neurotransmitters. It is speculated that increasing local amounts of the catecholestrogens lead, via inhibition of the catechol 0-methyltransferase, to a subsequent in-crease in catecholamine concentrations which in turn trigger the secretion of gonadotrophin-releasing hormone. In this concept the primary estrogens play only a role as inactive precursors, and it may be even conceivable that not only the primary estrogens but also 2-hydroxylated androgens have part in the genesis of 2-hydroxy-estrogens.

On the other hand there is another very important question which needs to be answered, namely, how does the above hypothesis coincide with the fact that high blood levels of gonadotrophins are found in postmenopausal or castrated women and in ovariectomized rats? With respect to this question the data reported on the plasma levels of 2-substituted estrogens in postmenopausal women (cf. Table 1) and in ovariectomized rats (366 $\pm$ 43 pg/ml; Kuppen, to be published) together with the local concentrations of 2-hydroxyestrone in the hypothalamus and pituitary of cycling and ovariectomized rats are of interest. In contrast to the concentrations of the primary estrogen estradiol, high levels of 2-substituted estrogens are found in plasma, as well as in the hypothalamus and pituitary; being of the same order of magnitude as the levels found in women during the reproductive phase, and female rats, respectively. Consequently, one can speculate that the effects of catecholestrogens may even be potentiated since the negative feedback effect on gonadotrophin release caused by estradiol itself is abolished.

During recent years many investigators have tested the biological action of 2-hydroxyestrogens with respect to the above discussed concept. In 1975, Naftolin et al. (1975) injected 50 or 100 μg of 2-hydroxyestrone in 35 day old male rats. These authors found a 4-7 fold rise in serum LH. In further experiments with the same model (Morishita et al., 1976) the effect of 2-hydroxyestrone and 2-hydroxyestradiol on LH and FSH was tested. Doses of 0.5 - 1 μ g of 2-hydroxyestradiol and 50-100 μ g of 2-hydroxyestrone elevated serum LH and FSH, whereas the primary estrogens lowered LH and FSH. Based on these positive findings many reports were published in the following years testing the biological action of 2-hydroxy-estrogens in different species and different models, in vitro as well as in vivo (for review cf. Ball and Knuppen, 1980). Summarizing the results of the reports on the biological and pharmacological testing of the catecholestrogens, it must be stated that the results of different authors contradict each other covering the wide spectrum from: not effective to positive and/or negative effective on LH and FSH release.

With regard to the many discrepancies between the results from different authors often using the same model, the following methodological points must be stressed:
1) Purity of the catecholestrogens used,
2) preparation and handling of the solutions and
3) use of special preparations.

With respect to point 1) - Special precautions have to be taken to ascertain the complete absence of primary estrogens and other impurities in the preparations used for biological tests. Since the catecholestrogens are mostly synthesized from estrone and estradiol, and the preparative separation of catecholestrogens from the starting material is laborious, many catecholestrogen preparations used are contaminated with primary estrogens thus leading to erroneous results.

With respect to point 2) - The catecholestrogens are exceptionally unstable compounds which undergo rapid autoxidation. A

114

solution of catecholestrogens which is allowed to stand for a short length of time, even at refrigerator temperatures, may already have decomposed. Therefore, only freshly prepared solutions should be used, the mixtures should contain antioxidants and when ever possible kept at an acidic pH and in the dark.

With respect to point 3) – The free catecholestrogens are excellent substrates for glucuronyl-, sulphate- and catechol-0-methyl-transferases, whereas monosubstituted esters or ethers are poor substrates for the glucuronyl- and sulphate transferases and no longer act as substrates for the catechol – 0-methyltransferases. Consequently, the biological half-life of the free catecholestrogens is very short. In contrast, high blood levels of free catecholestrogens were demonstrated over a long period of time when catecholestrogen monobenzoates were administered to rats; a similar state of affairs could be demonstrated with catecholestrogen monomethyl ethers. Therefore, the monoesters or monoethers are often more effective when administered in vivo than the corresponding free compound.

On the basis of the equivocal results of the biological testing described above, which may in part be due to methodological insufficiences, it seems difficult to prove the physiological importance of catecholestrogens in reproductive physiology. To my feeling another approach seems more rewarding, that is the determination of endogenous catecholestrogen concentrations in the brain, locally at estrogen and/or catecholamine target cells. However, I am well aware that even this approach may be very laborious as recent work in this analytical field has also led to contradictory results.

So, in 1977 Paul and Axelrod (1977a,b) published a radio-enzymatic assay of doubtful specificity and accuracy for measuring "total" catecholestrogens in tissue. The assay is based on converting catecholestrogens to the more stable monomethyl ethers by the use of labelled S-adenosyl-methionine. The authors reported that rat brain tissue concentrations of "total" catecholestrogens exceeded those in plasma and also exceeded, by at least ten times, those of their parent estrogens. In contrast, Fishman and Martucci (1979) using two independent methods – direct radioimmunoassay for 2-hydroxy-estrone and enzymatic conversion to stable 0-methylated derivatives followed by a radioimmunoassay for the latter – were unable to detect any measurable endogenous amounts of 2-hydroxyestrone in the female rat brain.

In the past few years we have developed highly specific methods for the quantitative determination of catecholestrogens in tissue in the lower picogram range, using radioenzymatic methods, radioimmunoassays and combined gas chromatography mass spectrometry with the technique of selected ion monitoring. First results with a highly specific radioenzymatic method including combined Sephadex LH-20 and reversed phase high performance liquid column chromatography (Knuppen et al., 1980) enabling the simultaneous determination of 2-hydroxyestrone and 2-hydroxyestradiol showed concentrations of about 10 pg 2-hydroxyestrone and <1 pg 2-hydroxyestradiol for 10 mg of pituitary tissue from the cycling female and the male rat. Recent studies using larger numbers of rats at different stages of the cycle resulted, however, in a high variation of 2-hydroxyestrone tissue concentrations ranging from 4.2 - 303 pg/10 mg, whereas in ovariectomized rats relative constant levels (mean 26 ± 5 pg/10 mg) were found; these values were obtained by two independent methods: radioimmunoassay and radioenzymatic method.

In summary, to answer the question whether catecholestrogens are involved in the regulation of gonadotrophin release, in the first place accurate and reproducible data on endogenous catecholestrogen tissue levles - if possible not only in whole organs but also in well-defined nuclear areas - have to be obtained. Moreover, correlations between the levels of catecholestrogens, primary estrogens, catecholamines, releasing hormones and gonadotrophins must be assessed, and finally these studies have to be performed during different phases and different day-times of the menstrual cycle. This is presently being investigated in our laboratories.

References

Ball P, Knuppen R (1978) Formation of 2- and 4-hydroxyestrogens by brain, pituitary, and liver of the human fetus. J Clin Endocrinol Metab 21:732-737.

Ball P, Knuppen R (1980) Catecholestrogens: Chemistry, biogenesis, metabolism, occurrence and physiological significance. Acta Endocrinol Suppl 232:1-127.

Ball P, Knuppen R, Breuer H (1971) Purification and properties of a catechol-O-methyltransferase of human liver. Eur J Biochem 21:517-525.

Ball P, Knuppen R, Haupt M, Breuer H (1972a) Kinetic properties of a soluble catechol-O-methyltransferase of human liver. Eur J Biochem 26:560-569.

Ball P, Knuppen R, Haupt M, Breuer H (1972b) Interactions between estrogens and catechol amines III. Studies on the methylation of catechol estrogens, catechol amines and other catechols by the catechol-O-methyltransferase of human liver. J Clin Endocrinol Metab 34:736-746.

Ball P, Haupt M, Knuppen R (1978a) Comparative studies on the metabolism of oestradiol in the brain, the pituitary and the liver of the rat. Acta Endocrinol 87:1-11.

Ball P, Emons G, Haupt O, Hoppen H-O, Knuppen R (1978b) Radioimmunoassay of 2-hydroxyestrone. Steroids 31:249-258.

Ball P, Reu G, Schwab J, Knuppen R (1979a) Radioimmunoassay of 2-hydroxyestrone and 2-methoxyestrone in human urine. Steroids 33:563-576.

Breuer H, Köster G (1974) Interaction between oestrogens and neurotransmitters at the hypophysial-hypothalamic level. J Steroid Biochem 5:961-967.

Emons G, Ball P, v.Postel G, Knuppen R (1979) Radioimmunoassay for 2-methoxyoestrone in human plasma. Acta Endocrinol 91:158-166.

Emons G, Mente C, Haupt O, Ball P (1980) Radioimmunoassay for 4-hydroxyoestrone in human urine. Acta Endocrinol Suppl 234:108-109.

Fishman J, Martucci C (1979) Absence of measurable 2-hydroxyestrone in the rat brain: evidence for rapid turnover. J Clin Endocrinol Metab 49:940-942.

Fishman J, Norton B (1975a) Brain catecholestrogens - Formation and possible function. In Raspe G (ed) Advances in the Biosciences 15, Schering Workshop on Central Actions of Estrogenic Hormones, Pergamon Press, Oxford, pp.123-131.

Fishman J, Norton B (1975b) Catechol estrogen formation in the central nervous system of the rat. Endocrinology 96:1054-1059.

Fishman J, Norton B (1977) Relative transport of estrogens into the central nervous system. In Garattini S, Berendes HW (eds) Pharmacology of Steroid Contraceptive Drugs, Raven Press, New York, pp.37-41.

Fishman J, Naftolin F, Davies IJ, Ryan KJ, Petro Z (1976) Catechol estrogen formation by the human fetal brain and pituitary. J Clin Endocrinol Metab 42:177-180.

Knuppen R, Ball P, Zietz E (1980) Determination of 2-hydroxyestrone and 2-hydroxyestradiol in rat brain tissue. Sixth Int Congr of Endocrinology, Melbourne, Abst.-no. 45.

Morishita H, Adachi H. Naftolin F, Ryan KJ, Fishman J (1976) Elevation of serum gonadotropins in male rats by catechol estrogens. Acta Obstet Gynaecol Jpn (Engl Ed) 23:325-326.

Naftolin F, Morishita H, Davies IJ, Todd R, Ryan KJ, Fishman J (1975) 2-Hydroxyestrone induced rise in serum luteinizing hormone in the immature male rat. Biochem Biophy Res Commun 64:905-910.

Paul SM, Axelrod J (1977a) Catechol estrogens: Presence on brain and endocrine tissues. Science 197:657-659.

Paul SM, Axelrod J (1977b) A rapid and sensitive radioenzymatic assay for catechol estrogens in tissues. Life Sciences 21:493-502.

Effects of Oestradiol-17β and 2-Hydroxy-oestradiol-17β on LH-concentration in Plasma and COMT Activities in Hypothalamic Nuclei of Rats

H. Breuer, H.T. Schneider, C. Doberauer, S. Grüter and W. Ladosky, Bonn and Recife

In previous experiments, it has been shown that the catechol-0-methyltransferase (COMT) of brain is inhibited competitively by catecholoestrogens (e.g. 2-hydroxy-oestradiol-17β, 17α-ethynyl-2-hydroxy-oestradiol-17β) under in vitro conditions (Breuer and Köster, 1974). Recently, evidence has been presented that this inhibition may also occur in vivo (Breuer et al., 1978). Thus, the amount of methylated metabolites of tritiated noradrenaline, injected intraventricularly, is significantly reduced in rats pretreated with 2-hydroxy-oestradiol-17β, as compared with animals which had received oestradiol-17β. These findings underline the significance of the interaction between 2-hydroxylated oestrogens and COMT, an enzyme which is involved in the biological inactivation of noradrenaline.

Since the physiological significance of COMT in brain is not yet fully understood, it seemed justified to study the local distribution of this enzyme in brain. In view of the great importance of the hypothalamus in reproductive processes in rats, it was decided to study first the occurrence and activity of COMT in this tissue.

Enzyme activity was measured according to Axelrod and Tomchick (1958) in the 30 000 x g supernatant of hypothalamic tissue in the presence of S-adenosyl-$[4-^{14}C]$methylmethionine, $MgCl_2$ and cystein with noradrenaline as substrate for 60 min. After extraction from the incubation medium with butanol, the monomethyl ether was measured by counting the radioactivity.

The results of these studies are shown in Fig. 1. COMT activity, expressed as μmol substrate methylated per mg wet weight per 60 min, was highest in hypothalamic tissue of intact female rats during estrus. Ovariectomy led to a decrease in COMT activity.

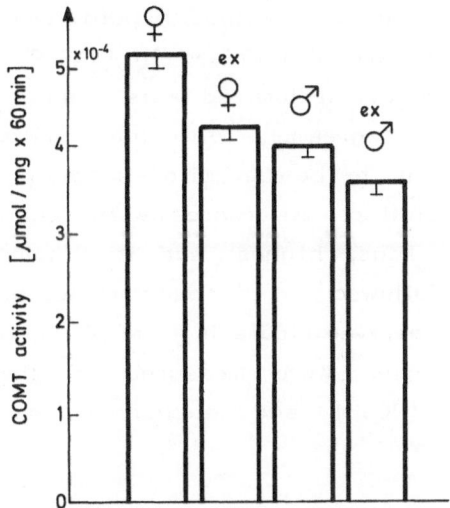

Figure 1: Activity of catechol-O-methyltransferase (COMT) in the hypothalami of intact and ovariectomized (ex♀) female rats and intact and
castrated (ex♂) male rats. Columns show the mean values obtained from
8-10 animals; standard errors are given.

Even less enzyme activity was observed in hypothalami of intact male
and castrated male rats. The differences between intact and
castrated female rats, and between castrated female and castrated
male rats were statistically significant ($p < 0.01$). These findings
suggest that COMT activity is highest in rats which are under the
influence of endogenous oestrogens. Removal of endogenous oestrogen
sources results in a decrease of enzyme activity, whereas removal of
endogenous androgen sources has no significant effect.

To obtain more detailed information about the occurrence of
COMT within the hypothalamic region, various nuclei were investigated. The procedure for removal of discrete structures from the
hypothalamus followed the technique described by Palkovitz (1974).
After decapitation, the brain is removed, frozen on a specimen holder
of a microtome with carbon dioxide and cut perpendicular to the
cortical surface. Sections (300 μm-thick) are cut at $-10°C$ and
mounted on glass slides. Hypothalamic nuclei are removed by
punching them out with a special needle under a stereomicroscope.
The tissue pellet is removed from the lumen by blowing out directly
on the tip of microhomogenizer. After homogenisation, the 10 000 x g
supernatant is assayed for COMT activity according to McCaman
(1965) in a slightly modified form.

The results of COMT determinations in the various hypothalamic nuclei of castrated male and female rats are summarised in Fig. 2. COMT activities were always higher in ovariectomized rats than in castrated male rats. This is in a good agreement with the results shown in Fig. 1. Although COMT seems to be ubiquitously distributed over the whole hypothalamus, distinct differences were found in the various hypothalamic nuclei. Thus, highest activities were present in the median eminence (ME), followed by the periventricular nucleus preopticus (POP), nucleus periventricularis (NPE) and nucleus arcuatus NA). Lowest activities were measured in the nucleus preopticus suprachiasmaticus (POSC) and nucleus supra-

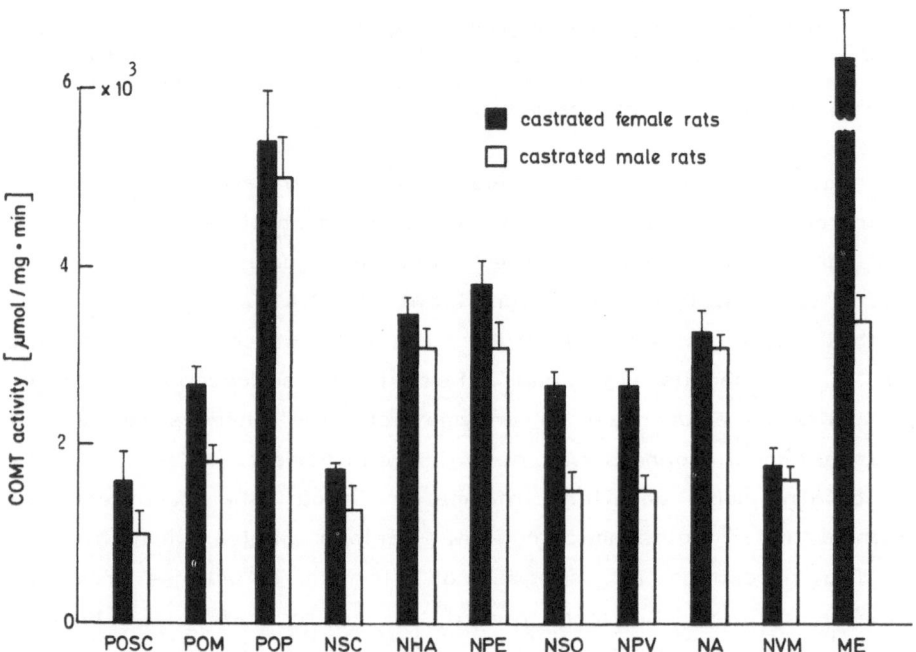

Figure 2: Activity of catechol-O-methyltransferase (COMT) in nuclei of hypothalamus of castrated female and male rats. Columns show the mean values obtained from 8-10 animals; standard errors are given. Designation of hypothalamic nuclei followed the atlas of König and Klippel (1963).
POSC = Nucleus preopticus pars suprachiasmaticus; POM = Nucleus preopticus pars medialis; POP = Nucleus preopticus pars periventricularis; NSC = Nucleus suprachiasmaticus; NHA = Nucleus hypothalamus anterior; NPE = Nucleus periventricularis; NSO = Nucleus supraopticus; NPV = Nucleus paraventricularis; NA = Nucleus arcuatus; NVM = Nucleus ventromedialis; ME = Eminentia mediana

chiasmaticus (NSC). It is interesting to note that COMT activity was highest in the median eminence, a part which also has the highest content of a large number of biologically active molecules: neurotransmitters, hypothalamic peptides and a variety of other active substances.

Similarly, COMT activity is very high in the periventricular region of the nucleus preopticus (POP) where a high density of oestrogen receptors has been observed. The observation that, even in the absence of gonads, different COMT activities exist between female and male rats may allow the conclusion that, at least to some extent, COMT activity in hypothalamus is influenced by other factors; a possible influence of hormones produced by the adrenal cortex cannot be ruled out.

The results described so far provide good evidence that COMT activity is regulated by oestrogens. In the following experiment, castrated female rats received implants of silastic capsules, containing 5 mg oestradiol-17β. 12 h later, COMT activity was measured in various hypothalamic nuclei. Fig. 3 reveals that, in castrated

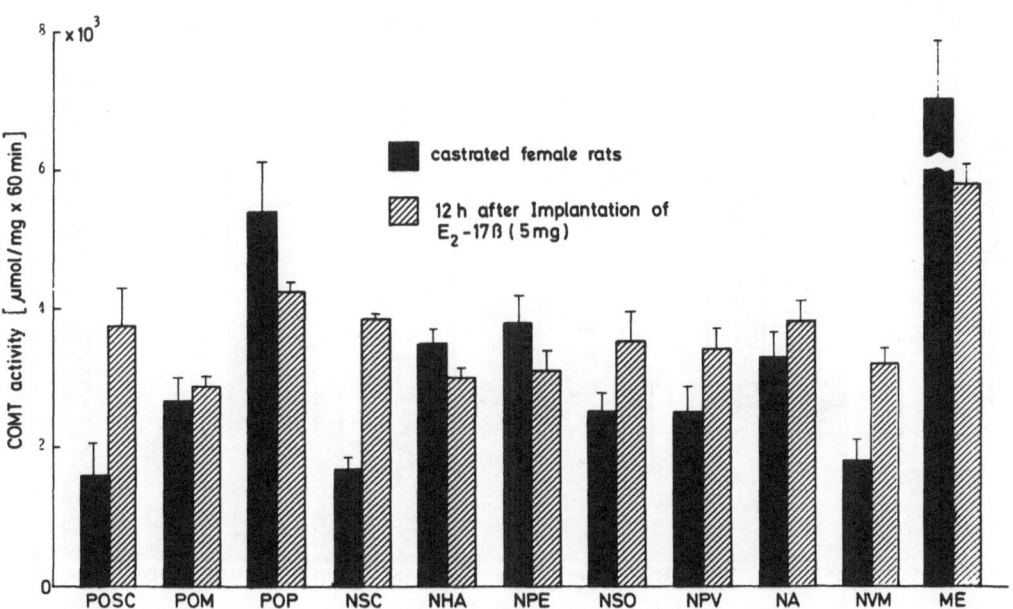

Figure 3: Activity of catechol-O-methyltransferase (COMT) in nuclei of hypothalamus of castrated female rats 12 h after subcutaneous implantation of 5 mg oestradiol-17β in silastic capsules. Columns show the mean values obtained from 8-10 animals; standard errors are given. For abbreviations, see legend to Fig. 2.

oestrogen–treated animals, COMT activities were significantly enhanced in the nucleus preopticus suprachiasmaticus (POSC), nucleus suprachiasmaticus (NSC), nucleus supraopticus (NSO), nucleus paraventricularis (NPV) and nucleus ventromedialis (NVM). No changes were observed in the nucleus preopticus medialis (POM) and nucleus arcuatus (NA), whereas a decrease of COMT after implantation of oestradiol–17β occurred in the remaining nuclei. A very pronounced drop in COMT activity was found in the median eminence. It would be interesting to speculate if the stimulation of COMT activity by oestrogens could be correlated to the density of oestrogen receptors or to the content and turnover of catecholamines – or both.

In view of the already mentioned interactions between COMT and 2-hydroxy-oestradiol–17β, the effect of this catecholoestrogen on COMT activity in hypothalamus was studied (Fig. 4). 12 h after

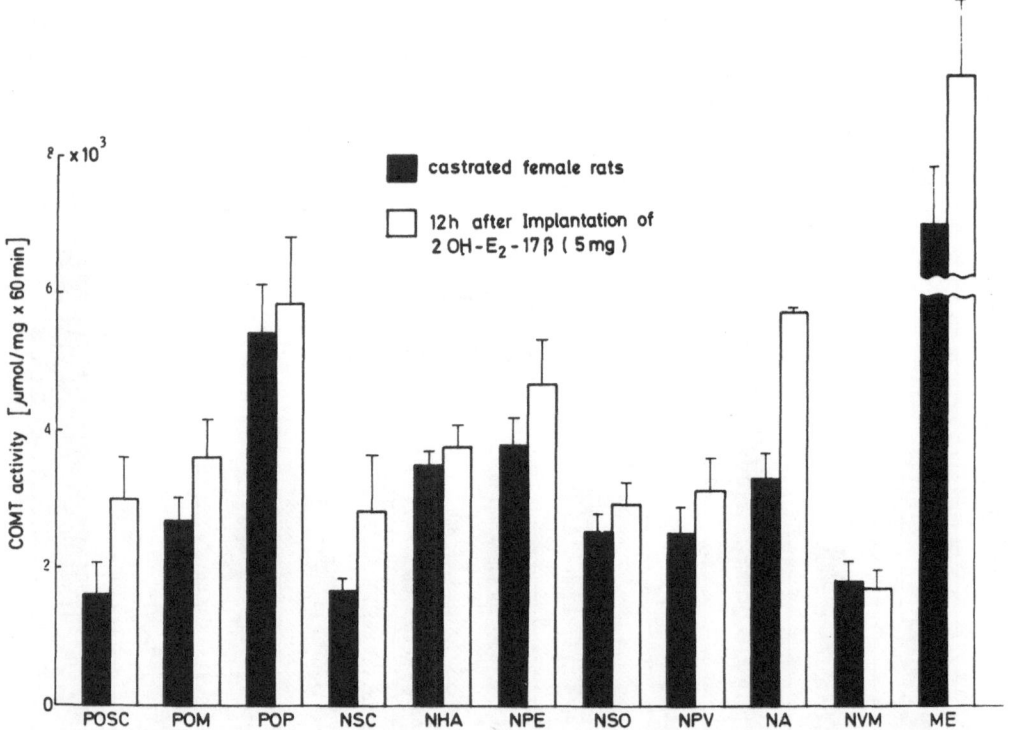

Figure 4: Activity of catechol–O–methyltransferase (COMT) in nuclei of hypothalamus of castrated female rats and castrated female rats 12 h after subcutaneous implantation of 5 mg 2-hydroxy-oestradiol–17β in silastic capsules. Columns show the mean values obtained from 8–10 animals; standard errors are given. For abbreviations, see legend to Fig. 2

implantation of 2-hydroxy-oestradiol-17β, COMT activity was, with
one exception (NVM), always higher than in control rats. Significant
differences were observed in nucleus preopticus suprachiasmaticus
(POSC), nucleus suprachiasmaticus (NSC), nucleus arcuatus (NA) and
median eminence (NE). These results leave no doubt that 2-hydroxy-
oestradiol-17β, when implanted into castrated female rats, has different effects in different hypothalamic nuclei on the COMT activity.

A comparison between oestradiol-17β and 2-hydroxy-oestradiol-
17β with respect to their action on COMT in hypothalamic nuclei is
shown in Fig. 5. In the nucleus suprachiasmaticus (NSC) and in the
suprachiasmatic part of the nucleus preopticus (POSC), both oestra-
diol-17β and 2-hydroxy-oestradiol-17β had a stimulatory influence on
COMT activity, the catecholoestrogen being less effective than oestra-
diol-17β. If the assumption is correct that in the suprachiasmatic
area light-dependent modulations of LH-release occur, then it seems

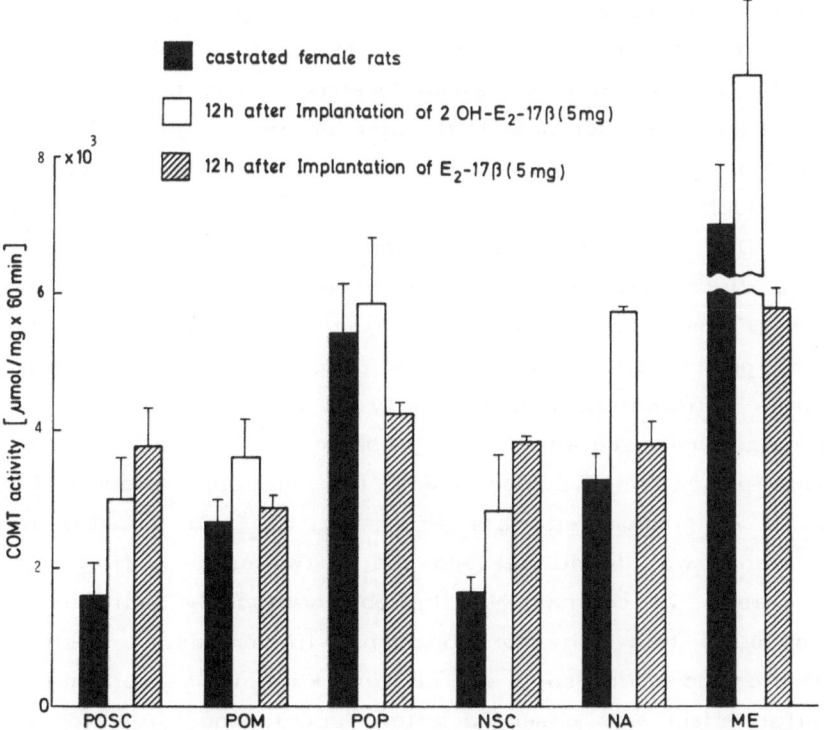

Figure 5: Activity of catechol-O-methyltransferase (COMT) in six nuclei
of hypothalamus of castrated female rats and castrated female rats 12 h
after subcutaneous implantation of 5 mg oestradiol-17β or 5 mg 2-hydroxy-
oestradiol-17β, respectively. Columns show the mean values obtained from
8-10 animals; standard errors are given. For abbreviations, see Fig. 2

not unreasonable to assume that, in addition to oestradiol-17β, also 2-hydroxy-oestradiol-17β may be involved in this process (which, of course, also requires progesterone).

In the nucleus arcuatus (NA) and nucleus preopticus medialis (POM) 2-hydroxy-oestradiol-17β was more effective than oestradiol-17β. In rats, the nucleus arcuatus has been named as the site of action for the negative feedback of oestrogen, whereas positive feedback has been localized in the preoptic area. The observation that 2-hydroxy-oestradiol-17β has a pronounced effect on COMT activity in this hypothalamic region leads to the question if and by which mechanism catecholestrogens are involved in the regulation of LH-release. Accordingly, the effect of 2-hydroxy-oestradiol-17β on the LH-concentration in plasma was studied under various experimental conditions.

Before discussing these experiments in detail, it should be made clear that 2-hydroxy-oestradiol-17β when given systemically undergoes a rapid metabolism (Breuer and Knuppen, 1960). Therefore, the actual concentration of catecholoestrogens in the brain is not known; it cannot be excluded that part of the original dose of 2-hydroxy-oestradiol-17β may reach the brain as methylated metabolite, thereby reducing the amounts of biologically effective catecholoestrogens. On the other hand, since it has been shown that oestradiol-17β is hydroxylated to 2-hydroxy-oestradiol-17β by hypothalamic tissue (Fishman and Norton, 1975) the possibility must be considered that oestradiol-17β exerts its effects partly in lower concentration than anticipated, and/or partly as catecholoestrogen.

When given intramuscularly, 10 μg oestradiol-17β as well as 10 μg 2-hydroxy-oestradiol-17β decreased the elevated plasma LH concentrations in ovariectomized rats after 30, 60, and 90 min; no significant difference was found between the two steroids (Fig. 6). These findings stand in contrast to the observation by Gethman et al. (1978) who found that 2-hydroxy-oestrone, in contrast to oestradiol-17β-3-benzoate, does not suppress LH and FSH plasma concentrations. A similar effect was observed after subcutaneous injection of both oestradiol-17β and 2-hydroxy-oestradiol-17β. However, whereas oestradiol-17β had a pronounced and long-acting effect (until 24 h) on LH concentration in plasma, 2-hydroxy-oestradiol-17β was less effective (Fig. 7). A significant decrease of LH was measurable 2

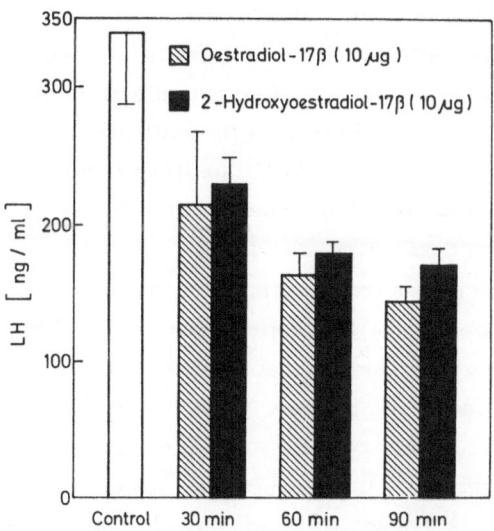

Figure 6: LH concentration in plasma of ovariectomized rats before and after intramuscular injection of 10 μg oestradiol-17β or 10 μg 2-hydroxy-oestradiol-17β, respectively. Columns show the mean values obtained from 6-8 animals; standard errors are given.

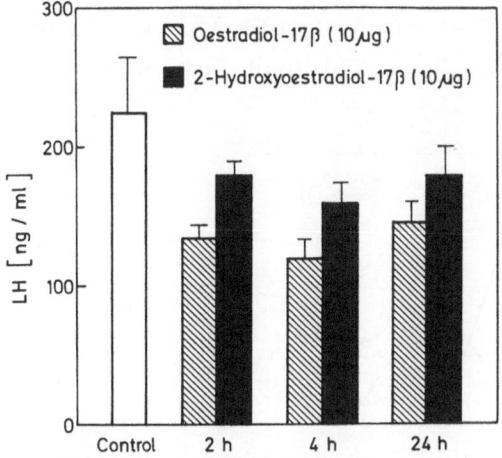

Figure 7: LH concentration in plasma of ovariectomized rats before and after subcutaneous injection of 10 μg oestradiol-17β, respectively. Columns show the mean values obtained from 6-8 animals; standard errors are given.

and 4 h after injection of 2-hydroxy-oestradiol-17β; 24 h after injection, plasma LH levels of 2-hydroxy-oestradiol-17β treated rats approached control values, probably because of the rapid disappearance of the biologically active steroid. These results, obtained under two different experimental conditions, leave no doubt that not only oestradiol-17β, but also 2-hydroxy-oestradiol 17β are capable of suppressing the elevated plasma LH concentrations in ovariectomized rats.

In further experiments, the pattern of plasma LH concentrations of ovariectomized rats between 55 and 58 h after implantation of silastic capsules of 5 mg oestradiol-17β or 2-hydroxy-oestradiol-17β, respectively, were studied (Fig. 8). As already known (Legan et al., 1975), in oestradiol-treated ovariectomized rats, the oestradiol-induced neural signal leads to a peak in LH concentration in the late afternoon (about 5 p.m.). Of particular interest is the effect of 2-hydroxy-oestradiol-17β. Here, a peak in plasma LH concentration was also observed, but this one occurred 1 1/2 h earlier than the peak induced by oestradiol-17β. A second, but somewhat lower peak was found 2 h after the first peak. These findings again confirm the observation that 2-hydroxy-oestradiol-17β, when administered systemically to ovariectomized rats, does have a definitive effect on LH. Under the present conditions, the LH peaks recorded are the result of neural signals which, however, lead to different time-dependent reactions after implantation of oestradiol-17β and 2-hydroxy-oestradiol-17β. Similar results were obtained previously with

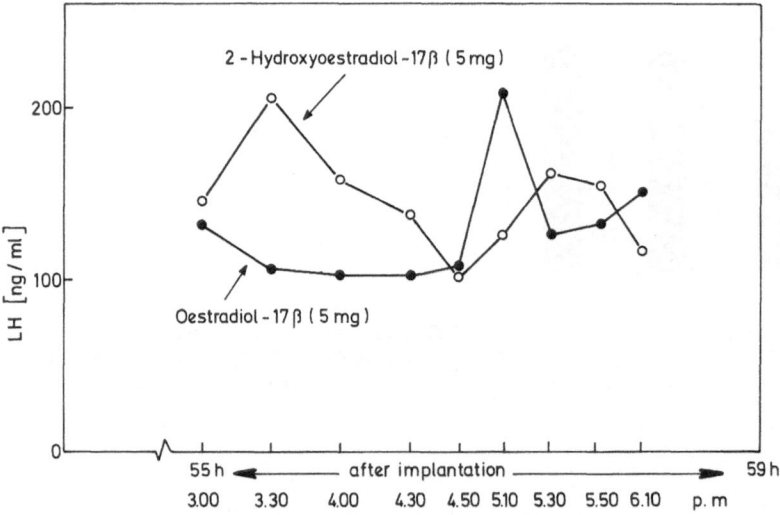

Figure 8: LH concentration in plasma of ovariectomized rats 55-59 h after implantation of 5 mg oestradiol-17β or 2-hydroxy-oestradiol-17β in silastic capsules, respectively. Points show the mean values obtained from 6-8 animals

ovariectomized rats which had been primed with oestradiol–17β–3–benzoate (Gethman et al., 1978; Gethman and Knuppen, 1976).

Nagle and Rosner (1976) have observed that the oestrogen–induced neural signal which leads to the LH peak in the afternoon is correlated with an increased concentration of noradrenaline in plasma. In view of this finding it seemed of interest to study COMT activities in hypothalamic tissues before and during the oestrogen–induced LH peak. As can be seen from Fig. 9, 52 h after intramuscular administration of 5 µg of oestradiol–17β–3–benzoate at 8 a.m., the expected low LH levels were measured; 4 h later (in the afternoon), the well–known LH peak was observed. Low LH levels corresponded with high COMT activity in hypothalamic tissue, whereas the LH peak corresponded with low COMT activity. Our finding that COMT activity is low at the time of the LH peak is compatible with the observation by Nagle and Rosner (1976) who found high noradre–naline values in plasma during the LH peak. Moreover, Ladosky and Wandscheer (1975) observed a decrease of plasma LH in rats, in which the noradrenaline content in the median eminence was reduced after intraventricular injection of 6–hydroxydopamine. With all reservations, it may be concluded that the LH peak is caused by an

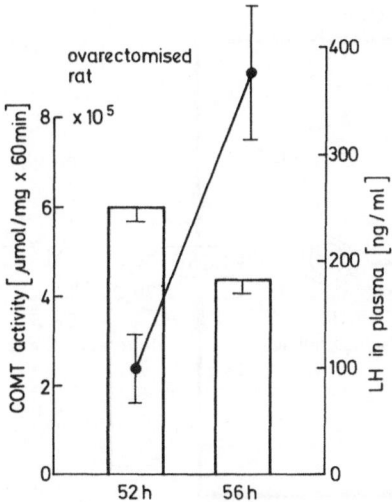

Figure 9: Activity of catechol–0–methyltransferase (COMT) in hypo–thalamus (columns) and LH concentration in plasma (dots) of ovarectomised rats after intramuscular administration of 5 µg oestradiol–17β–3–ben–zoate. Columns and dots represent the mean values obtained from 6–8 animals; standard errors are given

increase of noradrenaline in hypothalamus, and furthermore that this increase is somehow connected with the reduced activity of COMT.

Summarizing the results presented here, the following concept emerges (Fig. 10). The neurosecretion of LH-RH and the release of LH are influenced by oestrogens. As was demonstrated, systemically administered oestradiol-17β as well as 2-hydroxy-oestradiol-17 β have similar effects; both steroids inhibit LH secretion in ovariectomized rats and are capable of inducing neural signals. It may be speculated that the differences, observed in the effects of the two oestrogen, are the result of metabolic conversions, e.g. 2-hydroxyla-tion of oestradiol-17β. In addition to oestrogens, noradrenaline has also been shown to effect LH secretion. Since noradrenaline is methylated by COMT to normetanephrine, it is very likely that the activity of this enzyme is one of the factors influencing LH release. It was shown that both oestradiol-17 β and 2-hydroxy-oestradiol-17 β have an effect on COMT activity in hypothalamus. The differences which were observed in the various hypothalamic nulcei could per-haps be explained by some differences in the mode of action of the two oestrogens. Oestradiol-17β has most probably an indirect effect

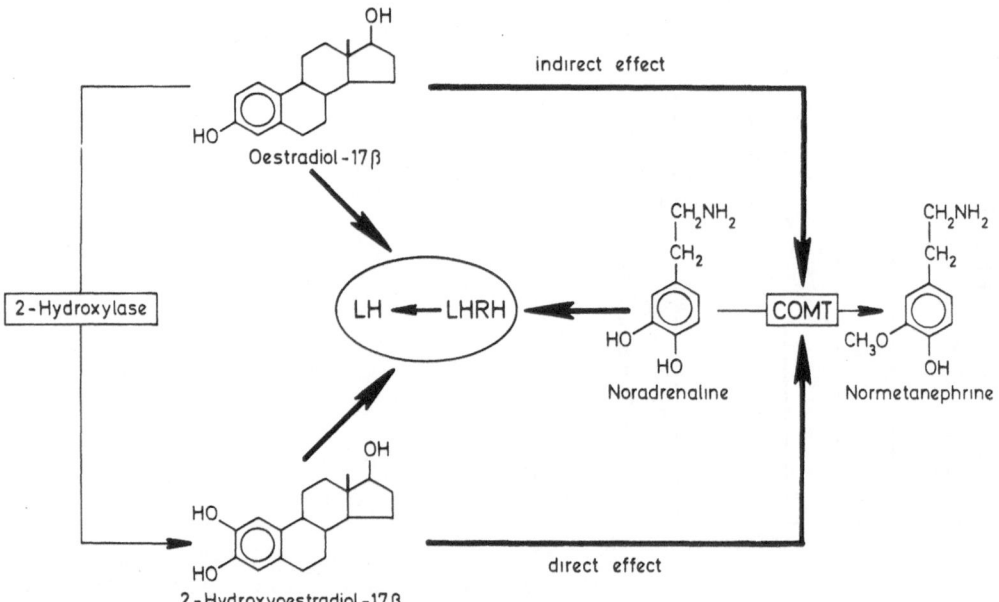

Figure 10: Present concept (1980) of actions and interactions of humoral and neuronal system

on COMT activity, whereas 2-hydroxy-oestradiol-17β is likely to act directly on the enzyme under in vivo conditions. This concept provides an explanation for the mechanisms of action of cate-choloestrogens and catecholamines in neural tissue.

Acknowledgement

The present study was supported by the Deutsche Forschungsgemeinschaft, Deutscher Akademischer Austauschdienst and Conselho Nacional de Pesquisa, Brasil.

References

Axelrod J, Tomchick R (1958) Enzymatic O-methylation of epinephrine and other catechols. J Biol Chem 233:702-705.

Breuer H, Knuppen R (1960) Biogenese von 2-Methoxyoestradiol-(17β) in der menschlichen Leber. Naturwissenschaften 47:280-281.

Breuer H, Köster G (1974) Interaction between oestrogens and neurotrans-mitters at the hypophyseal-hypothalamic level. J Steroid Biochem 5:961-967.

Breuer H, Köster G, Schneider HT, Ladosky W (1978) Interactions between Estrogens and Neurotransmitters: Effect of Estrogens on the Enzymatic Methylation of Noradrenaline in Brain. Brain-Endocrine Interaction III. Neural Hormones and Reproduction. 3rd Int Symp, Würzburg 1977, Karger, Basel, pp.274-285.

Fishman J, Norton B (1975) Catecholestrogen formation in the central nervous system of the rat. Endocrinology 96:1054-1059.

Gethman U, Knuppen R (1976) Effect of 2-Hydroxyoestrone on Lutropin (LH) and Follitropin (FSH) Secretion in the Ovarectomized Primed Rat. Hoppe-Seyler's Z Physiol Chem Bd 357:1011-1013.

Gethman U, Ball P, Knuppen R (1978) Effect of 2-hydroxyoestrone on gonadotropin secretion in the ovariectomized rat. Acta Endocrinol Suppl 215:102.

König JFR, Klippel RA (1963) The Rat Brain. A Stereotaxis Atlas of the Forebrain and Lower Parts of the Brain Stem. Williams & Wilkins Co., Baltimore.

Ladosky W, Wandscheer DE (1975) Interaction between Estrogen and Biogenic Amines in the Control of LH Secretion. Journal of Steroid Bio-chemistry, Vol. 6, pp.1013-1020.

Legan SJ, Coon GA, Karsch FJ (1975) Role of Estrogen as Initiator of Daily LH Surges in the Ovariectomized Rat. Endocrinology 96:50-56.

McCaman RE (1965) Microdetermination of Catechol-O-Methyl-Transferase in Brain. Life Sciences, Vol. 4, pp.2353-2359.

Nagle CA, Rosner JM (1976) Plasma Norepinephrine during the Rat Estrous Cycle and after Progesterone Treatment to the Ovariectomized Estro-gen-Primed Rat. Neuroendocrinology 22:89-96.

Palkovits M (1974) Isolated Removal of Hypothalamic Nuclei for Neuro-endocrinolocial and Neurochemical Studies Anatomical Neuroendo-crinology, Int Conf Neurobiology of CNS-Hormone Interactions, Chapel Hill, pp.72-80.

Gonadal Steroids and Brain Monoamines: How do they Interact?

W. Wuttke and T. Mansky, Göttingen

The preovulatory LH surge in the rat involves many complex processes. The responsivity of LH producing cells to a given LHRH stimulus is highest during proestrus, which is due to the sensitizing effects of estradiol. This appears to be the major component for the regulation of preovulatory LH release in the rhesus monkey and in the human (see Knobil, 1980, and this volume). As in these species, the rat hypothalamus appears to release LHRH surges in approximately hourly intervals (Gay and Sheth, 1972). The circhorally appearing LH peaks in ovariectomized animals including rats seem to be the consequence of such LHRH surges. Possibly because of the strict daytime locked ovulation in the rat, the timing of preovulatory LH surges needs additional central nervous system information. Until recently it was accepted that brain stem noradrenergic neurons play an essential role in stimulating LHRH release (for review s. Wuttke, 1976 and Weiner and Ganong, 1978) although the absolute necessity of the noradrenergic system for preovulatory LH release has been questioned (Nicholson et al., 1978; Clifton and Sawyer, 1979).

In the rat the LHRH producing neurons are located in the anterior hypothalamic medial preoptic-septal area (Ajika, 1979; Flerkó, 1980). Among other brain structures axon terminals from these neurons are found in the median eminence. Hence, by the punch technique (Palkovits, 1975) the pericaryal and terminal structures can be easily separated. This is quite different for the prolactin regulating system. Here most detailed studies have been performed on the inhibitory effect of dopamine (DA) on prolactin release and DA is considered to be a PIF. The hypothalamus contains dopaminergic neurons, the so called tuberoinfundibular DA

130

(TIDA) nerve cells, which innervate the hypothalamus and many axons terminate in the median eminence (Fuxe and Hökfelt, 1966). From these terminals DA is released into the portal capillaries, and depending on the endocrine status of the animal varying amounts of DA reach the anterior pituitary to act as a PIF at the lactotrophs (Ben-Jonathan et al., 1977). Other PIF's (GABA for example) and PRF's (TRH, VIP for example) have been postulated, but little is known about the localization of cells producing these factors. It is the aim of this chapter to briefly review the available data on the regulatory mechanisms of LHRH release and on the control system which governs pituitary prolactin release.

The involvement of catecholamines in preovulatory LH release was first suggested by the pioneering work of Sawyer et al. (1947) who blocked ovulation in animals by using the adrenergic blocking agent dibenamine. Much later Anton-Tay et al. (1968) and Coppola (1969) gave evidence that catecholamines, particularly norepinephrine (NE), are involved in regulating pituitary LH secretion. Later on Fuxe and coworkers (1976) using the histofluorescence technique suggested that norepinephrine may stimulate LHRH release by an action in the median eminence, and Löfström et al. (1977) extended these studies by demonstrating that preoptic NE may also participate in stimulating LHRH release. The serious limitation of the histo-fluorescence technique, i.e. the inability to quantify catecholamines and to differentiate between NE, DA and epinephrine (E), makes interpretation of these data difficult. In the late 70s, data accumulated from catecholamine turnover studies under a variety of endocrine conditions. In these studies catecholamines were measured radioenzymatically (Simpkins et al., 1979; Crowley et al., 1978; Honma and Wuttke, 1980). These studies indicated that NE turnover in the medial preoptic area (MPO) correlated well with serum LH levels. Both turnover and LH are low in diestrous (D) and ovariectomized (ovx)-estradiol (OE) treated animals and high in proestrous (P) and ovx animals (Fig. 1). Measurement of NE turnover in structures in close proximity to the MPO revealed that this pattern is only observed in the MPO. In the anterior part of the mediobasal hypothalamus (AMBH) for example (see Fig. 5) NE turnover is low in ovx animals. Such differential behavior of NE turnover in neighboring structures is hard to reconcile with the

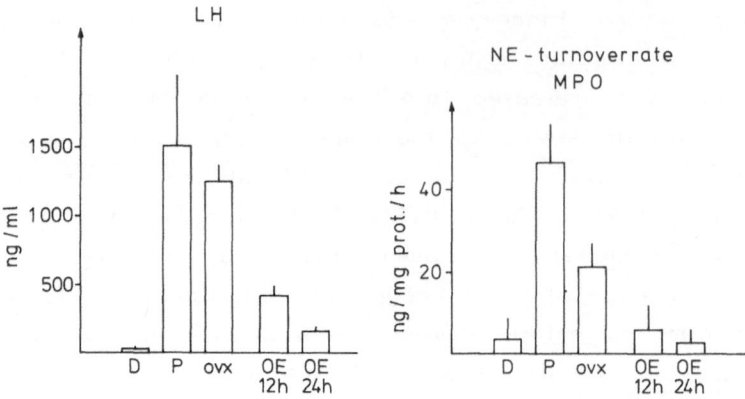

Figure 1: Serum LH levels and medial preoptic NE turnoverrates correlate well in diestrous (D), proestrous (P), ovariectomized (OVX) and OVX animals treated with estradiol-benzoate (OE) 12 h or 24 h prior to decapitation. Means ± SEM are shown

morphological and electrophysiological findings of the distribution of NE innervation (for review see Moore and Bloom, 1979). The perikarya of NE producing neurons are exclusively located in the brain stem and a few thousand NE cells innervate the entire CNS. Some of the NE neurons are also estrogen receptive as demonstrated by simultaneous autoradiography and immuno-staining of dopamine-β-hydroxylase (Sar and Stumpf, 1980). There is however, no indication that such estrogen sensitive NE neurons project to selected parts of the brain or to hypothalamic substructures. In fact, based on morphological and electrophysiological findings it is clear that brain stem NE neuronsproject diffusely to many areas of the CNS. Therefore we asked ourselves the following question: How can such a diffusely projecting system exert selective actions in circumscribed areas of the brain? Theoretically steroids may modulate NE turnover locally by several mechanisms. 1) By a direct action at the axon terminals to reduce or increase NE turnover. So far, there is no evidence that axon. terminals have estrogen binding sites. 2) Estrogens may be converted into catechol-estrogens which interfere with catecholamine metabolism (s. Breuer et al. and Knuppen et al., this volume). This possibility can explain some, but not all, estrogen feedback actions. 3) Estrogens may act at estrogen receptive cells which interact presynaptically with NE axon terminals. This alternative can explain all estrogen feedback actions but it is experimentally hard to verify. Estrogen receptive neurons have been demonstrated in areas where monoamine turnover is affected by estrogens (s. Stumpf, this volume). A possible neurotransmitter candidate involved in presynaptic interactions is GABA which was shown to mediate presynaptic inhibition in the spinal cord (Schmidt, 1971). It was therefore of interest to measure GABA concentrations and turnover rates in estrogen receptive areas under different steroid feedback situations. The technical details and difficulties in measuring this parameter is reported elsewhere. (Mansky et al., 1980; Mansky and Wuttke, this volume). Fig. 2

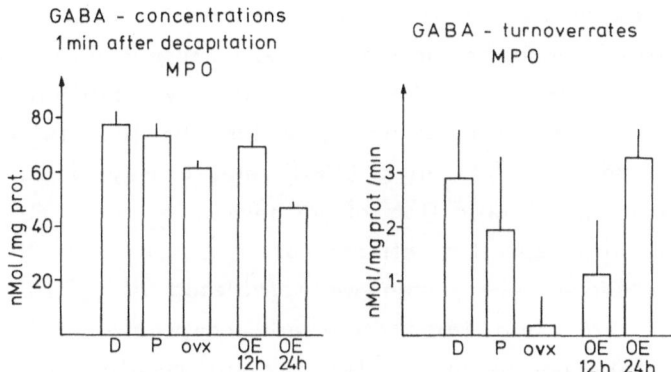

Figure 2: Under absent or present negative feedback action of estradiol (i.e. in OVX, D and OE animals) the turnoverrates of GABA in the medial preoptic area are inversely correlated to serum LH levels and medial preoptic NE turnover (see Fig. 1). This negative correlation cannot be demonstrated in P animals. The comparatively high concentrations of GABA in the MPO support the view that it plays an important role as a neurotransmitter in this region

shows GABA concentrations and turnover rates in the MPO. The concentrations of this neurotransmitter tend to be lower in ovx rats when compared to D or P rats. Estrogen replacement does not restore the GABA stores within 24 hrs. GABA turnover rates in the MPO show clear changes in association with the endocrine situation. They are high in D and in the estradiolbenzoate treated animals and low in ovx rats. Hence, the negative feedback action of estrogens increases GABA turnover, and absent feedback action results in low GABA turnover. Thus, with the exception of P rats GABA turnover in the MPO is inversely correlated with NE turnover and consequently it also correlates inversely with serum LH levels. These results suggest that some estrogen receptive neurons which mediate the negative feedback message are located in the MPO and that they may be GABA-ergic. In this context, it must be mentioned that intraventricular GABA injections into pentobarbital treated male and ovx female rats stimulated LH release which was interpreted such that GABA has a stimulatory effect on LHRH release (Vijayan and McCann, 1978a). Later on Pass and Ondo (1977) showed that such effects were only demonstrable in pentobarbital anesthetized but not in unanesthetized animals. Baseline LH levels in intact male rats remained unaffected, which would fit into our hypothesis because in these animals the negative feedback action of testosterone is fully functional, hence GABA turnover may be high and any additional GABA therefore ineffective. The mechanism by which the postulated E_2-receptive, GABA-ergic neurons influence LHRH release may be an indirect one through presynaptic inhibition of NE terminals. This may also explain the local and specific effects of estrogens on NE turnover in the MPO. Several years ago we speculated along this line (Wuttke and Höhn, 1978) and later Fuxe and coworkers (1979) came to similar theoretical conclusions. The present results give, according to our knowledge, the first experimental evidence for the involvement of GABA in the negative feedback action of estrogens. This challenges also the concept of general effects of the noradrenergic system as proposed by Moore and Bloom (1979) who discuss the NE system: "...the projections are widespread, the topography of projections apparently diffuse, and the function, thereby, general."

It is interesting that the positive feedback action of estradiol also involves a noradrenergic (Fig. 1) but apparently no GABA-ergic component (Fig. 2). This leads to the suggestion that other estrogen receptive neurons exist which respond to high estrogen concentrations. The neurotransmitter quality of these neurons remains to be established.

The role of DA in regulating LHRH release is much less clear. In vitro coincubation of DA with hypothalamic fragments points to a stimulatory effect of this amine on LHRH release (Rotsztejn et al.,

1977). Injection of DA or DA receptor stimulating drugs slightly increase serum LH levels (Vijayan and McCann, 1978b). The majority of physiological, pharmacological and neurochemical experiments however, indicate that DA is inhibitory to LH release (Fuxe et al., 1976, 1978; Beck and Wuttke, 1977; Beck et al., 1977, 1978). The possibility arises therefore that different DA systems may be involved in the regulation of LHRH secretion. One such system is the tuberoinfundibular DA cell cluster which innervates the basal hypothalamus and the median eminence. The other is the incerto-hypothalamic system which innervates the septal-preoptic complex, (Björklund et al., 1975). Hence, studies of DA turnover rates in the MBH and MPO in correlation with serum LH levels may add to the understanding of the action of DA on LH release. As shown below (Fig. 4) DA turnover in the mediobasal hypothalamus of P, D, ovx and ovx in estrogen treated animals does not correlate with serum LH levels. A number of investigators demonstrated that increased serum prolactin levels stimulated hypothalamic DA turnover (Gudelsky et al., 1976; Höhn and Wuttke, 1978) and also that hyperprolactinemia reduced serum LH levels (Wuttke, 1976; Beck et al., 1977) and it was concluded that the increase activity of the TIDA neurons was inhibitory to LH release. Meanwhile we demonstrated that other neurotransmitter systems, such as the noradrenergic and GABA-ergic (Höhn and Wuttke, 1978; Mansky and Wuttke, 1980) also change their activity in response to high serum prolactin levels which may also explain reduced serum LH levels. Hence, the feedback action of prolactin on pituitary LH release may not necessarily involve an inhibitory action of TIDA neurons on LHRH release. In view of the recently shown effects of endogenous opioids on TIDA turnover (Deyo et al., 1979; Versteeg et al., 1978) the involvement of these neurons in controlling LHRH release becomes even more questionable. Endogenous opioids reduce hypothalamic DA turnover but they also reduce serum LH levels. Hence, we face the situation that two experimental manipulations, i.e. induction of hyperprolactinemia and treatment with endogenous opioids result in reduced serum LH levels. However, the former manipulation increases while the latter decreases hypothalamic DA turnover. The effect of both treatments on DA turnover is much more meaningful in view of resulting changes in pituitary prolactin release because hyperprolactinemia reduces, whereas β -

135

endorphin administration increases release of this hormone, which points again to the importance of DA in regulating pituitary prolactin secretion.

Besides the well documented direct inhibitory action of DA on prolactin release, GABA has increasingly attracted neuroendocrine prolactin research. This amino acid stimulates pituitary prolactin release after intraventricular injection but has a direct inhibitory action at the lactotrophs (Ondo and Pass, 1976; Mioduszewski et al., 1976; Locatelli et al., 1979). In the third part of this report we will address this problem.

The question arises whether GABA-ergic neurons, in the hypothalamus also show cycle stage dependant changes in GABA turnover. Fig. 3 shows GABA concentrations and turnover rates in the anterior

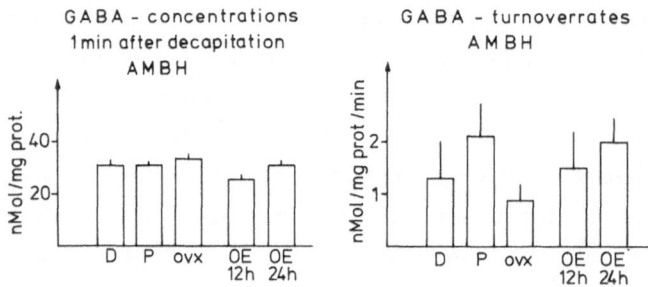

Figure 3: GABA turnoverrates in the AMBH seem to correlate with serum prolactin levels. The observed changes, however, are not significantly different

part of the mediobasal hypothalamus (AMBH). The concentrations in this part of the hypothalamus are much lower than in the MPO and do not change following endocrinological manipulations. GABA turnover in the AMBH was highest in P and in estradiol treated ovx rats and lowest in D and ovx animals. Although at the borderline of statistical significance these data may indicate that GABA might be involved in the control of ·pituitary prolactin release. GABA has been shown to have a direct inhibitory effect at the lactotrophs. Intraventricular administration however, stimulates pituitary prolactin release. Our results lend support to this stimulatory effect of GABA and the possibility arises that GABA inhibits DA release.

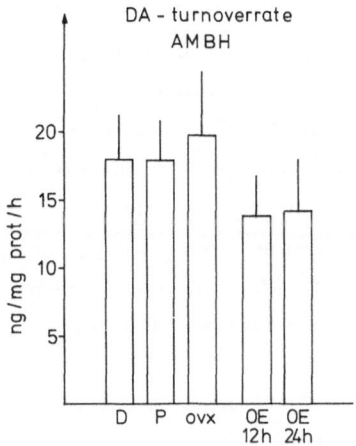

Figure 4: DA turnoverrates in the AMBH are not significantly different between the animal groups

In this case DA turnover should inversely correlate with GABA turnover. This is apparently not the case. Fig. 4 shows DA turnover rates in the AMBH and no reduction of DA turnover can be seen in P or estrogen treated ovx rats which is in good agreement with results published by Crowley et al. (1978), Simpkins et al. (1979) and Barraclough et al. (this volume). Although the latter authors observed decreased DA turnover in P rats they were unable to demonstrate reduced DA turnover in ovx-estrogen primed-pro-gesterone treated animals which also have high prolactin levels. All of these turnover results deriving from experiments in which catechol-amine synthesis was blocked apparently need cautious interpretation because Pilotte et al. (1980) demonstrated recently that minor changes of DA concentrations in the portal blood of female rats do not necessarily reflect catecholamine turnover changes in the median eminence. On the other hand, results published earlier by this group which were obtained in female rats indicate that portal blood DA concentrations are appparently much higher in female rats (Ben-Jonathan et al., 1977). They measured approximately 1 ng/ml in P and 4 ng/ml of portal blood in D rats. At a flow rate of 5-10 μl/min roughly 300-600 μl of portal blood are collected per hour wich correspond to 0.33-0.66 ng of DA in P and 1.3-2.6 ng/ml in D rats. Both values come close or exceed the reported total DA content of the median eminence. On the basis of this calculation one may conclude that the total content of DA is being released into the portal blood within 60 min or less. Such dramatic effects should be readily picked up 60 min following blockade of catecholamine synthesis. As mentioned above neither others nor ourselves were able to demonstrate such dramatic effects in D or P rats (Fig. 4) which may indicate that other than DA mechanisms are involved in controlling preovulatory and other prolactin surges. Hence, we suggest that GABA may stimulate prolactin release via mechanisms which do not exclusively involve inhibition of DA release. Since GABA is known to have generally inhibitory effects it may be assumed that it inhibits the release of a PIF.

Pharmacological experiments suggest that NE is also involved in the regulation of pituitary prolactin release (Donoso et al., 1971; Fenske and Wuttke, 1976; Carr et al., 1977). The turnover rate of NE in the AMBH is shown in Fig. 5. Low NE turnover in D and ovx

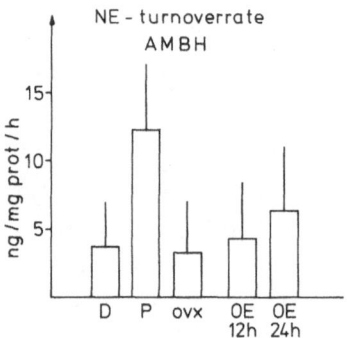

Figure 5: NE turnoverrates in the AMBH appear to parallel serum prolactin levels

and high turnover in P and ovx E_2-treated animals suggests that NE correlates with serum prolactin levels which may indicate that this amine has also a stimulatory function on pituitary prolactin release which is in agreement with the available pharmacological evidence. As in the case of GABA, this monoamine does not act via dopaminergic mechanisms because DA turnover in the MBH is not significantly reduced at times of high NE turnover. Possibly NE acts to stimulate a prolactin releasing factor.

The results presented in this report give evidence that preoptic NE turnover correlates with serum LH levels under a number of experimentally manipulated endocrine situations. The negative but not the positive feedback action of estrogens on LH release appears to involve GABA-ergic neurons in the MPO which may presynaptically specify NE release. The good correlation of the NE and GABA turnover in the AMBH with serum prolactin levels suggests that these neurotransmitters are involved in prolactin controlling mechanisms. It should be emphasized however, that correlations do not necessarily mean functional significance. Clearly, more work, using combined morphological, electrophysiological and neurochemical methods is needed to further elucidate how neurotransmitters control adeno-hypophysial hormone release.

References

Ajika K (1979) Simultaneous localization of LH-RH and catecholamines in rat hypothalamus. J Anat 128:331-347.

Anton-Tay F, Pelham RW, Wurtman RJ (1969) Increased turnover of ^{3}H-norepinephrine in rat brain following castration or treatment with ovine follicle-stimulation hormone. Endocrinology 84:1489-1492.

Beck W, Wuttke W (1977) Desensitization of the dopaminergic inhibition of pituitary luteinizing hormone release by prolactin in ovariectomized rats. J Endocr 74:67-74.

Beck W, Hancke JL, Wuttke W (1978) Increased sensitivity of dopaminergic inhibition of luteinizing hormone release in immature and castrated female rats. Endocrinology 102:837-841.

Beck W, Engelbart S, Gelato M, Wuttke W (1977) Antigonadotrophic effect of prolactin in adult castrated and immature female rats. Acta endocr (Kbh.) 84:62-71.

Ben-Jonathan N, Oliver C, Weiner HJ, Mical RS, Porter JC (1977) Dopamine in hypophysical portal plasma of the rat during the estrous cycle and throughout pregnancy. Endocrinology 100:452-457.

Björklund A, Lindvall O, Nobin A (1975) Evidence of an incerto-hypo-thalamic dopamine neurone system in the rat. Brain Res 89:29-42.

Carr LA, Conway PM, Voogt JL (1977) Role in norepinephrine in the release of prolactin induced by suckling and estrogen. Brain Res 133:305-314.

Clifton DK, Sawyer CH (1979) LH release and ovulation in the rat following depletion of hypothalamic norepinephrine: chronic vs. acute effects. Neuroendocrinology 28:442-449.

Coppola JA (1969) Turnover of hypothalamic catecholamines during various states of gonadotrophin secretion. Neuroendocrinology 5:75-80.

Crowley WR, O'Donohue TL, Wachslicht H, Jacobowitz DM (1978) Effects of estrogen and progesterone on plasma gonadotropins and on catechol-amine levels and turnover in discrete brain regions of ovariectomized rats. Brain Res 154:345-357.

Deyo SN, Swift RM, Miller RJ (1979) Morphine and endorphine modulate dopamine turnover in rat median eminence. Proc Natl Acad Sci USA 76:3006-3009.

Donoso AO, Bishop W, Fawcett CP, Krulich L, McCann SM (1971) Effects of drugs that modify brain monoamine concentrations on plasma gonadotropin and prolactin levels in the rat. Endocrinology 89:774-784.

Fenske M, Wuttke W (1976) Effects of intraventricular 6-hydroxydopamine injection on serum prolactin and LH levels: Absence of stress-induced pituitary prolactin release.Brain Res 104:63-70.

Flerkó B (1980) The hypophysical portal circulation today. Neuroendocrinology 30:56-63.

Fuxe K, Löfström A, Eneroth P, Gustafsson J-A, Hökfelt T, Skett P, Wuttke W (1976) Interactions between hypothalamic nerve terminals and LRH containing neurons. Further evidence for an inhibitory dopaminergic and facilitory noradrenergic influence. Exc Med Int Congr Ser 374:165-177.

Fuxe K, Hökfelt T (1966) Further evidence for the existence of tuberoinfundibular dopamine neurons. Acta Physiol Scand 66:245-246.

Fuxe K, Andersson K, Löfström A, Hökfelt T, Ferland L, Agnati LF, Pérez de la Mora M, Schwarcz R, Eneroth P, Gustafsson G-A, Skett P (1978) Neurotransmitter mechanisms in the control of the secretion of hormones from the anterior pituitary. In: Fuxe K, Hökfelt T, Luft R (eds) Central regulation of the endocrine system. Plenum Press, New York, pp.349-380.

Gay VL, Sheth NA (1972) Evidence for a periodic release of LH incastrated male and female rats. Endocrinology 90:158-162.

Gudelsky GA, Simpkins G, Mueller GP, Meites J, Moore KE (1976) Selective actions of prolactin on catecholamine turnover in the hypothalamus and on serum LH and FSH. Neuroendocrinology 22:206-215.

Höhn KG, Wuttke W (1978) Changes in catecholamine turnover in the anterior part of the mediobasal hypothalamus and the medial preoptic area in response to hyperprolactinemia in ovarietomized rats. Brain Res 156:241-252.

Honma K, Wuttke W (1980) Norepinephrine and dopamine turnover rates in the medial preoptic area and the mediobasal hypothalamus in the rat brain after various endocrinological manipulations. Endocrinology 106:1848-1853.

Knobil E (1980) Neuroendocrine control of the menstrual cycle. Rec Prog Horm Res 36:53-88.

Locatelli V, Cocchi D, Frigerio C, Betti R, Krogsgaard-Larsen P, Racagni G, Müller EE (1979) Dual γ -aminobuyric acid control of prolactin secretion in the rat. Endocrinology 105:778-785.

Löfström A, Eneroth P, Gustafsson J-A, Skett P (1977) Effects of estradiol benzoate on catecholamine levels and turnover in discrete areas of the median eminence and the limbic forebrain, and on luteinizing hormone, follicle stimulating hormone and prolactin concentrations in the ovariectomized female rat. Endocrinology 101:1559-1569.

Mansky T, Mestres-Ventura P, Wuttke W (1980) Involvement of GABA in the feedback action of estradiol on gonadotropin and prolactin release: Hypothalamic GABA and catecholamine turnover rates. Brain Res, in press.

Mioduszewski R, Grandison L, Meites G (1976) Stimulation of prolactin release in rats by GABA. Proc Soc Exp Biol Med 151:44-46.

Moore RY, Bloom FE (1979) Central catecholamine neuron systems: Anatomy and physiology of the norepinephrine and epinephrine systems. Ann Rev Neurosci 2:113-168.

Nicholson G, Greeley G, Humm J, Youngblood W, Kizer GS (1978) Lack of effect of noradrenergic denervation of the hypothalamus and medial preoptic area on the feedback regulation of gonadotropin secretion and the estrous cycle of the rat. Endocrinology 103:559-56.

Palkowits M (1975) Isolated removal of hypothalamic nuclei for neuro-endocrinological and neurochemical studies. In: Stumpf WE, Grant LD (eds) Anatomical Neuroendocrinology, Karger, Basel, pp.72-80.

Pass KA, Ondo JG (1977) The effects of γ-aminobutyric acid on prolactin and gonadotropin secretion in the unanesthetized rat. Endocrinology 100:1437-1442.

Pilotte N, Gudelsky GN, Porter JC (1980) Relationship of prolactin secretion to dopamine release into hypophysial portal blood and dopamine turnover in the median eminence. Brain Res 193:284-288.

Rotsztein WH, Charli GL, Patton E, Kordon C (1977) Stimulation by dopamine of luteinizing hormone-releasing hormone (LHRH) release from the mediobasal hypothalamus in male rats. Endocrinology 101:1475-1483.

Sar M, Stumpf WE (1980) Localization of ^{3}H-estradiol and dopamine-β-hydroxylase in cells of locus ceruleus by a combined autoradiographic and immunohistochemical technique. Abstr VI Inter Congr Endocrinol p.252.

Sawyer CH, Markee JE, Hollinshead WH (1947) Inhibition of ovulation in the rabbit by the adrenergic-blocking agent dibenamine. Endocrinology 41:395-402.

Schmidt RF (1971) Presynaptic inhibition in the vertebrate central nervous system. Ergebn Physiol 63:20.

Simpkins GW, Huang HH, Advis JP, Meites J (1979) Changes in hypothalamic NE and DA turnover resulting from steroid-induced LH and prolactin surges in ovariectomized rats. Biol Reproduct 20:625-632.

Vijayan E, McCann SM (1978a) The effects of intraventricular injection of γ-aminobutyric acid (GABA) on prolactin and gonadotropin release in conscious female rats. Brain Res 155:35-42.

Vijayan E, McCann SM (1978b) The effect of systemic administration of dopamine and apomorphine on plasma LH and prolactin concentrations in conscious rats. Neuroendocrinology 25:221-235.

Weiner RJ, Ganong WF (1978) Role of brain monoamines and histamine in regulation of anterior pituitary secretion. Physiol Rev 58:905-976.

Wuttke W (1976a) Regulation of prolactin release. Exc Med Int Congr Ser 409:287-292.

Wuttke W (1976b) Neuroendocrine mechanisms in reproductive physiology. Rev Physiol Biochem Pharmacol 76:59-101.

Wuttke W, Höhn KG (1978) Ontogeny of preoptic and hypothalamic catecholamine turnover rates and the relation to prolactin and gonadotropin levels. In: Dörner G, Kawakami M (eds) Hormones and brain development. Elsevier, Amsterdam, pp.341-349.

Steroid Effects on Hypothalamic-gonadotropin Interactions

S.M. McCann, A. Negro-Vilar, S.R. Ojeda, J.P. Advis, M. Lumpkin, W.K. Samson and
E. Vijayan, Dallas

The hypothalamic stimulatory control over gonadotropin release is
mediated by the decapeptide, LHRH, which exercises minute to minute
control over the release of LH from the pituitary. The decapeptide
has been found to release FSH under certain circumstances, particularly with prolonged exposure of the gland to the neurohormone.
This has prompted the conclusion that LHRH is gonadotropin releasing
hormone and that there is no separate FSH-releasing factor (FSH-RF)
(McCann, 1980). Certain evidence, which we will review, suggests
that indeed there probably is an FSH-RF distinct from the decapeptide. In this communication we will briefly review the steroid-
hypothalamic-pituitary interactions with particular reference to the
interplay between steroids and brain monoamines.

1. Actions of Steroids Directly on the Pituitary to Inhibit or Augment Gonadotropin Release

Gondadal steroids have complex actions directly at the pituitary to
modulate release of gonadotropins. In the ovariectomized female
minute doses of estradiol can inhibit LH release and this is
accompanied by a diminished responsiveness of the pituitary to the
decapeptide. The inhibitory effect was maximal at two hours and
had largely disappeared by four hours. At six hours after injection
of estradiol there was an enhanced responsiveness to LHRH. Similar
results were obtained for FSH. Thus, there is a biphasic response
to estrogen at the pituitary level in the ovariectomized rat (Libertun
et al., 1974): First, an inhibitory effect and then an augmentation

142

of the release of gonadotropins in response to LHRH. This negative feedback effect of estrogen is important in maintaining gonadotropin secretion in check in the intact animal. Progesterone synergizes with estrogen to hold LH secretion in check in the luteal phase of the cycle (McCann, 1962). The stimulatory effect is important in the proestrous or preovulatory discharge of gonadotropins. The response to LHRH on the afternoon of proestrus is further magnified by the so called self-priming action of LHRH (Castro-Vazquez and McCann, 1975; Aiyer et al., 1974).

In the castrate animal, LH and FSH release is augmented by removal of negative feedback of gonadal steroids which augments responsiveness to the decapeptide at the pituitary level. In addition, there is increased pulsatile release of the decapeptide in the castrate animal as evidenced by increase in peripheral circu-lating LHRH (Wheaton and McCann, 1976), and increased LHRH pulses in portal blood (Sakar and Fink, 1980). Release apparently exceeds synthesis and the content of LHRH in the hypothalamus decreases (Wheaton and McCann, 1976). On proestrus, there is enhanced release of LHRH induced by estradiol released from the preovulatory follicles. The evidence for this statement is increased titers of LHRH in peripheral (Wheaton and McCann, 1976) and portal blood (Fink, 1979) at this time of the cycle. The initial LHRH released may prime the gland to the subsequently released decapeptide by its self-priming action.

2. Catecholaminergic Control of LHRH Release

In vivo studies: The evidence for a stimulatory noradrenergic control over LH release is now overwhelming. For example, injection of microgram doses of norepinephrine or epinephrine into the third ventricle of ovariectomized steroid-primed animals leads to a release of LH. The effect is dose-related and the response to epinephrine is greater than that to norepinephrine (Vijayan and McCann, 1978b). The action can also be demonstrated in ovariectomized animals but is less pronounced. Inhibitors of catecholamine synthesis or alpha blockers block gonadotropin release. The site of the presumed stimulatory noradrenergic synapse is probably located in the pre-

143

optic-anterior hypothalamic area since stimulation of LH release by preoptic stimulation can be blocked by inhibitors of norepinephrine synthesis (Kalra and McCann, 1973). The cell bodies of the noradrenergic neurons concerned with gonadotropin release are probably located in the brain stem since injections of 6-hydroxy-dopamine into the ventral noradrenergic tract can block the release of LH in response to progesterone and also the preovulatory release (Clifton and Sawyer, 1979; Martinovic and McCann, 1977; Wuttke et al., 1980). Recovery occurs which may be due to the failure to denervate the hypothalamus completely, or to supersensitivity to the remaining norepinephrine.

The role of dopamine in the control of LH release has been controversial. In the ovariectomized, steroid-primed animal intra-ventricular dopamine clearly stimulates LH release (Vijayan and McCann, 1978a). The action is difficult to demonstrate in the ovariectomized animal and in this situation, large doses of dopamine or apomorphine given i.p. can inhibit LH release (Vijayan and McCann, 1978b). This action appears to be via suppression of LHRH release since responsiveness to the decapeptide is similar to that in ovariectomized controls. Thus, dopamine appears to be capable of either stimulating LHRH release or inhibiting its release depending on the steroid environment.

In vitro studies: We have confirmed the ability of cate-cholamines to release radioimmunoassayable LHRH from median eminence fragments incubated in vitro and a dose-response relation-ship existed. The release induced by norepinephrine was blocked by the alpha adrenergic receptor blocker, phentolamine, whereas that induced by dopamine was blocked by the dopamine receptor blocker, pimozide (Negro-Vilar et al., 1979). Addition of low doses of norepinephrine and of higher doses of dopamine to the fragments incubated in vitro provoked release of prostaglandins of the E series as determined by radioimmunoassay. We have strong evidence for an obligatory role of prostaglandins in the catecholaminergic stimulation of LH release since the release of LHRH by both norepinephrine and dopamine was blocked by indomethacin, an inhibitor of prostaglandin synthesis. Indomethacin failed to block the LHRH release induced by added prostaglandin E_2. Consequently, we postulate that the cate-cholamines release prostaglandin E_2 which in turn releases LHRH from

144

the terminals of the LHRH neurons in the median eminence (Ojeda et al., 1979b).

The in vitro studies confirmed the steroid dependence of the sensitivity of LHRH release to catecholamines. The responsiveness to either dopamine or norepinephrine was an order of magnitude less in ovariectomized animals than in ovariectomized, estrogen progesterone-treated animals (Ojeda et al., 1979a).

Not only can dopamine release LHRH from median eminence fragments but we have recently demonstrated that dopamine can also release LHRH from synaptosomes prepared from medial basal hypothalamus of the rat (Samson et al., 1980a).

3. Mechanism of Circhoral LH Release

That dopamine may be involved in the pulsatile release of LH which occurs in castrates appears likely from recent studies which we have carried out. We have obtained sequential blood samples from ovariectomized animals bearing cannulae in the jugular vein. The animals were then sacrificed and hypothalamic LRH, DA, and NE concentrations were determined by suitable assays. The time course of LH release could then be plotted and related to the concentrations LRH and catecholamines within the hypothalamus. Just prior to pulsatile release of LH, there was a decline in LRH and dopamine content in the median eminence, but no change in the content of norepinephrine. This suggests that dopamine release triggers LRH release which in turn evokes a pulsatile discharge of the gonadotropin. Furthermore, in these castrates, injection of L-dopa elevated LH even if conversion of dopamine to norepinephrine was blocked by the prior administration of diethyl-dithiocarbamate, an inhibitor of dopamine beta oxidase. Therefore, dopamine appears to stimulate pulsatile LRH release (Negro-Vilar, et al., unpublished). There may be involvement of norepinephrine as well since alpha adrenergic receptor blockers lower plasma LH in castrates. We would postulate that the central excitatory state of LRH neurons is maintained by noradrenergic drive so that pulsatile release can be induced by release of dopamine.

Considerable evidence also suggests a role for acetylcholine in pulsatile LH release. In recent studies third ventricular injection of acetylcholine resulted in elevation of plasma LH (Vijayan and McCann, 1980). The effect could be blocked by the muscarinic antagonist, atropine. The cholinergic link appears to involve the tuberoinfundibular dopaminergic tract since injection of pimozide to block dopamine receptors blocked the response to intraventricular acetylcholine. Consequently, we postulated that pulsatile LH release involves at least several steps: (1) Discharge of cholinergic neurons in the arcuate region which would synapse with the tuberoinfundibular dopaminergic neurons in the arcuate nucleus and trigger the release of dopamine; (2) Dopamine released from terminals in axo-axonal contact with LRH terminals in the median eminence would then depolarize these terminals resulting in release of LRH which would evoke the pulsatile release of LH; (3) As indicated above, noradrenergic tone would be necessary to maintain the central excitatory state of the LRH neurons.

4. Changes in Dopamine and Norepinephrine Metabolism After Castration and Estradiol Treatment

Studies involving measurements of monoamine content and turnover further support the role of catecholaminergic activity in the maintenance of elevated gonadotropin release in the castrate (Advis et al., 1980). Not only content but also turnover of norepinephrine was markedly elevated in female castrates. A new finding from these experiments was the fact that the increased turnover of norepinephrine was not limited to the basal tuberal region which has been thought to be a primary site of negative feedback of gonadal steroids, but was also present in the suprachiasmatic-preoptic region, which suggests that the region concerned with negative feedback of gonadal steroids may include not only the basal tuberal region but also the preoptic area. The dramatic increases in norepinephrine turnover rate were completely reversed two hours after treatment with estradiol.

Changes in dopamine turnover were less marked on a relative basis and a significant increase in turnover rate was only seen at

10 days in both median eminence and preoptic-suprachiasmatic area. Because the absolute turnover rate was much greater for dopamine than for norepinephrine the absolute increase in turnover at 10 days was greater for dopamine than for norepinephrine. Estradiol reversed the increased dopamine turnover.

5. Role of Serotonin in Control of LH

Serotonin injected into the ventricle can inhibit LH release in the castrate (Schneider and McCann, 1970) suggesting an inhibitory serotonergic drive on LRH, but it is not clear as yet if this plays a physiological role. Kordon and his associates (Hery et al., 1976) have shown that inhibition of serotonin synthesis by parachlorophenyl-alanine will block estrogen-induced LH release which suggests the possibility that serotonergic tone may be necessary for preovulatory release of LH induced by steroids.

6. Hypothalamic Action of Inhibin

In collaborative studies with Franchimont's group, we have tested the effects of various inhibin preparations supplied by them. We have shown that the intraventricular injection of inhibin in castrates can suppress FSH release in the face of normal responsiveness of the pituitary to a challenge with LHRH (Lumpkin, Negro-Vilar, and McCann, unpublished). Consequently, we have evidence that inhibin acts not only at the pituitary to suppress FSH but also at the hypothalamus to suppress the release of LHRH or possibly FSH-RF. Since the action was limited specifically to FSH release, inhibin may have suppressed the release of FSH-RF.

7. Possible Existence of an FSH-RF

There is evidence that the dorsal anterior hypothalamic area may play a selective role in control of FSH release perhaps via release of an FSH-RF. Lesions in this area are followed by a selective

147

lowering of FSH and not LH, whereas stimulation of the area either electrically or by implantation of prostaglandin E_2 gives selective release of FSH (see McCann, 1980 for references). This led us to evaluate the FSH-releasing action of hypothalamic extracts. Although the dorsal anterior hypothalamic area contained greater gonadotropin-releasing activity than could be accounted for by the content of LHRH as determined by RIA, no evidence for selective FSH release was obtained (Lumpkin et al., 1980). Subsequent experiments assaying gonadotropin-releasing activity by measuring FSH and LH release from dispersed pituitary cells revealed selective FSH release from extracts of the organum vasculosum lamina terminalis (Samson et al., 1980b).

It occurred to us that it had been relatively easy to detect an FSH-RF separate from LHRH when the activities were detected by bio- rather than immunoassay of gonadotropins. This prompted us to examine fractions from the same Sephadex G-25 column originally used to separate FSH-RF from LHRH. Aliquots of the fractions were added to male rat hemipituitaries incubated in vitro. FSH in the media was measured by bioassay by the Steelman-Pohley assay and by RIA. LH and LHRH were measured by RIA. Bioassayable FSH-RF was contained within the same fractions previously shown to contain it (Dhariwal et al., 1965). Bioactive FSH-RF eluted from the column prior to LHRH. We believe these data provide evidence for a bioassayable FSH-RF distinct from LHRH.

8. Conclusions

A) Steroidal control of gonadotropin release is complex. There are inhibitory as well as stimulatory actions of estrogen directly on the pituitary. In addition, progesterone synergises with estrogen to maintain negative feedback in the latter half of the cycle. The stimulatory action of estrogen is important in sensitizing the gland to the action of LHRH on proestrus. Additionally, the self-priming action of LHRH is important in increasing responsiveness to the gland at this time.

B) Feedback actions also occur at the hypothalamic level. Removal of negative feedback of gonadal steroids augments release of

LHRH which occurs in pulsatile form in the castrate. On proestrus there is augmented release of LHRH induced by estrogen and progesterone can similarly increase release of the decapeptide.

C) These actions are the result of a complex interplay between the steroids and monoamines. There is a stimulatory noradrenergic control of LHRH release and this is magnified under the influence of gonadal steroids. The role of dopamine is controversial, both stimulatory and inhibitory actions of LHRH release can be demonstrated. The stimulatory actions are observed in intact males and in ovariectomized steroid-primed females. In the ovariectomized female it is much more difficult to show the stimulatory action and in this situation large doses of dopamine appear to inhibit the release of LHRH. Nonetheless, dopamine may have a facilitatory action on the circhoral release of LH as demonstrated by declines in hypothalamic dopamine coincident with declines in LHRH on the rising limb of the LH release cycle. Acetylcholine may initiate the pulsatile release of LHRH via a dopaminergic step.

D) There is evidence for separate control of FSH release by an FSH-RF and via inhibin which acts not only at the pituitary but also at the hypothalamus to inhibit FSH release.

References

Advis JP, McCann SM, Negro-Vilar A (1980) Evidence that catecholaminergic and peptidergic (LHRH) neurons in suprachiasmatic-medial preoptic, medial basal hypothalamus and median eminence are involved in estrogen negative feedback. Endocrinology (in press).

Aiyer MS, Fink G, Greig F (1974) Changes in the sensitivity of the pituitary gland to luteinizing hormone releasing factor during the oestrous cycle of the rat. J Endocr 60:47-64.

Castro-Vazquez A, McCann SM (1975) Cyclic variations in the increased responsiveness of the pituitary to luteinizing hormone-releasing hormone (LHRH) induced by LHRH. Endocrinology 97:13-19.

Clifton DK, Sawyer CH (1979) LH release and ovulation in the rat following depletion of hypothalamic norepinephrine: chronic vs. acute effects. Neuroendocrinology 28:442-449.

Dhariwal APS, Nallar R, Batt M, McCann SM (1965) Separation of FSH-releasing factor from LH-releasing factor. Endocrinology 76:290-294.

Fink G (1979) Feedback actions of target hormones on hypothalamus and pituitary, with special reference to gonadal steroids. Ann Rev Physiol 41:571-586.

Hery M, Laplante E, Kordon C (1976) Participation of serotonin in the phasic release of LH. I. Evidence from pharmacological experiments. Endocrinology 99:469-503.

Kalra SP, McCann SM (1973) Effect of drugs modifying catecholamine synthesis on LH release from preoptic stimulation in the rat. Endocrinology 93:356-362.

Libertun C, Orias R, McCann SM (1974) Biphasic effect of estrogen on the sensitivity of the pituitary to luteinizing hormone-releasing factor (LRF). Endocrinology 94:1094-1100.

Lumpkin MD, Vijayan E, Ojeda SR (1980) Does the hypothalamus of infantile female rats contain a separate follicle-stimulating hormone releasing factor? Neuroendocrinology 30:25-32.

Martinovic JV, McCann SM (1977) Effect of lesions in the ventral noradrenergic tract produced by microinjection of 6-hydroxydopamine on gonadotropin release in the rat. Endocrinology 100:1206-1213.

McCann SM (1962) Effect of progesterone on plasma luteinizing hormone activity. Amer J Physiol 202:601-604.

McCann SM (1980) Control of anterior pituitary hormone release by brain peptides. Neuroendocrinology (in press).

Negro-Vilar A, Ojeda SR, McCann SM (1979) Catecholaminergic modulation of luteinizing hormone-releasing hormone release by median eminence terminals in vitro. Endocrinology 104:1749-1757.

Ojeda SR, Negro-Vilar A, McCann SM (1979a) Effect of catecholaminergic transmission blockade on prostaglandin E (PGE) release by the median eminence (ME) and modulatory effect of ovarian steroids on PGE-induced LHRH release in vitro. Prog 61st Endocr Soc Mtg. #446 (Abstr.).

Ojeda SR, Negro-Vilar A, McCann SM (1979b) Release of prostaglandin Es (PGE) by hypothalamic tissue: Evidence for their involvement in catecholamine-induced LHRH release. Endocrinology 104:617-624.

Samson WK, Koenig J, Reeves J, McCann SM (1980a) Vasoactive intestinal peptide stimulates LHRH release from hypothalamic synaptosomes. Prog 62nd Endocr Soc Mtg # 746 (Abstr.).

Samson WK, Snyder G, Fawcett CP and McCann SM (1980b) Chromatographic and biologic analysis of ME and OVLT LHRH. Peptides 1:97-102.

Sakar DK, Fink G (1980) Luteinizing hormone releasing hormone in pituitary stalk plasma from long-term ovariectomized rats and effects of steroids. Prog 62nd Endocr Soc Mtg # 648 (Abstr.).

Schneider HPG, McCann SM (1970) Mono- and indolamines and control of LH secretion. Endocrinology 86:1127-1133.

Vijayan E, McCann SM (1978a) Re-evaluation of the role of catecholamines in control of gonadotropin and prolactin release. Neuroendocrinology 25:150-165.

Vijayan E, McCann SM (1978b) The effect of systemic administration of dopamine and apomorphine on plasma LH and prolactin concentrations in conscious rats. Neuroendocrinology 25:221-235.

Vijayan E, McCann SM (1980). Effect of blockade of dopaminergic receptors on acetylcholine (Ach)-induced alterations of plasma gonadotropin and prolactin (Prl) in conscious ovariectomized rats. Brain Res Bull 5:23-29.

Wheaton JE, McCann SM (1976) Luteinizing hormone-releasing hormone in peripheral plasma and hypothalamus of normal and ovariectomized rats. Neuroendocrinology 20:296-310.

Wuttke W, Honma K, Hilgendorf W (1980) Neurotransmitter-neuropeptide interaction. In: Wuttke W, Weindl A, Voigt KH, Dries RR (eds) Brain and Pituitary Peptides, Karger, Basel, pp.190-201.

Differences in Negative and Positive Feedback of Gonadal Steroids on Release of Gonadotropins and Prolactin in Young and Old Rats

J. Meites, H.H.H. Huang and R.W. Steger, East Lansing

Both male and female rats show a decline in reproductive functions with aging. In the aging female this is manifested first by the onset of irregularity of cycles (lengthened), followed by a persistent estrous syndrome with failure to ovulate, by prolonged pseudo-pregnancies with active corpora lutea, and in the final stages of life by anestrus with ovarian shrinkage and presence of undeveloped follicles (Meites et al., 1976, 1978). Aging male rats show a reduction in circulating testosterone levels and perhaps a decrease in total number of spermatozoa. The causes for the reproductive decline appear to lie predominantly in the hypothalamus, but the pituitary, gonads, and possibly other endocrine glands also are involved. The gonads, pituitary and hypothalamus of aging rats show a remarkable plasticity throughout their lifespan, and can be reactivated to normal or near normal function even late in life. An exception is the old anestrous rat, with a pituitary tumor, but even in these rats, the ovaries can be reactivated.

1. Gonadotropic and Gonadal Hormone Secretion in Old and Young Rats

In early work, bioassays of pituitary hormone concentration by our laboratory showed that old Sprague-Dawley constant estrous rats (20–24 months old), contained more FSH and prolactin and less LH in their pituitaries than young rats (3–4 months old) on the day of estrus (Clemens and Meites, 1971). A comparison of serum concentrations of LH and prolactin in old (23–30 months) and young (4–6 months) female Long-Evans rats, without regard to their reproductive states, showed that LH values were about the same in both groups, but serum prolactin levels were about six-fold greater in the old rats (Shaar et al., 1975). Serum concentrations of LH and prolactin in old constant estrous rats were higher than in old pseudopregnant rats (Wuttke and Meites, 1973).

In a recent study by our laboratory (Huang et al., 1978), basal serum levels of LH, FSH, estradiol and progesterone of old Long-Evans, constant estrus and pseudopregnant rats (20-30 months old) were found not to differ from values in young rats (4-5 months old) in estrus or diestrus. However, the young rats exhibited a surge of these hormones every four days, whereas the hormone levels remained relatively unchanged in the old rats. It was concluded that the failure of old rats to show a cyclic surge of these hormones every 4-5 days constituted the biggest difference between the two age groups. In a more recent study by our laboratory (Steger, Huang and Meites, unpublished), and also by Estes et al. (1980), it was found that even basal secretion of LH and FSH was lower in old than in young female rats. When rats were ovariectomized and blood was collected frequently in an undisturbed state via atrial cannula, pulsatile release of LH was found to be only about 1/3 as much in old as in young rats. It can be concluded therefore, that old female rats secrete less LH and FSH and more prolactin than young female rats.

Comparisons between old and young male rats have shown similar differences to those between old and young female rats. Serum LH and FSH values were lower and serum prolactin was higher in old than in young male rats (Simpkins et al., 1977; Bruni et al., 1977; Shaar et al., 1975). In addition, serum testosterone levels in old males were only about 1/5 to 1/2 of those present in young males (Simpkins et al., 1977; Bruni et al., 1977). No changes were found in testicular LH binding or in the spermatogenic cycle in old (22 months) as compared with young (4 months) rats, although a total sperm count was not made (Steger et al., 1979).

2. Negative and Positive Feedback of Gonadal Steroids on Gonadotropin and Prolactin Release in Old and Young Rats

Marked differences in old and young rats have been demonstrated in both negative and positive feedback by gonadal steroids on secretion of gonadotropins and prolactin. Although basal serum LH values in old (23-30 months) and young (4-6 months) female rats did not differ, as indicated by single assays, ovariectomy resulted in serum LH increases several-fold greater in young than in old rats (Shaar et al., 1975). Huang et al. (1976) found that seven weeks after ovariectomy, young rats (4-5 months) showed a 26-fold rise in serum LH, whereas old rats (22-24 months) exhibited only about a 3-14 fold increase in serum LH. LH did not rise in the old anestrous rats, and the levels remained undetectable. The old rats also exhibited a smaller rise in serum FSH after ovariectomy. Estrogen produced a relatively smaller inhibition of LH and FSH release in old than in young rats. Shaar et al. (1975) found that young male rats showed basal serum LH values about four times greater than in old male rats, and LH levels rose significantly more in the young males after castration.

Basal serum prolactin levels were about six times greater in old than in young female rats, and exhibited a greater fall after ovariectomy in the old than in the young rats (Shaar et al., 1975). Estrogen administration increased serum prolactin more in old than in young rats. The latter is in agreement with the finding of Aschheim (1976), who observed that the prolactin response to estrogen gradually increased with aging. Huang et al. (1976) found that old anestrous rats had much higher serum prolactin levels than old constant estrous or pseudopregnant rats, and all categories of old rats had greater serum prolactin concentrations than young rats. Ovariectomy had no effect on serum prolactin levels in the old anestrous rats, since the ovaries of these rats produce almost no estrogen. The old persistent estrous, pseudopregnant and young rats showed a fall in serum prolactin values after ovariectomy.

The positive feedback of estrogen and/or estrogen and progesterone also has been tested in old and young ovariectomized rats. Cycling rats 60-70 days of age and persistent estrous rats 10-11 months of age were ovariectomized, and at 25 to 52 days after ovariectomy they were each injected with 8 µg estradiol benzoate/100 g body weight, followed 72 hours later by an injection of 0.8 mg progesterone. Serum LH rose significantly higher in the young than in the old rats (Lu et al., 1977). In another study, Steger et al. (1980) showed that mid-aged irregular cycling rats and persistent estrous rats (10–12 months old) showed a reduced positive LH feedback response to estrogen followed by progesterone, when compared with young rats (4–5 months old). Older constant estrous rats (18–20 months) showed no positive LH feedback response to the steroid hormone treatment. This suggests that aging female rats exhibit a progressively reduced positive LH feedback response to ovarian steroid stimulation.

3. Relation of Hypothalamic Neurotransmitters to Secretion of Gonadotropins and Prolactin

It is apparant hat there is reduced secretion of gonadotropins and increased secretion of prolactin in old rats of both sexes, and a decreased capacity to release LH after castration. Old female rats also release less LH in response to the positive feedback of ovarian steroids. These differences could be accounted for by (a) changes in hypothalamic function, including reduced ability to release LHRH into the portal circulation of the pituitary, (b) reduced responsiveness of the pituitary to LHRH stimulation, (c) other causes, including reduced gonadal hormone secretion, and lower thyroid function (Huang et al., 1980). The pituitary of old male rats does show a definite reduction in LH and FSH responsiveness to repeated injections of synthetic LHRH (Bruni et al., 1977), and the pituitary of old female rats appears to exhibit a decreased LH response to a single injection of LHRH. However, since the pituitary of old rats does respond to LHRH stimulation, any decrement in the pituitary capacity to release LH in old rats can be ruled out as a major factor responsible for the reproductive decline.

Much of the work from our laboratory, as well as that of others (Aschheim, 1976; Finch, 1978) points to the hypothalamus as mainly responsible for the low gonadotropin and high prolactin

154

secretion seen in old rats. LHRH is present in the hypothalamus of old rats (Steger et al., 1978), but apparently the neural signal to release it cyclically is lost in old female rats. The cause(s) for this loss in ability to release LHRH cyclically by old female rats appears to be related to the changes in hypothalamic neurotransmitters that regulate the release of LHRH from its nerve terminals in the median eminence into the hypophysial portal vessels. There is considerable evidence that catecholamines, particularly norepinephrine (NE) is stimulatory, whereas serotonin (5-HT) is inhibitory to gonadotropin release in rats (Meites et al., 1977). Our laboratory has reported that dopamine (DA) and NE concentration and metabolism are reduced in the hypothalamus of old male and female rats, whereas hypothalamic 5-HT metabolism is increased (Simpkins et al., 1977; Meites et al., 1978). We recently found that the hypothalamus of old male rats also contains significantly more methionine-enkephalin, a brain opiate, than the hypothalamus of young male rats (Steger et al., 1980b). The low DA in the hypothalamus of old rats, as well as the increased serotonin activity could be responsible for the increase in serum prolactin, whereas the reduction in NE and the increase in 5-HT could account in part at least, for the decreased release of gonadotropins by the old rats. Methionine enkephalin inhibits gonadotropin release and stimulates prolactin release (Meites et al., 1979).

We have shown that increasing hypothalamic CAs by administering L-DOPA or iproniazid, and other central acting drugs and hormones, can induce ovulation and reinitiate cycling in old constant estrous rats (Quadri et al., 1973; Huang and Meites, 1975). In addition, we have observed that chronic administration of L-DOPA to old female rats increases LH release in response to ovariectomy and to the feedback by ovarian steroids (Forman and Meites, unpublished).

In addition to possible changes in hypothalamic neurotransmitters that modulate release of LHRH, gonadotropins and prolactin in aging rats, there also is evidence for reduced uptake by the hypothalamus of old rats of estrogen (Peng and Huang, 1972), and for a reduction in neurons in the median eminence and anterior hypothalamus (Hsu and Peng, 1978). Other changes in hypothalamic function may occur during aging that contribute to the reduction in feedback by gonadal hormones on gonadotropin release, and the increase in feedback by estrogen on prolactin release.

Acknowledgements

Meites aided in part by research grants AG00416 from the National Institute of Aging, AM 04784 from the National Institute on Arthritis, Metabolism and Digestive Diseases, CA 10771 from the National Cancer Institute, and the Michigan Agricultural Experiment Station (Journal Article No.).
Steger aided by post-doctoral fellowship AG05062 from the National Institute on Aging.

References

Aschheim P (1976) Aging in the hypothalamic-hypophseal-ovarian axis in the rat. In: Everitt AV, Burgess JA (eds) Hypothalamus, Pituitary and Aging, Chas. C. Thomas, Springfield, Ill., pp.376-418.

Bruni JF, Huang HH, Marschall, S, Meites J (1977) Effects of single and multiple injections of synthetic GnRH on serum LH, FSH and testosterone in young and old male rats. Biology of Reproduction 17:309-312.

Clemens JA, Meites J (1971) Neuroendocrine status of old constant estrous rats. Neuroendocrinology 7:249-256.

Estes KE, Simpkins JW, Chen CL (1980) Alteration in pulsatile release of LH in aging female rats. Proc Soc Exp Biol Med 163:384-387.

Finch CE (1978) Reproductive senescence in rodents: factors in the decline of fertility and loss of regular cycles. In: Schneider EL (ed) The Aging Reproductive System, Raven Press, New York, pp.193-212.

Hsu HK, Peng MT (1978) Hypothalamic neuron number of old female rats. Gerontology 24:434-440.

Huang HH, Meites J (1975) Reproductive capacity of aging female rats. Neuroendocrinology 17:289-295.

Huang HH, Steger RW, Bruni JF, Meites J (1978) Patterns of sex steroid and gonadotropin secretion in aging female rats. Endocrinology 103:1855-1859.

Huang HH, Steger RW, Meites J (1980) Capacity of old versus young male rats to release thyrotropin (TSH), thryoxine (T_4) and triiodothyronine (T_3) in response to different stimuli. Experimental Aging Research 6:3-12.

Huang HH, Marshall S, Meites J (1976) Capacity of old versus young female rats to secrete LH, FSH and prolactin. Biology of Reproduction 14:538-543.

Lu KH, Huang HH, Chen HT, Kurcz M, Mioduszewski R, Meites J (1977) Positive feedback by estrogen and progesterone on LH release in old and young rats. Proc Soc Exp Biol and Med 154:82-85.

Meites J, Huang HH, Riegle, GD (1976) Relation of the hypothalamo-pituitary-gonadal system to decline of reproductive functions in aging female rats. In: Labrie F, Meites J, Pelletier G (eds) Hypothalamus and Endocrine Functions, Plenum, New York, pp.3-20.

Meites J, Huang HH, Simpkins JW (1978) Recent studies on neuroendocrine control of reproductive senescence in rats. In: Schneider EL (ed) The Aging Reproductive System, Raven Press, New York, pp.213–236.

Meites J, Bruni JF, Van Vugt DA, Smith AF (1979) Relation of endogenous opioid peptides and morphine to neuroendocrine functions. Life Sciences 24:1325–1336.

Peng MT, Huang HH (1972) Aging of hypothalamic–pituiatry–ovarian function in the rat. Fertility and Sterility 23:535–542.

Quadri SK, Kledzik GS, Meites J (1973) Reinitiation of estrous cycles in old constant estrous rats by central acting drugs. Neuroendocrinology 11:807–810.

Shaar CJ, Euker JS, Riegle GD, Meites J (1975) Effects of castration and gonadal steroids on serum luteinizing hormones and prolactin in old and young rats. J Endocrinol 66:45–51.

Simpkins JW, Mueller GP, Huang HH, Meites J (1977) Evidence for depressed catecholamine and enhanced serotonin metabolism in aging male rats: possible relation to gonadotropin secretion. Endocrinology 100:1672–1678.

Steger RW, Peluso JJ, Bruni JF, Hafez ESE, Meites J (1979) Gonadotropin binding and testicular function in old rats. Endokrinologie 73:1–5.

Steger RW, Huang HH, Chamberlain DS, Meites J (1980a) Changes in control of gonadotropin secretion in the transition period between regular cycles and constant estrus in aging female rats. Biology of Reproduction 22:595–603.

Steger RW, Van Vugt DA, Huang HH, Meites J (1980b) Reduced ability of naloxone to stimulate LH and testosterone release in aging male rats; Possible relation to increase in hypothalamic met[5]-enkephalin. Life Sciences (in press).

Gonadal Steroids and the Control of Gonadal Function in Seasonally Breeding Species

B.T. Donovan and B. Gledhill, London

In a seasonally breeding species such as the sheep it is quite clear that the gonadal hormones limit the secretion of gonadotrophin during the period of sexual quiescence, as well as during the breeding season. Ovariectomy enhances gonadotrophin secretion in the anoestrous ewe, and the sensitivity of the hypophysis toward the negative feedback action of oestradiol is much greater during the season of anoestrus than during the breeding season (Foster and Ryan, 1979; Turek and Campbell, 1979; Karsch et al., 1980). In fact, the seasonal change in the ability of oestradiol to inhibit tonic luteinizing hormone (LH) secretion has been used as a key observation in arguing that it is the seasonal difference in response to oestradiol that imparts seasonality to the reproductive process (Karsch et al., 1980). This view is akin to those advanced concerning the timing of puberty (Donovan and van der Werff ten Bosch, 1959a), for a change in the sensitivity of the hypothalamo-hypophysial system to oestrogen is evident in infancy (Ramirez and McCann, 1963), but takes no account of possible changes in the secretion of follicle-stimulating hormone (FSH). Further, the fundamental question remains to be resolved: what generates the change in the level of restraint to allow secretion of the additional amounts of gonadotrophin necessary for follicular maturation – if such a change in gonadotrophin secretion occurs? One suggestion (Foster et al., 1975; Lincoln, 1976) is that the frequency of episodic gonadotrophin secretion increases on the approach of the breeding season, so that any inhibitory action on the part of the gonadal hormones is overridden. The neural stimulus derived from changes in environmental lighting would provide the drive for an increased frequency of gonadotrophin surges. However, episodic hormone secretion can itself be affected by gonadal hormones, so complicating interpretation.

The changes outlined above could simply reflect the differences in sexual status of the sheep and are not necessarily the prime movers in the generation of seasonal reproductive periodicity. Caution in this respect is prompted by current work in the ferret. Many years ago Bissonnette (1932) demonstrated that anoestrous ferrets exposed to extra light during the winter came into oestrus several months before controls kept in natural daylight, and this species has since been used frequently in laboratory studies of periodicity. Unlike the sheep, the ferret does not experience oestrous cycles during the breeding season but remains in heat until ovulation is induced by coitus. Thus, the assessment of hormonal interactions is simplified by the absence of those reciprocal ex- changes between the gonads and the brain that generate oestrous cycles in other species.

The passage of the seasons in the ferret is clearly imprinted upon the genital tract. During anoestrus, the uterus is of small diameter with the endometrium being regressed, inactive, and showing no signs of hormone action. As oestrus approaches the uterus enlarges, with hypertrophy and differentiation of the endometrium, so that uterine weight provides an excellent index of the level of ovarian activity. Ovarian weight alone, by contrast, is of little value because the gonads of the anoestous female frequently weigh more than those of the oestrous ferret, but only small follicles are present and the stroma may be made up of a mass of plump cells. The ovaries of the oestrous ferret are characterized by the presence of large follicles, with the stromal tissue seemingly being reduced in amount by comparison with the anoestrous condition.

Such distinct morphological differences in the ovaries and uterus would be expected to reflect differing levels of gonadotrophin secretion during the breeding and non-breeding seasons, or between oestrus and anoestrus, especially as the circulating levels of FSH and LH may be raised during exposure to stimulatory photoperiods in other species, including trout, sparrows, quail, hamsters and sheep (Turek and Campbell, 1979). Accordingly, radioimmunoassays for FSH (using an anti-ovine gonadotrophin antiserum generated and generously supplied by Dr. J.Th. Uilenbroek) and for LH (using an anti-ovine gonadotrophin antiserum generated and generously supplied by Dr. G. Niswender) were set up and validated by Donovan and ter Haar (1977a). Using these procedures the plasma concentrations of FSH and LH in anoestrous ferrets have been compared with those during oestrus. On one occasion all of the ferrets in our colony were anaesthetized with sodium pentobarbitone and blood samples collected by cardiac puncture (Donovan and ter Haar, 1974, unpublished). In twenty-two anoestrous females the plasma FSH concentrations ranged between 277–711 ng NIH–FSH RP1/ml and for eight oestrous females between 229–320 ng/ml, with the mean for the former group being 454 ± 30 (S.E.M.) ng/ml and for the latter 270 ± 12 ng/ml. The difference between the means was statistically significant (P< 0.01). For the same anoestrous females the plasma LH concentrations ranged between non-detectable and 2.37 ng/ml, and for the oestrous ferrets between non-detectable and 0.51 ng/ml, with the respective means (calculated after assigning a value of 0.1 ng/ml to the samples in which the hormone was not detectable) being 0.50 ± 0.12 and 0.24 ± 0.05 ng/ml and not being statistically significant (P <0.3). While the use of anaesthesia and the occurrence of episodic gonadotrophin secretion limits deduction from this sampling exercise it is hard to avoid the impression that the plasma FSH concentration in anoestrous females can be higher than that during oestrus, and is not distinctly lower. The same feeling is gleaned from consideration of the findings for LH, where values above the maximum of 0.51 ng/ml for the oestrous group were found in six of the twenty-two anoestrous females. A raised plasma gonadotrophin level during anoestrus could be physiologically important, for Richards (1980) suggests that over-exposure to gonadotrophin may impede follicular growth.

It proved equally difficult to discern any change in FSH and LH secretion when animals bled weekly or bi-weekly were transferred from short to long days in order to advance oestrus, although there was a trend for the plasma FSH and LH concentrations to decline with the onset of vulval swelling, which is an index of the action of oestrogen (Donovan and ter Haar, 1974, unpublished). A complication in work of this kind is that some weeks elapse between the time of transfer from short to long days and the occurrence of genital changes, so that abrupt changes in the pattern of gonadotrophin secretion upon shifts of environmental lighting are unlikely. Changes in daylength altered the serum concentration of LH in castrated rams (Pelletier and Ortavant, 1975), but not in spayed ewes (Legan et al., 1977). There was no seasonal change in plasma LH levels in castrated red deer stags (Lincoln and Kay, 1979), while falls in gonadotrophin secretion in castrated hamsters occurred after transfer from long to short days, but were lacking when the animals were in breeding condition before castration and transfer (Ellis and Turek, 1980).

Attempts to trace seasonal changes in gonadotrophin secretion by the collection of single weekly, twice-weekly or daily blood samples are clearly unsatisfactory, although such procedures have proved valuable in other species. Short-term but significant alterations in hormone release may occur outside the sampling period and remain undetected, or may take place at night. As yet it has not proved practicable to plot the changes in episodic hormone secretion during anoestrus and oestrus, and it is difficult to collect serial blood samples from conscious animals without disruption of the normal patterns of existence of this small and very mobile creature. However, we have no evidence that barbiturate anaesthesia alters the pattern of episodic FSH and LH release in this species.

Hypothalamic lesions provide an alternative means of modifying gonadal function in the ferret, and of verifying that the assays being used are capable of detecting changes in plasma gonadotrophin level. Lesions placed in the anterior hypothalamus during the winter period of sexual quiescence advance the onset of oestrus (Donovan and van der Werff ten Bosch, 1959b), so that when lesions were placed at the end of December or early January, oestrus set in within three weeks and was sustained for months. Despite this reaction to the lesion, the hypothalamic control of gonadotrophin secretion did not appear to be adversely affected, for lesioned animals mated and readily became pregnant. It was argued that oestrus was advanced in these animals by destruction of or interference with an area normally inhibiting the secretion of gonadotrophin secretion, but recent work has cast doubt upon that view. In one experiment (Donovan and ter Haar, 1976, unpublished) lesions were placed in the hypothalamus of anoestrous ferrets and single blood samples collected under pentobarbitone anaesthesia twice weekly for three months in an effort to track any changes in gonadotrophin secretion that resulted. None were found. While an inappropriate blood sampling regime may have missed subtle changes in gonadotrophin secretion, there is an alternative explanation for the seeming lack of effect upon gonadotrophin release – though not for the onset of oestrus. In another study (Donovan and ter Haar, 1980) acute changes in gonadotrophin secretion were followed in animals serially bled at 15 min intervals before and for some hours after the hypothalamus was damaged. Passage of the lesioning current was associated with an immediate increase in LH output, but a raised plasma concentration of this gonadotrophin was never sustained overnight; the secretion of FSH was not altered consistently. There was also no consistent difference between the response of the anoestrous or oestrous females. It would seem that any change in gonadotrophin secretion in the ferret produced by damage to the hypothalamus is of limited duration, thus adding to the mystery surrounding the endocrine events taking place between the placement of hypothalamic lesions and the onset of oestrus several weeks later.

Despite the lack of understanding of the mode of action of hypothalamic lesions in enhancing ovarian activity in the ferret, and the evident inadequacy of any explanation based solely upon interference with the feedback action of gonadal hormones, there is good reason to presume that gonadal–hypophysial interaction occurs both during oestrus and anoestrus. Hemiovariectomy in ferrets causes compensatory hypertrophy of the remaining organ in anoestrous, as well as in oestrous, animals (Donovan, 1967), and we have since found no difference between anoestrous and oestrous ferrets in the rate of increase of gonadotrophin secretion after ovariectomy. The hypothalamo–hypophysial system is responsive to gonadal steroids, for prolonged treatment with oestradiol inhibited gonadotrophin secretion in anoestrous as well as in oestrous females, as shown by the absence of antral follicles in the ovaries. Interference with the feedback action of ovarian hormones has also been assayed by treatment with an anti-oestrogenic drug, clomiphene citrate (Donovan, 1971). Inhibition of gonadotrophin secretion in anoestrous females was produced by large doses, but could not be achieved in oestrous ferrets with amounts that exerted a notable oestrogenic action upon the uterus.   Occasionally, clomiphene induces ovulation in oestrous ferrets, as did oestradiol in earlier work.

Little information is available concerning the hormones produced by the ovaries of the ferret.   In one trial (Donovan and ter Haar, 1974, unpublished) the plasma concentrations of progesterone, oestradiol, testosterone, dihydrotestosterone and androstenedione were followed in three anoestrous littermate females transferred from short to long days and brought into oestrus.   Progesterone was measurable in only two of 15 samples from one female (one collected before and the other after the onset of oestrus) and in none from the other ferrets.   Marked changes in plasma androgen set in upon transfer to long days, with sharp falls in androstenedione and dihydrotestosterone (DHT) being noted before swelling of the vulva.   The changes in plasma testosterone were much smaller.   Oestradiol was frequently not detectable, despite the occurrence of marked vulval swelling. The significance of these changes is not understood, although Richards (1980) quotes evidence to the effect that DHT prevents the hormonal induction of LH receptors in developing antral follicles of immature intact rats and appears to alter the ability of follicles to respond to oestradiol.   Nazian and Mahesh (1980) suggest that androstenedione interferes with the maturation of the negative feedback system controlling LH secretion in the young male rat, and with the self-priming effect of multiple injections of GnRF upon gonadotrophin secretion.   If comparable effects were to be produced in the ferret by these steroids the reason for the fall in plasma concentration of these steroids with change of lighting remains to be determined.

A differential feedback action of gonadal hormone upon gonadotrophin secretion in the ferret might well be reflected in the response to electrical stimulation of the hypothalamus, where the anoestrous female showed a greater increase in FSH and LH release than did the oestrous ferret (Donovan and ter Haar, 1977b).   In this instance the gonadal secretions appeared to limit gonadotrophin release in the oestrous female, perhaps through an alteration in the sensitivity of the hypophysis to hypothalamic gonadotrophin releasing factor (GnRF), for the output of gonadotrophin in response to an injection of 4 μg GnRF is likewise greater during anoestrus than during oestrus (Donovan and ter Haar, 1977a).   Since ovariectomised females released LH after GnRF treatment in a manner characteristic of anoestrous females, and treatment of spayed females with oestrogen depressed the response to the factor, these findings provide evidence for the feedback action of an oestrogen upon the sensitivity of the hypophysis to GnRF, but do not explain how gonadotrophin secretion is held in check during anoestrus. A non-oestrogenic hormone could be utilized.

The reaction of the hypophysis to a long-acting analogue of GnRF, D-Ser (TBU)^6 LH-RH-ethylamide (HOE 766 or buserelin), differs from that to the native product in that the gland of the oestrous female releases both FSH and LH as readily as that of the anoestrous animal, although the pattern of release differs (Gledhill and Donovan, 1980). In a closer analysis of the response to this peptide, ferrets were pretreated with cycloheximide to block the synthesis of gonadotrophin by the hypophysis and distinct differences in the response of anoestrous and oestrous ferrets emerged, with the surge of LH secretion induced in the anoestrous females steadily waning, whereas in oestrous females the initial increase in LH secretion was minimal but increased steadily over the ensuing hours. The pattern of FSH secretion in these animals broadly matched that of LH. The basis of this differential response is not understood, but since the GnRF analogue must be acting directly upon the hypophysis these observations indicate that the factor responsible must also be acting directly upon the pituitary gland.

One complication in consideration of the feedback action of gonadal hormones upon gonadotrophin secretion is that the hypophysis may change the form of hormone secreted under different circumstances. Evidence for this phenomenon has been presented for the rat (Bodganove et al., 1975), monkey (Peckham and Knobil, 1976) and man (Dufau et al., 1976). The circulatory survival of gonadotrophins in hypophysectomized spayed ferrets is extremely long, with a half-life for FSH in excess of three hours, and for LH of some 100 minutes. The half-life of FSH in ferrets given HOE 766 to acutely raise gonadotrophin secretion before hypophysectomy and the subsequent serial bleeding was about 75 minutes for anoestrous females and about two hours during oestrus. In the anoestrous ferrets given HOE 766 the half-life of LH was approximately 15 minutes. Pretreatment of anoestrous ferrets with GnRF instead of HOE 766 did not affect the half-life of FSH or LH. Although the possibility remains that different metabolic clearance rates for a constant molecular species may account for such differences, these observations undoubtedly give rise to questions concerning the biological activity of the various hypophysial products, for the FSH and LH activity detected radioimmunologically need not necessarily reflect biological function. In short, the concentration of gonadotrophin detected during anoestrus, or even after spaying, may be meaningless from the point of view of the target organ. Here, some old observations may take on a new significance. In rats it is well known that autotransplantation of ovarian tissue to the spleen of spayed rats results in marked enlargement of the grafts, even to the extent of tumour formation (Donovan, 1966). This change ensues through loss of the feedback action of gonadal steroids by inactivation in the liver of the steroids produced by the grafts before they can reach the peripheral ciculation. When this procedure was applied to the ferret no hypertrophy of the spleen-engrafted ovarian tissue occurred and follicular development was poor (Donovan, 1969). It was presumed that the hypophysis of the ferret responded sluggishly to withdrawel of gonadal hormone, but that conclusion is evidently incorrect. An alternative suggestion is that the increased concentrations of gonadotrophic hormone to which the ovarian grafts were exposed may have lacked biological potency.

On the basis of the information available the idea that seasonal reproductive periodicity arises as the inhibitory action of gonadal hormones upon gonadotrophin secretion is opposed, and at times favoured, by the waxing and waning of day length does not seem to be applicable to the ferret. It could be an attractive hypothesis when applied to the sheep and hamster, where there is evidence for the continuation of subthreshold gonadal cycles during the anoestrous phase (Seegal and Goldman, 1975), but then common ground has to be found for the parallel action of short days in the sheep and long days in the hamster. Alternative mechanisms thus merit consideration, for seasonal reproductive quiescence may be produced by mechanisms other than a straightforward depression of plasma gonadotrophin concentration. Indeed, exposure to short days has failed to increase the secretion of FSH and LH in the ewe (Walton et al., 1980), in contrast to the ram. Richards (1980) points out that follicular growth may be prevented either because serum concentrations of gonadotrophin are markedly suppressed, or because a sustained increment is never achieved. Further, anoestrus in the Syrian hamster is characterized by daily surges of gonadotrophins (Seegal and Goldman, 1975) and these could desensitise ovarian follicular cells and so prevent a recovery phase necessary for continuous follicular growth.

The secretion of prolactin is known to be affected by changing daylength (Tindal, 1978) and in view of the close relationship between prolactin release and the level of gonadal activity (McNeilly, 1980) the primary control of the level of reproductive function could be exercised through this pituitary factor. Thus, the testicular atrophy in hamsters that occurred after transfer from a long to a short photoperiod could be delayed by the transplantation of homologous pituitary tissue to a kidney capsule, and Bartke et al. (1980) have concluded that the effect is due to the maintenance of testicular LH receptors by the prolactin released from the grafts. Chen and Reiter (1980) concurred with this view, and made the point that in blind male hamsters with regressed testes twice daily injections of GnRF failed to restore testicular and accessory organ weights to normal, although the plasma levels of FSH and LH were raised by this treatment. On the other hand, normal testis and accessory organ weights were recorded in similarly treated blind hamsters provided with two homografted pituitary glands. However, the reports that plasma gonadotrophin levels change in gonadectomized hamsters after transfer from long to short days (Ellis and Turek, 1980) indicate the operation of a gonad-independent process. Hyperprolactinaemia is characteristically seen in anoestrous sheep, but reduction of plasma prolactin concentrations in anoestrous ewes by treatment with bromocriptine had little effect upon the secretion of FSH or LH, or upon the proportion of ewes ovulating in response to an injection of oestradiol benzoate (Land et al., 1980; Walton et al., 1980). No direct evidence on the relationship between prolactin and oestrus or anoestrus in the ferret is available.

It is clear that there are great difficulties in constructing an hypothesis accounting satisfactorily for the changes in gonadotrophic hormone release in three seasonally breeding species, let alone one of general application. In part this inability reflects a lack of

166

knowledge of the basic mechanisms concerned, as is illustrated with particular reference to the ferret, where the absence of oestrous cycles should facilitate analysis. Nevertheless, the first step in any scientific endeavour is the delineation of those areas where more information is needed. That step is being taken.

References

Bartke A, Goldman BD, Bex FJ, Kelch RP, Smith MS, Dalterio S, Doherty PC (1980) Effects of prolactin on testicular regression and re-crudescence in the golden hamster. Endocrinology 106:167-172.
Bissonnette TH (1932) Modification of mammalian sexual cycles; reactions of ferrets with both sexes to electric light added after dark in November and December. Proceedings of the Royal Society, Series B 110:322-336.
Bogdanove EM, Nolin JM, Campbell GT (1975) Qualitative and quantitative gonad-pituitary feedback. Recent Progress in Hormone Research 31:567-619.
Chen HJ, Reiter RJ (1980) The combination of twice daily luteinizing hormone-releasing factor administration and renal pituitary homo-grafts restores normal reproductive organ size in male hamsters with pineal-mediated gonadal atrophy. Endocrinology 106:1382-1385.
Donovan BT (1966) The regulation of the secretion of follicle-stimulating hormone. Harris GW, Donovan BT (eds) The Pituitary Gland, Butterworths, London, 2:49-98.
Donovan BT (1967a) The feedback action of ovarian hormones in the ferret. Journal of Endocrinology 38:173-179.
Donovan BT (1969) The functional capacity of ovarian tissue transplanted to the spleen or kidney in the ferret. Journal of Endocrinology 45:91-97.
Donovan BT (1971) The action of clomiphene in the ferret. Journal of Endocrinology 51:387-391.
Donovan BT, ter Haar MB (1977a) Effects of luteinizing hormone releasing hormone on plasma follicle-stimulating hormone and luteinizing hormone levels in the ferret. Journal of Endocrinology 73:37-52.
Donovan BT, ter Haar MB (1977b) Stimulation of the hypothalamus and FSH and LH secretion in ferret. Neuroendocrinology 23:268-278.
Donovan BT, ter Haar MB (1980) Acute effects of hypothalamic lesions upon gonadotrophin secretion in the ferret. Journal of Endocrinology, in press.
Donovan BT, van der Werff ten Bosch JJ (1959a) The hypothalamus and sexual maturation in the rat. Journal of Physiology 147:78-92.
Donovan BT, van der Werff ten Bosch JJ (1959b) The relationship of the hypothalamus to oestrus in the ferret. Journal of Physiology 147:93-108.
Dufau ML, Beitins IZ, McArthur JW, Catt KJ (1976) Effects of luteinizing hormone releasing hormone (LHRH) upon bioactive and immunoreactive serum LH levels in normal subjects. Journal of Clinical Endocrinology and Metabolism 43:658-667.
Ellis GB, Turek FW (1980) Photoperiodic regulation of serum luteinizing hormone and follicle-stimulating hormone in castrated and castrated-adrenalectomized male hamsters. Endocrinology 106:1338-1344.
Foster DL, Lemons JA, Jaffe RB, Niswender GD (1975) Sequential patterns

of circulating luteinizing hormone and follicle-stimulating hormone in female sheep from early postnatal life through the first estrous cycles. Endocrinology 97:985-994.

Foster D, Ryan K (1979) Mechanisms governing onset of ovarian cyclicity at puberty in the lamb. Ann Biol anim Biochem Biophys 19(4):1369-1380.

Gledhill B, Donovan BT (1980) Changes in gonadotrophin secretion in the ferret induced by teatment with a long acting LH-RH analogue (HOE 766). Proceedings of the Annual Conference of the Society for the Study of Fertility, 13.

Karsch FJ, Goodman RL, Legan SJ (1980) Feedback basis of seasonal breeding: test of an hypothesis. Journal of Reproduction and Fertility 58:521-535.

Land RB, Carr WR, McNeilly AS, Preece RD (1980) Plasma FSH, LH, the positive feedback of oestrogen, ovulation and luteal function in the ewe given bromocriptine to suppress prolactin during seasonal anoestrus. Journal of Reproduction and Fertility 59:73-78.

Legan SJ, Karsch FJ, Foster DL (1977) The endocrine control of seasonal reproductive function in the ewe: a marked change of response to the negative feedback action of estradiol on luteinizing hormone secretion. Endocrinology 101:818-824.

Lincoln GA (1976) Seasonal variation in the episodic secretion of luteinizing hormone and testosterone in the ram. Journal of Endocrinology 69:213-226.

Lincoln GA, Kay RNB (1979) Effects of season on the secretion of LH and testosterone in intact and castrated red deer stags (Cervas elaphus). Journal of Reproduction and Fertility 55:75-80.

McNeilly AS (1980) Prolactin and the control of gonadotrophin secretion in the female. Journal of Reproduction and Fertility 58:537-549.

Nazian SJ, Mahesh VB (1980) Delay in some aspects of the sexual maturation of the male rat induced by androstenedione. Biology of Reproduction 22:451-458.

Peckham WD, Knobil E (1976) The effects of ovariectomy, estrogen replacement, and neuroaminidase treatment on the properties of the adenohypophysial glycoprotein hormones of the rhesus monkey. Endocrinology 98:1054-1060.

Pelletier J, Ortavant R (1975) Photoperiodic control of LH release in the ram. I. Influence of increasing and decreasing light photoperiods. Acta Endocrinologica 78:435-441.

Ramirez DV, McCann SM (1963) Comparison of the regulation of luteinizing hormone (LH) secretion in immature and adult rats. Endocrinology 72:452-464.

Richards JS (1980) Maturation of ovarian follicles: actions and interactions of pituitary and ovarian hormones on follicular cell differentiation. Physiological Reviews 60:51-89.

Seegal RF, Goldman BD (1975) Effects of photoperiods on cyclicity and serum gonadotrophins in the Syrian hamster. Biology of Reproduction 12:223-231.

Tindal JS (1978) Control of prolactin secretion. Jeffcoate SL, Hutchinson JSM (eds) The Endocrine Hypothalamus. Academic Press, London, pp.333-360.

Turek FW, Campbell CS (1979) Photoperiodic regulation of neuroendocrine-gonadal activity. Biology of Reproduction 20:32-50.

Walton JS, Evins JD, Fitzgerald BP, Cunningham FJ (1980) Abrupt decrease in daylength and short-term changes in the plasma concentrations of FSH, LH and prolactin in anoestrous ewes. Journal of Reproduction and Fertility 59:163-171.

Influence of Estradiol and Other Gonadal Steroids on Central Effects of Lisuride and Comparable Ergot Derivatives

R. Horowski and R. Dorow, Berlin and Bergkamen

The activity of the CNS is influenced in different ways by the gonads and their hormones. This applies to the well documented feedback mechanisms of these hormones on the hypothalamus or their modulation of anterior pituitary function. One classical example is the influence of estrogens on the production and secretion of prolactin.

In many cases, the CNS is supposed to have a regulatory effect on the endocrine system, as in the case of the transmission of environmental factors such as the day-night periods triggering circadian rhythmicity or, as another example, the influence of different 'stress' factors on hormonal systems.

In addition to this regulatory role of CNS systems on circulating hormone levels, the strong influence of gonadal hormones on behaviour is well-known. This applies, e.g., to the far-reaching behavioural consequences of castration which, in male domestic animals, is used because of its taming and antiaggressive effect since many centuries. It is not surprising, that sexual behaviour seems to depend especially on gonadal function, but recently, also profound interactions have been found between estrogens and motor function in some laboratory animals.

In this situation, we decided to look on the influence of gonadal steroids, and especially estrogens, on central effects caused by ergot derivatives, since these compounds have specific effects on hormonal systems, but are also well-known to have behavioural effects and to affect the motor system. We used different ergot derivatives with different patterns of CNS effects but focused our interest on lisuride which has been shown by our group to be a potent dopamine agonist with prolactin-lowering effects (Horowski and Wachtel, 1976; Gräf et al., 1976), but which also influences the motor system and, finally, causes a unique behavioural effect in rats which apparently cannot be distinguished from normal sexual male behaviour in this species (Da Prada et al., 1977).

Lisuride is a semi-synthetic ergot derivative which by pharmacological (Horowski and Wachtel, 1978), biochemical (Kehr, 1977; Pieri et al., 1978), and electrophysiological (Rogawski and Aghajanian, 1979) methods has been shown to be a potent dopamine agonist, but which also has a high affinity to serotonin receptors where it may act as an agonist or, especially at higher concentrations, as an antagonist. At very high concentrations, also α-adrenolytic and β-receptor blocking properties have been described which are of no practical relevance but show the broad potential of ergot effects (Cote et al., 1979). Under in vitro-conditions, lisuride has been shown to displace ^{3}H-spiroperidol binding at lower concentrations than haloperidol or apomorphine (Fujita et al., 1978). ^{3}H-lisuride binding seems to be quite similar to spiroperidol binding, and here again, high specifity and affinity has been demonstrated (Fujita et al., 1979). In rodents, lisuride concentration in the brain is in a similar order of magnitude as plasma levels, whilst the pituitary has 5-10-fold higher concentrations (Hümpel et al., 1981). Since it is well-known that lisuride acts at the pituitary level as a prolactin-lowering compound, and since prolactin cells have dopamine receptors or concentrate dopamine (Gudelsky and Porter, 1979), it is tempting to speculate that the high concentration of lisuride in the pituitary reflects its binding on prolactin cells.

Since lisuride is a compound with intense spontaneous fluorescence, its high affinity for monoamine and especially dopamine receptors may led to its use for localisation of lisuride binding and, thus, monoaminergic receptors in in vitro or even in vivo-situations. In preliminary experiments, we have indeed observed that after incubation of pituitary slices or cell suspensions with solutions of lisuride and repeated washing, a few cells maintain a prominent fluorescence whilst most others do not. If it can be demonstrated that the fluorescent cells correspond to the known prolactin-producing cells of the pituitary, lisuride fluorescence may become a very valuable tool for morphological investigation. In addition, we have

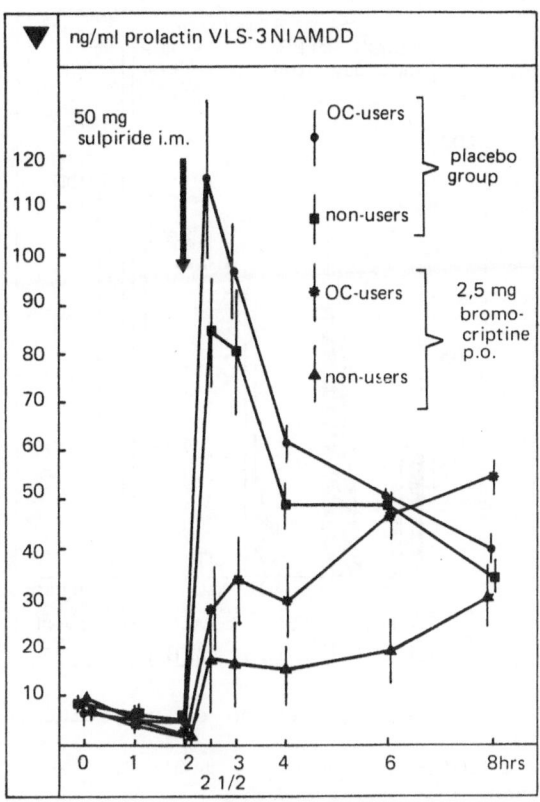

Figure 1: Serum prolactin levels in 2 groups of 6 healthy female volunteers aged 20-35 who received bromocriptine 2.5 mg or placebo at time 0 on a radomized double-blind basis; after 2 hours, all women had an i.m. injection of sulpiride 50 mg as a stimulus for prolactin secretion. OC-users were continuously on oral contraceptives containing estrogens whilst non-users had other methods of contraception

observed that granulocytes of human blood display an intense flouorescence when slides have been incubated with fresh solutions of lisuride and subsequently washed.

In agreement with many others, we have observed that treatment with functional dopamine antagonists such as reserpine, sulpiride or spiroperidol results in higher prolactin concentrations in adult female than in male rats; this applies also to the inhibitory effects of lisuride or bromocriptine which result in lower prolactin concentrations in male or ovariectomized female rats, when compared with intact or estrogen-substituted female animals (data not shown, for ref. see Gräf et al., 1976; Horowski and Gräf, 1976).

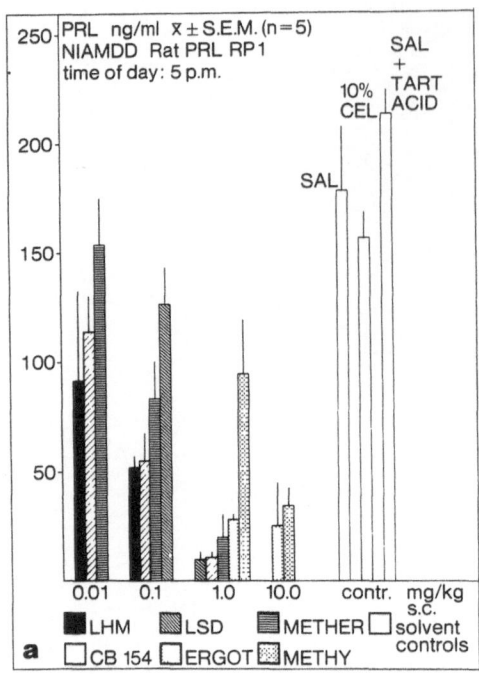
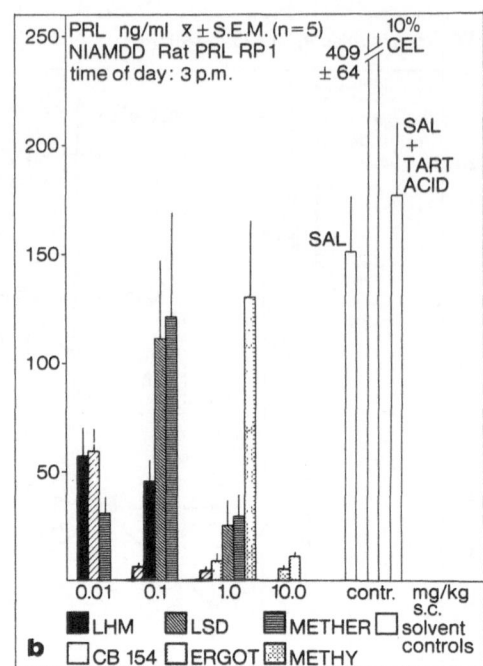

Figures 2a and 2b: Influence of ergot derivatives on serum prolactin
levels in rats.
a) Intact female rats were pretreated with reserpine (2 mg/kg i.p._20-24
   hrs before testing) and subsequently received s.c. injections of
   various ergot derivaties or vehicles 6 hours before testing (for
   methods see Gräf et al., 1976).
b) Ovariectomized female rats primed with one single injection of
   estradiol benzoate (25 μg/kg s.c.) were treated with various ergot
   derivatives 2 days after estradiol injection and 6 hours before
   testing.
LHM = lisuride hydrogen maleate, CB 154 = bromocriptine, LSD = lyser-
gamid, ERGOT = ergotamine, METHER = methergoline, METHY = methysergide

These differences are interpreted as being due to the presence of
estrogens in female rats. The relevance of these results is stressed
by our similar observation in humans where healthy female
volunteers, taking ostrogen-containing oral contraceptives, not only
had slightly, but significantly higher prolactin levels after injections of the dopamine antagonist sulpiride (25 mg i.m.), but
where also after additional treatment with bromocriptine, serum
prolactin levels were clearly higher than in similar groups of women
who did not use oral contraception (Fig. 1). For further studies we
have developed an estrogen model for testing the prolactin-lowering

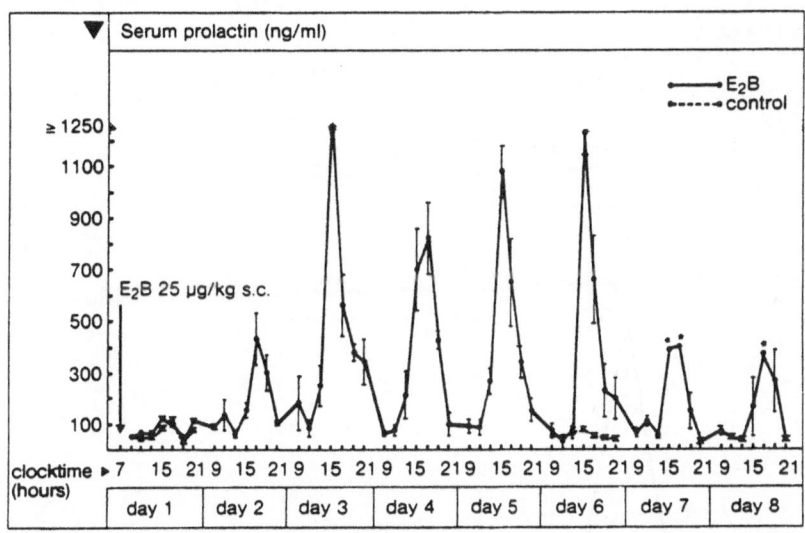

Figure 3: Effect of a single s.c. injection of 25 µg/kg E$_2$B (given at 7:00 h on day 1) on PRL-levels (mean S.E.M.; n = 5 animals/time) sampled every two hours between 9:00 h and 21:00 h. All animals were exposed to a photoperiod lasting from 6:00 h to 18:00 h every day (L/D). Controls (day 1 and day 6) were treated with the vehicle (sesame oil) only. Bar indicated PRL values > 1250 mg/ml

effect of ergot derivatives (Gräf et al., 1976). Ovariectomized female rats were treated with one single s.c. injection of 25 µg/kg of estradiol benzoate which results in pronounced circadian rhythms of PRL lasting for more than one week (Fig. 2) and a daily maximum at 5 p.m. which depends, however, on the light-dark cycle since it can be switched to an opposite maximum at 5 a.m. by an inverse day-night-rhythm (Fig. 3). This and additional results (Dorow et al., 1980) are an indication that very low concentrations of estradiol trigger an unknown, most probably central mechanism which, under physiological conditions, is responsible for the very similar proestrous afternoon surge in blood prolactin concentration. Other, non-estrogenic steroids such as testosterone (1 mg/kg), progesterone (1 mg/kg), dihydrotestosterone (1 mg/kg) and norethisterone enanthate (10 mg/kg), all given s.c., have been unable, in our hands, to elicit a similar phenomenon (data not shown). This strong, definite, specific and highly reproducible estrogen effect can be considered as a good tool for studying central mechanisms which

173

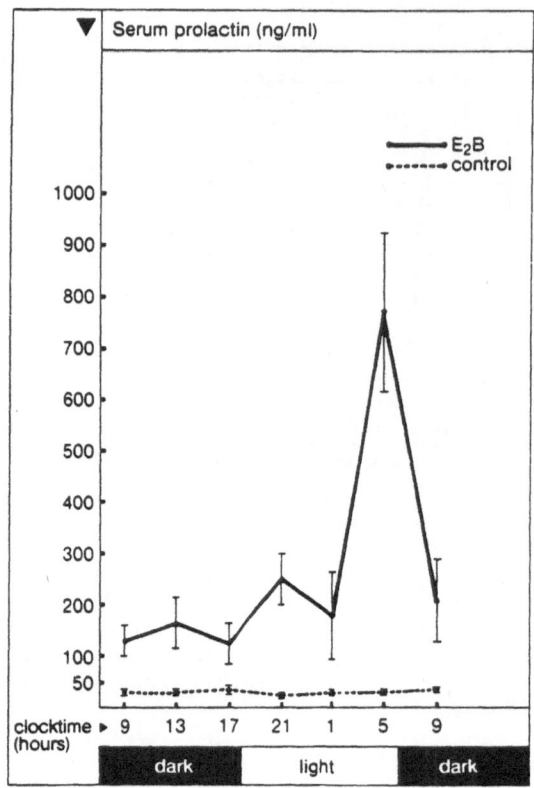

Figure 4: Circadian profile of prolactin (PRL) secretion in ovariectomized rats after a single injection of 25 µg/kg s.c. E_2B or sesame oil 2 days before decapitation. Fourteen days prior to decapitation the animals were housed at an inversed light-dark schedule with a 12 hour photo-period, light starting at 18:00 h (D/L). Each point is the mean ± S.E.M. (n = 10/group)

regulate prolactin rhythms in the rat; in addition, we have used this model in order to compare different ergot derivatives with known or suspected dopaminergic activity in their prolactin-lowering activity as we did in another test system (Gräf et al., 1976), where intact female rats had been pretreated with a low dose of reserpine (2 mg/kg i.p., 20-24 hours before test). As can be seen from the differences between Fig. 4a and 4b, there is the same order of potency in both groups with lisuride, bromocriptine and d-LSD being the most potent compounds; however, higher doses of ergots are necessary in the rats primed with estradiol to achieve a clear reduction of prolactin levels as compared with the reserpinized rats.

174

Whilst the dopamine depletion caused by reserpine may have produced some supersensitivity of dopamine receptors, the differences between both models are also in favour of our suggestion that the presence of estrogens can modulate the prolactin-lowering effects of ergot derivatives. This is not surprising since oestrogens have been shown for a long time to affect the activity and number of prolactin cells at the pituitary level.

Another system for studying CNS-gonadal interactions is the pronounced mounting behaviour caused by lisuride in rats. This behaviour can be induced by a single injection of 0.5 mg/kg lisuride subcutaneously to groups of rats without any pretreatment or specific conditions for observation, and it has been claimed that this unique phenomenon is due to the potent stimulation of dopamine receptors and, at the same time, a central functional antagonism of serotoninergic neurotransmission by this drug which is due to a preferential stimulation of presynaptic serotonin receptors by lisuride (Da Prada et al., 1977). In agreement with this, lisuride-induced mounting behaviour can be inhibited by dopamine antagonists as well as by serotonin agonists. It therefore could be used as a pharmacological screening test for the development of new and more specific serotonin agonists. In contrast to other effects of lisuride, the presence of endogeneous monoamines is a prerequisite for lisuride-induced mounting behaviour since pretreatment with reserpine and α-methyl-p-tyrosine reduces this behaviour, whereas it can be enhanced by MAO inhibitors and especially by d-amphetamine (see Table 1).

We as well as others have observed that lisuride-induced mounting behaviour strongly resembles effects which can be induced by prolonged treatment of young male rats with pCPA + a dopamine agonist, and also cannot be distinguished from normal male sexual behaviour in adult rats (Da Prada et al., 1977; Horowski and Wachtel, 1978; Benkert and Eversmann, 1972). Quite surprisingly, the same behaviour can be induced as well in juvenile female rats in a highly reproducible dose-dependent way, with maximal effects shown after a single dose of 0.5 mg/kg lisuride given s.c.

When this doses of lisuride is injected to groups of juvenile female rats kept in a normal acrylic glass rat cage, within the first minute some explorative and stereotyped behaviour – mainly consisting of licking – can be observed. This is followed rapidly by

Table 1: Influence of various neuropharmacological treatments on lisuride-induced mounting behaviour in juvenile female rats (weight 60-80 g, groups of 5, observation period 90 mins after simultaneous injection of test drug and lisuride 0.5 mg/kg s.c.):

Inhibition		Enhancement		No chance	
haloperidol	1 mg/kg i.p.	d-amphetamine	0.5 mg/kg i.p.	methysergide	1 mg/kg s.c.
sulpiride	50 mg/kg i.p.	nialamide	50 mg/kg i.p.	methergoline	1 mg/kg s.c.
reserpine	10 mg/kg i.p.		(2 hours before lisuride)	pCPA	100 mg/kg i.p.
	(20 hours before lisuride)				(over 3 days)
reserpine as above					
+ α-methyl-p-tyrosine	250 mg/kg i.p.				
	(2 1/2 hours before lisuride)				
d-LSD	0.5 mg/kg s.c.				
BOL 148	0.5 mg/kg s.c.				
5-HTP	10 mg/kg i.p.				
+ RO 4-4602	50 mg/kg i.p.				
	2 1/2 hours before lisuride)				

176

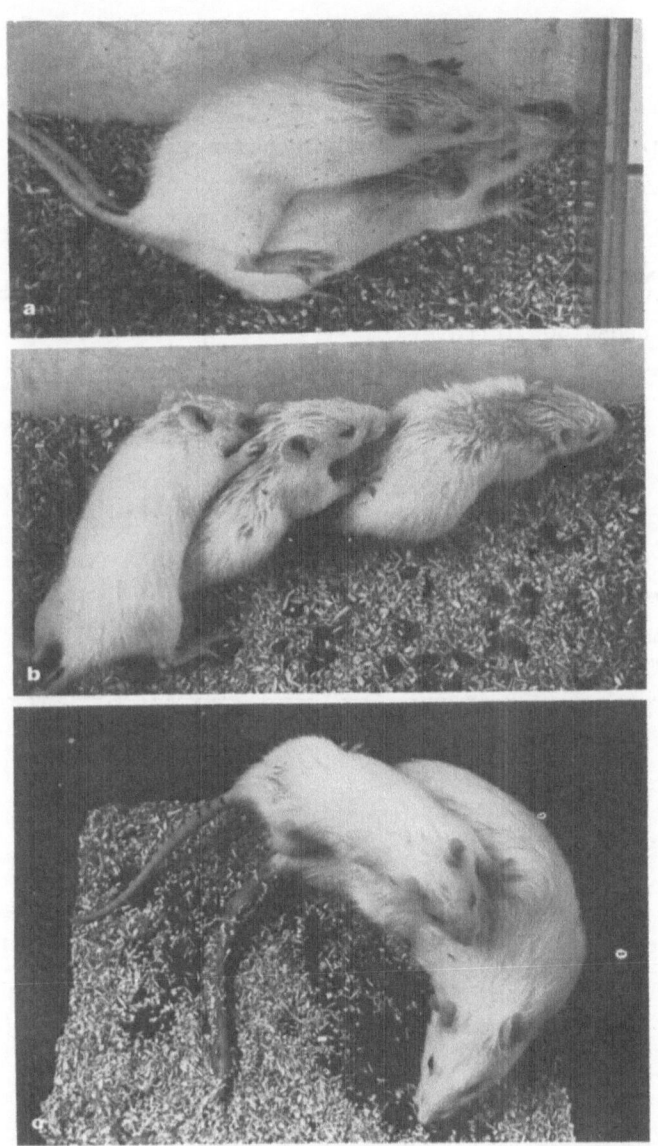

Figures 5a, 5b, and 5c: Mounting episodes in juvenile female rats
treated with lisuride 0.5   g/kg s.c.
Whilst in Fig. 5a and 5b all animals were female, in Fig. 5c a juvenile
female rat (weight 80 g) mounts an adult male (weight 350 g)

frequent mountings of 2 or more animals, a behaviour which lasts for
90 to 120 minutes.   About 200-300 mountings per group can be
observed with a maximal effect at 40-60 minutes after injection.

177

Mounting is often preceeded by genital sniffing or licking of the neck and is associated with forepaw spreading, ptosis, pinna adduction and sometimes pelvic thrushing movements (see Fig. 5). The animals also display piloerection and increased salivation. Rarely, offensive-defensive postures can be observed.

Table 2: Endocrine situations and manipulations which did not influence lisuride-induced mounting behaviour in rats:

---

male animals
prepuberal status
castration
castration and substitution with testosterone
testosterone treatment
treatment with cyproterone acetate
    prenatal treatment with cyproterone acetate
    postnatal treatment with androgens

---

female rats
prepuberal status
ovariectomy
ovariectomy and substitution with estradiol
testosterone treatment

As can be seen from this table, all these endocrine manipulations which are well-known to affect physiological sexual behaviour in rats had no influence on the mounting caused by treatment with lisuride

We used this particular behaviour as a tool for investigating the presence of central-nervous mechanisms related to sexuality and tested it in various endocrine conditions as shown in Table 2.

Indeed, the only situation in which the mounting-inducing effect of lisuride was clearly reduced, was increasing age (or weight) of the animals in both sexes, as can be seen from one experiment where female rats born at the same time were tested randomly at 2 week intervals with the standard dose of 0.5 mg/kg lisuride s.c.:

178

Whilst young females at an age of 3 weeks displayed no mountings at all, 2 weeks later already a full response (with 340 mountings over a period of 90 mins in a group of 5 animals) was observed. This high frequency was maintained at an age of 7 weeks (351 mountings) and then slowly declined to 269 (9 weeks), 259 (11 weeks), 122 (13 weeks), 60 (15 weeks), and 42 (17 weeks of age). A similar development could be seen with male animals, so that a body weight of $\leqslant 250$ g or an age of $\leqslant 12$ weeks seems to be important to obtain a full response.

Another interesting observation was that repeated treatment with lisuride greatly enhanced the mounting activity, and that also doses as low as 0.025 mg/kg s.c. which were completely inactive in the acute test caused a pronounced mounting activity after 2 weeks' treatment or longer (Horowski and Wachtel, 1978).

From these results it can be concluded that hormonal influences are very important for the expression of sexual behaviour under physiological conditions; however, the neuronal basis for male-type sexual behaviour in its complexity must be present in all animals, male or female, at least up to an age of about 12 weeks, and even before puberty. It seems that e.g. prenatal androgenic priming may be decisive for the way male sexual behaviour is expressed or not during adult life; however, the neuronal networks and monoamine receptors coordinating this behaviour do not disappear in female rats but can be activated by appropriate pharmacological stimulation, and then, the total male-type sequence of behavioural patterns is displayed in a well-coordinated form, however, highly independent on the sex of the partner.

That lisuride can produce the entire sequence of behavioural events also in the absence of the gonads has recently been demonstrated by Ahlenius and his co-workers (Ahlenius et al., 1980). In their studies, treatment with lisuride in castrated male rats not only restored mounting behaviour, but also intromission and ejaculation in a dose-dependent way and thereby permitted normal mating with receptive females.

Finally, the motor effects induced by dopaminergic ergot derivatives which seem to be mediated through an action within the nucleus accumbens, seem to differ quantitatively between male and female rats, when spontaneous motor activity is recorded using photocell motility cages (H. Wachtel, personal communication). Using a running-wheel, we could confirm the old observations that running-wheel activity is highly dependent on the ovarian cycle and greatly reduced by ovariectomy. Preliminary results suggest that effects of ergot derivatives on motor activity are influenced by the cycle situation and the test system used, and we therefore propose a further investigation of the motor activity influenced by these compounds as another test for studying CNS effects of estrogens. This is in agreement with recent observations from Silbergeld and Hruska that ^{3}H-spiroperidol binding within the CNS is influenced by estrogens.

In conclusion, our studies demonstrate various forms of the interaction between the CNS and hormones and the value of ergot derivatives as a tool to investigate this interaction. Whilst the importance of estrogens for the regulation of pituitary hormones such as prolactin is well-known, more work is needed for the elucidation of the influence of estrogens on motor activity in rats. Finally, lisuride-induced mounting behaviour is an example that even within the sexual field, central actions can be quite independent from the hormonal situation within the body.

Acknowledgements

We want to thank Mrs. C. Riedel and R. Zimmermann for their excellent technical assistence, and Mr. H. Bender in his most valuable help in preparing this manuscript.
We are indebted to the NIAMDD Pituitary Hormone Distribution Program, and to Prof. F. Neumann, Dr. K.J. Gräf and Dr. H. Wachtel for their helpful comments and assistance.

References

Ahlenius S, Larsson K, Svensson L (1980) Stimulating effects of lisuride on masculine sexual behaviour of rats. Eur J Pharmacol 64:47-51.
Benkert O, Eversmann T (1972) Importance of the antiserotonin effect for mounting behaviour in rats. Experientia 72:352.
Cote TH, Munemura M, Kebabian J (1979) Lisuride hydrogen maleate: An ergoline with β-adrenergic antagonist activity. Eur J Pharmacol 59:303-306.
Da Prada M, Bonetti EP, Keller HH (1977) Induction of mounting behaviour in female and male rats by lisuride. Neurosci L 6:349-353.

Dorow R, Neumann F, Horowski R (1980) Evidence for light-dependent prolactin secretion in estrogen-primed ovariectomized female rats. Acta Endocrinol (Kbh), submitted.

Fujita N, Saita K, Yonehara N, Yoshida H (1978) Lisuride inhibits ^{3}H-spiroperidol binding to membranes isolated from striatum. Neuropharmacology 17:1089-1091.

Fujita N, Saito K, Yonehara N, Watanabe Y, Yoshida H (1979) Binding of ^{3}H-lisuride hydrogen maleate to striatal membranes of rat brain. Life Sciences 25:969-974.

Gräf K-J, Neumann F, Horowski R (1976) Effect of the ergot derivative lisuride hydrogen maleate on serum prolactin concentrations in female rats. Endocrinology 98:598-605.

Gudelsky GA, Porter CJ (1979) Release of dopamine from tuberoinfundibular neurons into pituitary stalk blood after prolactin or haloperidol administration. Endocrinology 106:526-529.

Horowski R, Wachtel H (1976) Direct dopaminergic action of lisuride hydrogen maleate, an ergot derivative, in mice. Eur J Pharmacol 36:373-383.

Horowski R, Gräf K-J (1976) Influence of dopaminergic agonists and antagonists on serum prolactin concentration in the rat. Neuroendocrinology 22:273-286.

Horowski R, Wachtel H (1979) Pharmacological effects of lisuride in rodents mediated by dopaminergic receptors: Mechanism of action and influence of chronic treatment with lisuride. In: Fuxe K, Calne DB (eds) Dopaminergic ergot derivatives and motor function. Proceedings of an intern. symposium held in the Wenner Gren Center, Stockholm, July 24-25, 1978. Pergamon Press, Oxford and New York.

Hümpel M, Toda T, Oshino N, Pommerenke G (1981) The pharmacokinetics of lisuride hydrogen maleate in rat, rabbit and rhesus monkey. Eur J Pharmacology, submitted.

Kehr W (1977) Effect of lisuride and other ergot derivatives on monoaminergic mechanisms in rat brain. Eur J Pharmacol 41:261-273.

Pieri L, Keller HH, Burkhard W, da Prada M (1978) Effects of lisuride and LSD on cerebral monoamine systems and hallucinosis. Nature 272:278-280.

Rogawski MA, Aghajanian GK (1979) Response of central monoaminergic neurons to lisuride: comparison with LSD. Life Science 24:1289-1298.

Regulation of Prolactin Secretion at the Pituitary Level

M. Ruberg, A. Enjalbert, S. Arancibia and C. Kordon, Paris

Prolactin is a multifunctional hormone affecting a number of tissues. Best known for its role in lactation, it also affects reproduction, growth, metabolism and the central nervous system. Disfunctional regulation of the hormone is associated with several pathological conditions, such as galactorrhea, ammenorrhea, some mammary tumors, and certain behavioral disturbances. Prolactin secretion varies rhythmically both with the nyctemere and the estrous cycle. Acute increases in circulating prolactin levels occur during lactation and in response to stress. It can thus be supposed that prolactin secretion is subject to complex, probably multifactorial regulation.

Some elements of this regulation have been rather well documented; the participation of serotonin in the suckling reflex, for example, or the tonic inhibition of the prolactin cell by tuberoinfundibular dopamine (Review in Weiner, 1979).

Data has accumulated implicating a number of other substances endogenous to the hypothalamus in the regulation of prolactin secretion either within the central nervous system or at pituitary level. Among these are GABA, histamine, noradrenalin, met–enkephalin, β–endorphin, arginine vasotocin, neurotensin, substance P, vasoactive intestinal peptide, somatostatin, TRH, histydyl-proline-diketopiperazine. The effects of these substances are, in some cases, unconfirmed and their levels of action and the interactions among them far from clear.

The level of regulation most accessible to study is the pituitary where the inhibitory or stimulatory effects of suspected regulatory factors can be observed in isolation. The following

remarks will be addressed to the subject of pituitary level regulation of prolactin secretion other than that exerted by dopamine.

1. Non-dopaminergic Prolactin Inhibiting Factors

Experiments with hypothalamic extracts from which dopamine had
been eliminated by adsorption on alumine oxide have shown that
the mediobasal hypothalamus, unlike other dopamine containing
regions of the brain, retains prolactin inhibiting activity
(Enjalbert et al., 1977a,b). Much work has been done to identify
the factors responsible.

A. GABA

Schally and his collaborators isolated the amino acid GABA from a
fraction of hypothalamic extract having prolactin inhibiting activity, and demonstrated in vivo and in vitro that it was indeed
capable of inhibiting secretion of the hormone (Schally et al.,
1976, 1977). Inhibition in vitro was confirmed by Lamberts and
MacLeod (1978), but, because the GABA antagonist picrotoxin did
not block the effect of GABA in their in vitro experiments, the
inhibition was suspected to be non-specific. In vivo, these
authors reported that although the amino acid inhibited stimulated
release, it did not affect the basal activity of the prolactin cell.
Stimulation of prolactin secretion or both stimulation and inhibition
were reported by others (Mioduzewski et al., 1976; Ondo and Pass,
1976; Vijayan and McCann, 1978).

The dose-dependence of GABA inhibition of prolactin secretion
and its sensitivity to picrotoxin has since been demonstrated in
vitro (Enjalbert et al., 1979d). The results of these experiments
are presented in Figure 1. Maximum inhibition of about 30% was
obtained with a concentration of 10^{-5}M, the half maximal dose
being 10^{-6}M which may be considered on approximation of the
affinity of GABA for its recognition site on the prolactin cell. It
should be noted that GABA is 100 times less active than dopamine
in this respect, and its maximum effect is inferior.

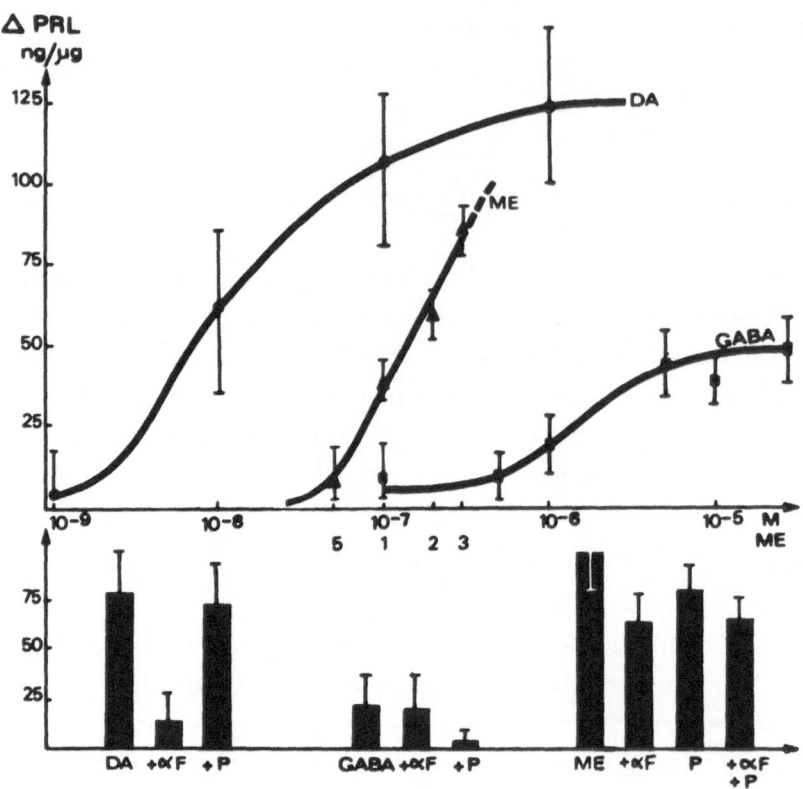

Figure 1: Inhibition of prolactin secretion from rat hemi-pituitaries by dopamine, GABA and extract of mediobasal hypothalamus containing the median eminence. Upper half: Dose response curve. Lower half: Effects of dopamine antagonist α-flupentixol (10^{-6}M) and GABA antagonist picrotoxin (10^{-5}M) on inhibition of prolactin secretion by dopamine (10^{-7}M), GABA (10^{-6}M) and extract (equivalent of 3 hypothalami). Experimental procedure: Paired control and experimental hemi-pituitaries from male Wistar rats were pre-incubated twice for 45 min then incubated for 1 hour in 1 ml of medium (pH 7.4) at 37°C in a shaking water bath under an atmosphere of O_2-CO_2 (95%-5%). Prolactin in the medium and in the tissue were assayed by RIA. Expression of Results: Effects on prolactin secretion were calculated as the difference between control and experimental half pituitaries (ΔPRL) according to the following formula:

$$\Delta\text{PRL} = \left[\frac{\text{PRL medium (ng)}}{\text{PRL tissue + medium (μg)}}\right]_{\text{control}} - \left[\frac{\text{PRL medium (ng)}}{\text{PRL tissue + medium (μg)}}\right]_{\text{exp.}}$$

Values represented are the mean $\pm$ SEM of 6 pituitaries

Maximum inhibition by GABA could be reversed by the presence of 10^{-5}M picrotoxin which alone had no effect on basal release. The pituitary dopamine receptor is not involved in GABA inhibition of prolactin release, as evidenced by the inability of the dopamine receptor antagonist α-flupentixol to block the effect. Picrotoxin is conversely inactive on the dopamine receptor.

These in vitro data have been confirmed by other groups using the GABA agonist muscimol and the antagonists picrotoxin and bicuculline (Grandison and Guidotti, 1979; Locatelli et al., 1979), and the presence of pituitary GABA binding sites with characteristics similar to those of the GABA receptor in brain demonstrated (Grandison and Guidotti, 1979). The independence of the GABA and dopamine receptors was also confirmed, and the effects of the two substances are additive at least when dopamine inhibition is submaximal.

In vivo, data reported by the above authors, however, indicate that while GABA can act peripherally to inhibit prolactin secretion, in the central nervous system it seems to facilitate release of the hormone.

Physiologically, it is not impossible that GABA intervenes both centrally and peripherally in the regulation of prolactin secretion since two hypothalamic GABA neuron systems have been described, one projecting to the mediobasal hypothalamus behind the pituitary stalk, the other from the mediobasal hypothalamus to the median eminence (Tappaz et al., 1977a,b). GABA found in the pituitary has been demonstrated to originate in the hypothalamus (Racagni et al., 1979), although it is not clear which of the two possible GABA-ergic structures is the source of the amino acid.

If GABA represents the non-dopaminergic prolactin-inhibiting activity detected in hypothalamic extracts, a combination of GABA and dopamine receptor antagonists should block all inhibitory activity of the extract on the pituitary. Figure 1 shows that this is not the case. While α-flupentixol reduced prolactin inhibition by an extract known to contain both dopamine and GABA by approximately 50%, picrotoxin had a lesser effect which was not statistically significant, and the effect of the two antagonists together did not differ from the effect of α-flupentixol alone. It is possible, as the results of Grandison and Guidotti (1979) suggest, that in the presence of maximal dopamine inhibition, the prolactin cell is less sensitive to GABA. In any case, another prolactin inhibiting factor is also present in the hypothalamus.

B. Histidylproline-diketopiperazine (DKP)

It has been found that histidylproline-diketopiperazine (DKP), formed by enzymatic degradation of thyreotropin releasing hormone (TRH) in both the hypothalamus and the pituitary, inhibits prolactin release (Bauer et al., 1978). Figure 2 shows the dose-dependence of its effect on incubated half-pituitaries (Enjalbert et al., 1979a). The apparent affinity of DKP for a putative receptor, deduced from the dose-response curve, in on the order of 10^{-9}M. This figure is comparable to the affinities of other peptide hormones for which a receptor has been identified; TRH, for example, stimulates prolactin secretion from GH_3 cells with a half-maximal effective dose in the low nanomolar range. Similar results were obtained with prolactin tumor cells of the GH_3 line in culture (Bauer et al., 1978).

The diketopiperazine acts independently of dopamine receptors, being unaffected by a variety of dopamine antagonists (Enjalbert et al., 1979a). Confirmation of the existence of a specific DKP receptor has not yet been obtained by direct binding studies, but the inability of two related dipeptides also derived from TRH (his-pro-OH and his-pro-NH$_2$) to inhibit prolactin secretion under the same conditions (Enjalbert et al., 1979a) provides preliminary evidence of the specificity of the effect. Also, DKP was shown to antagonize stimulation of prolactin secretion by TRH without affecting TSH, the primary target of the neurohormone both in vivo and in vitro (Bauer et al., 1978).

This suggests that the effect of DKP is specific to the prolactin cell and due to properties intrinsic to the molecule rather than to a structural homology with TRH.

Whether the active molecule originates in the hypothalamus or the pituitary has yet to be determined.

C. Others

At the present time, dopamine, GABA and DKP are the only prolactin-inhibiting factors supported by a substantial body of evidence.

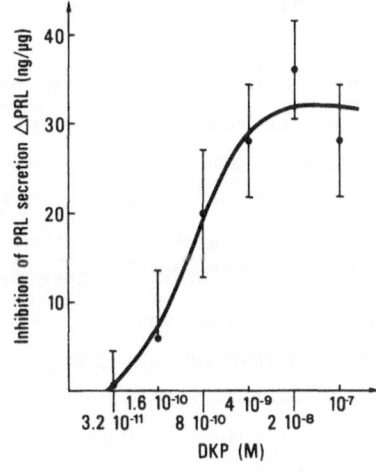

Figure 2: Inhibition of prolactin secretion from rat hemi-pituitaries by increasing concentrations of histidylproline-diketopiperazine (DKP). Δ PRL: see Figure 1

Somatostatin has also been reported to inhibit prolactin secretion at the pituitary level (Vale et al., 1974), but others have not been able to confirm this result.

2. Prolactin Stimulating Factors

As far as prolactin-stimulating factors are concerned, TRH has been demonstrated to stimulate release of the hormone from GH_3 cells (Tashjian et al., 1971; Gourdjil et al., 1966), dissociated pituitary cells (Nakano et al., 1976) and whole pituitaries (Mueller et al., 1973), and in vivo under particular physiological conditions (Blake et al., 1974; Noel et al., 1974), but prolactin stimulating activity distinct from TRH has also been detected in hypothalamic extracts (Valverde et al., 1972; Rivier and Vale, 1974; Boyd et al., 1976).

A. Morphine and Endogenous Opiate Peptides

Morphine and the morphinomimetic peptides met-enkephalin and β-endorphin have been observed to increase serum prolactin levels both clinically and in animal experiments (Bruni et al., 1977; Rivier et al., 1977; Shaar et al., 1977; Dupont et al., 1977; Cocchi et al., 1977; Grandison and Guidotti, 1977; Kato et al., 1978), although in vitro on pituitary preparations they were ineffective. It was con-

187

cluded that these substances act in the central nervous system to stimulate secretion of a PRF or inhibit a PIF.

In fact, these substances do act at the pituitary level, not to stimulate prolactin release directly, but to counteract dopamine inhibition (Enjalbert et al., 1979b,c). Figure 3 shows that while morphine and the endogenous opiates indeed have no effect by themselves, in the presence of dopamine they reversed its action, restoring hormone secretion. When the pituitary opiate receptors were blocked by naloxone, dopamine inhibition reappeared. The effect of naloxone is dose-dependent. These substances act then as indirect prolactin-releasing factors. The dose-response curve for met-enkephalin is reproduced in Figure 4. The peptide is maximally active at 10^{-6}M with an apparent affinity calculated to be about 4×10^{-8}, and exhibits simple non cooperative kinetics.

These experiments demonstrate indirectly that the prolactin cell possesses a functional opiate receptor. Direct evidence for the existence of this receptor in the pituitary and the absence of cross-recognition of opiates by the DA receptor have been provided by binding studies (Simantov and Snyder, 1977; Caron et al., 1978; Meltzer and So, 1979). Although the effect of morphine and the peptides is to block dopaminergic inhibition of prolactin secretion, the dopamine and opiate receptors are independent entities. The mechanism of their interaction, however, has not yet been elucidated. Neither is it known, under physiological conditions, which opioid

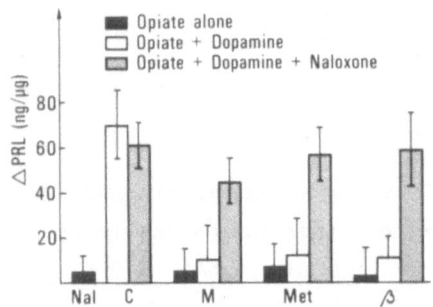

Figure 3: Effects of morphine, met-enkephalin and β-endorphin on basal and dopamine-inhibited prolactin secretion from rat hemi-pituitaries. Inhibition by naloxone of the effect of the opiates.

C: Control; M = Morphine (10^{-6}M); Met: Met-enkephalin (10^{-6}M); β-Endorphin (5×10^{-7}M); Nal: Naloxone (10^{-6}M). ΔPRL: see Figure 1

188

peptide intervenes in the regulation of prolactin secretion, met-enkephalin or β-endorphin of hypothalamic origin (Bloom et al., 1978) or β-endorphin secreted by pituitary ACTH producing cells (Bloom et al., 1977; Akil et al., 1978). A dual regulation at both hypophysial and hypothalmic levels cannot be excluded since met-enkephalin has been observed to decrease dopamine secretion in the hypothalamus concomitant with an increase in prolactin release (Ferland et al., 1977).

Login and MacLeod (1979) reported that they were unable to reproduce these results using morphine, met-enkephalin and its non-degradable analogue D-Ala-met-enkephalin at a concentration of 1.3×10^{-5}M againt 5×10^{-8}M dopamine. The incubations lasted 5 hours in these experiments during which unprotected met-enkephalin would have been degraded (bacitracin, a peptidase inhibitor, was included in the incubation medium in the experiments described

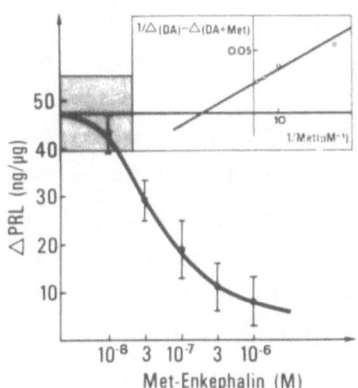

Figure 4:   Effect of increasing concentrations of met-enkephalin on the inhibition of prolactin secretion from rat hemi-pituitaries by dopamine (10^{-7} M). Shaded area: Inhibition of prolactin secretion by 10^{-7} M dopamine (mean ± SEM). Inset: Lineweaver-Burke double reciprocal plot of the dose-response curve.

$$\frac{I}{\Delta DA - \Delta(DA-MET)} = \frac{K}{\left[\Delta DA - \Delta(DA-MET)\right]_{max}} \times \frac{I}{[MET]} + \frac{I}{\left[\Delta DA - \Delta(DA-MET)\right]_{max}}$$

ΔPRL: see Figure 1

189

B. Vasoactive Intestinal Peptide

Direct stimulation of prolactin release has been observed in the case of vasoactive intestinal peptide (VIP) (Ruberg et al., 1978; Enjalbert et al., 1980). This peptide, originally isolated from the intestine, is also found in brain (Besson et al., 1979) and has been detected in portal blood (Saïd and Porter, 1978). The dose-response curve for VIP stimulation of prolactin secretion is presented in Figure 5. The effective concentrations of the peptide, reaching a maximum at 10^{-7}M, are not incompatible with an action on a specific receptor, although pharmacological characterization has not yet been possible. It has been possible, however, to demonstrate the independence of VIP's mechanism of action from that of dopamine. As the experiment presented in Figure 6 shows, dopamine alone inhibited prolactin secretion by 49% whereas VIP increased release by 14%. The effects of the two substances were additive resulting in a net inhibition of 28%. In the presence of the dopamine antagonist α-flupentixol, dopamine inhibition was blocked unmasking the stimulatory effect of VIP which was 22% above control secretion. VIP stimulation of prolactin secretion is also additive with that of TRH (Enjalbert et al., 1980) as is shown in Figure 7. These data strongly suggest the presence of a specific VIP receptor in the pituitary. Binding studies have been performed in the central nervous system where the related peptide secretin acts as a partial agonist and glucagon not at all (Robberecht et al., 1978). The effects of these two peptides on VIP stimulated prolactin secretion from the pituitary parallel their effects on the hypothalamic VIP receptor.

Vijayan et al. (1979), who have studied the effect of VIP on prolactin secretion both in vivo and in vitro, concluded it acts in the hypothalamus rather than in the pituitary. They were able to stimulate prolactin secretion by both peripheral and intraventricular injection of the peptide, the latter only with high concentrations, the former with only the intermediate concentrations among those tested. In vitro, VIP had no effect under their experimental conditions. A possible explanation of this failure is the length of their incubation period (2.5 hours). In vitro, once secretion

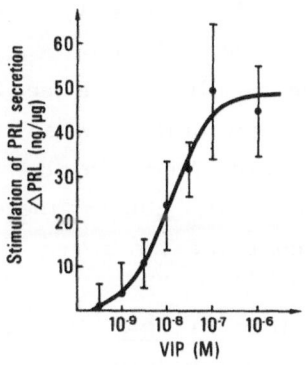

Figure 5: Stimulation of prolactin secretion from half-pituitaries by increasing concentration of vasoactive intestinal peptide (VIP). Δ PRL: see Figure 1

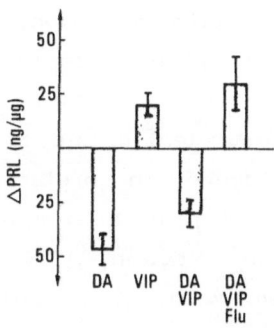

Figure 6: Inhibition by domine and stimulation by VIP of prolactin secretion from rat hemi-pituitaries are independent and additive processes. DA: Dopamine (10^{-7} M); VIP: Vasoactive intestinal peptide (10^{-7}M); Flu: α flupentixol, dopamine antagonist (10^{-6}M); C: Control. Δ PRL: see Figure 1

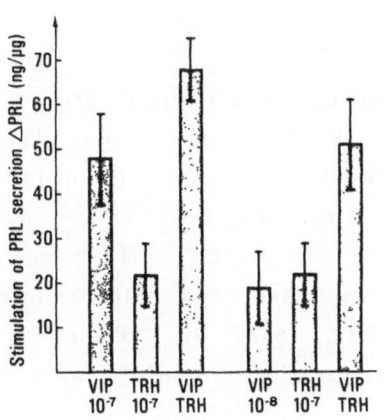

Figure 7: Stimulation of prolactin secretion from rat hemi-pituitaries by TRH and VIP are independent and additive processes

191

stabilizes, accumulation of prolactin in the incubation medium under uninhibited secretion conditions is linear for approximately two hours provided that the medium is changed every 30 minutes. Otherwise, feedback inhibition occurs with the result that after 2 hours prolactin in the medium represents less than half of what it would have been if linear secretion had been maintained (Enjalbert et al., unpublished results). It may be that, under these conditions, the release stimulus could not overcome the inhibition by prolactin of its own secretion.

Kato and his collaborators, who also obtained in vivo stimulation of prolactin by VIP, showed that L-DOPA and naloxone block the effect of the peptide. Both of these drugs increase dopamine inhibition, the former by increasing the amount of dopamine available, the latter by antagonizing enkephalin or endorphin suppression of dopamine inhibition (see above), thereby masking though not necessarily antagonizing VIP stimulation of prolactin secretion, a result which is compatible with the in vitro experiment described above.

Along with VIP and the opioid peptides, neurotensin had also been implicated by a growing body of evidence in prolactin regulation at the pituitary level where it seems to play a stimulatory role (Maeda and Frohman, 1978; Vijayan and McCann, 1979). It may also act in the central nervous system with an opposing inhibitory action. These data require confirmation in that stimulation in vitro was not dose-related in the case of Vijayan and MacCann, and Maeda and Frohman were unable to obtain stimulation of prolactin release from a dispersed cell preparation.

C. Others

Lastly, substance P has also been observed to stimulate prolactin release at pituitary level (Kato et al., 1976; Rivier et al., 1977; Vijayan and McCann, 1979), although others have not been able to reproduce these results (Maeda and Frohman, 1978; Enjalbert et al., unpublished results). Since substance P containing cells are not located in the over layer of the median eminence, but rather in the interior of the structure (Elde and Hökfelt, 1978) the role of this peptide in pituitary level prolactin regulation remains open to question.

3. Conclusion

In summary, serious evidence implicates dopamine, GABA, DKP, met-enkephalin and/or β-endorphin, VIP and neurotensin in pituitary level prolactin regulation. In all cases, transport of these substances from the hypothalamus to the pituitary is possible, and has been demonstrated in the case of dopamine, GABA and VIP. Alternatively, in situ pituitary sources of β-endorphin and DKP are known to exist. Also, recognition sites for dopamine, GABA and the morphinomimetic peptides have been identified in the pituitary and characterized. If DKP and VIP receptors have not been directly demonstrated, the dose-dependence of other actions and their effective concentrations strongly suggest the presence of specific recognition sites.

It remains to demonstrate their localization on the prolactin cell itself. Hormone specificity is, of course, good presumptive evidence. Several of these substances seem to act both peripherally and centrally to affect prolactin secretion. They also affect other hormones as well.

If appropriate physiological localization and the existence of specific receptor-effector mechanisms on the prolactin cell are necessary conditions defining regulatory factors, they are not sufficient to prove their participation in physiological regulation.

It is perhaps not superfluous to emphasize the difficulties encountered in studying the regulation of prolactin secretion with respect both to experimental design and the evaluation and comparison of results. Experimental conditions in which basal prolactin release is depressed by ovariectomy or increased by the administration of steroid hormones influence the effects of regulatory substances.

In vivo, peripheral injection can affect both the pituitary itself as well as the central nervous system; local injection in the CNS may or may not affect the periphery. Feedback regulation may transfer effects on one hormone to another (the relation between the gonadotropins and prolactin is a case in point). When interactions between regulatory factors are studied, especially if only the prolactin secreted is monitored, opposed but physiologically unrelated mechanisms may annul one another.

In vitro, incubation conditions, particularly the absence of

193

modulatory agents and the kinetics of spontaneous prolactin release, affect the results observed. Receptor binding kinetics also impose constraints.

Lastly, the effects of all other putative regulatory mechanisms must be considered in view of the tonic inhibition of prolactin secretion by dopamine under physiological conditions, either because they affect dopamine regulation (secretion of the catecholamine, its recognition by the prolactin cell or transduction of its "message"), because they act concomitantly with the amine adding to or decreasing its effect, or because simultaneous changes occur in dopaminergic regulation at the same time that other regulatory mechanisms are put into play.

Even without approaching the question of prolactin regulation within the central nervous system, that is to say the afferent pathways controlling the release of the putative neurohormones discussed above, regulation of prolactin secretion involves complicated interactions at the level of the prolactin cell itself. It has been seen that a number of substances act through independent receptors to affect the secretory activity of the cell.

It must be asked whether, under physiological conditions, these substances·act individually or in combination and whether a common intracellular effector or different mechanisms are activated by the various receptors present on the cell.

Given the tonic effect of dopamine, integration of multiple input by the mammotrophe must be envisaged. The interactions between dopamine and opiates, the additive effects of VIP and TRH and the opposing effects of VIP and DA described above indicate that this question is not gratuitous.

Data concerning this subject are as yet very fragmentary. Although prolactin secretion is an excytotic process, present knowledge of this process consists mainly of a phenomenological description, the underlying chemistry is largely unknown.

Research on the control of ions channels or "second messengers", the cyclic nucleotides for example, has, in the case of the prolactin cell, hardly begun.

Prolactin secretion is calcium-dependent, but unlike other endocrine cells, high potassium concentrations do not seem to enhance secretion.

194

The dopamine receptor has been said to be of the D_2 type (Schmidt and Hill, 1977; Kebakian and Calne, 1979) – not linked to an adenylate cyclase – but this is not certain. Dopamine has been reported both to stimulate cyclic AMP formation in the pituitary (Ahn et al., 1979) and to inhibit the adenylate cyclase in a prolactin secreting adenoma (De Camilli et al., 1979). In vivo, both Ojeda et al. (1974) and MacLeod (1976) report inhibition of prolactin secretion with dibutyril-cyclic AMP. Both TRH (Dannies et al., 1974) and VIP (Gourdji et al., 1979), on the other hand, do seem to stimulate cyclic AMP production, at least in GH_3 cells. It has been noted that depletion of GABA in the central nervous system causes accumulation of cyclic AMP in the pituitary, an effect which is blocked by the GABA agonist muscimol (Grandison and Guidotti, 1979). GABA may then exert an inhibitory control on TRH or VIP secreting cells.

All these questions concerning the intracellular mechanisms of prolactin secretion, of the utmost interest, await the development of a suitable research model. Isolated normal prolactin cells in sufficient number with reproducible behavior will undoubtedly provide the appropriate material with which to study the problem of cellular integration of multiple input, essential for understanding the regulation of prolactin secretion, but also a means by which to penetrate the mysteries of all secretory cells, glandular or neuronal.

References

Ahn HS, Gardner E, Makman MH (1979) Anterior pituitary adenylate cyclase: Stimulation by dopamine and other monoamines. Eur J Pharmacol 53(3):313–317.
Akil H, Watson S, Berger PA, Barchas JD (1978) Endorphins, β-LPH, and ACTH: Biochemical pharmacological and anatomical aspects. In: Costa A, Trabucchi M (eds) Advances in biochemical psychopharmacology. Raven Press, New York, pp.125–139.
Bauer K, Gräf KJ, Faivre-Bauman A, Beier S, Tixier-Vidal A, Kleinkauf H (1978) Inhibition of prolactin secretion by histidylproline-diketopiperazine. Nature 274:174–175.
Besson J, Rotsztejn W, Laburthe M, Epelbaum J, Beaudet A, Kordon C, Rosselin G (1979) Vasoactive intestinal peptide (VIP): Brain distribution, subcellular localization and effect of de-afferentation of the hypothalamus in male rats. Brain Res. 165:79–85.

Blake CA (1974) Stimulation of pituitary prolactin and TSH nerve release in lactating and proestrous rats. Endocrinology 94:503-508.

Bloom F, Battenberg E, Rossier J, Hing N, Guillemin R (1978) Neurons containing β-endorphin in rat brain exist separately from those containing enkephalin. Immunological studies. Proc Soc Natl Acad Sci (USA) 75:1591-1595.

Bloom F, Battenberg E, Rossier J, Ling N, Leppaluoto J, Vargo TM, Guillemin R (1977) Endorphins are located in the intermediate and anterior lobes of the pituitary gland, not in the neurohypophysis. Life Sci 20:43-48.

Boyd AE, Spencer E, Jackson I, Reichlin S (1976) Prolactin-releasing factor (PRF) in porcine hypothalamic extract distinct from TRH. Endocrinology 99:861-871.

Bruni J, Van Vugt D, Marshall S, Meites J (1977) Effects of naloxone, morphine and methionine enkephalin on serum prolactin, luteinizing hormone, follicle stimulating hormone, thyroid stimulating hormone. Life Sci 21:461-466.

Caron MG, Beaulieu M, Raymond V, Gagné B, Drouin J, Lefkowitz R, Labrie F (1978) Dopaminergic receptors in the anterior pituitary gland. J Biol Chem 253:2244-2253.

Cocchi D, Santogostino A, Gil-Ad I, Ferri S, Mueller E (1977) Leu-enkephalin stimulated growth hormone and prolactin release in the rat: Comparison with the effect of morphine. Life Sci 20:2041-2046.

Dannies PS, Gautvik KM, Tashjian AH (1976) A possible role of cyclic AMP in mediating the effects of thyrotropin-releasing hormone on prolactin release and on prolactin and growth hormone synthesis in pituitary cells in culture. Endocrinology 98:1147-1159.

De Camilli P, Macconi D, Spada A (1979) Dopamine inhibits adenylate cyclase in human prolactin-secreting pituitary adenomas. Nature 278:252-254.

Dupont A, Cusan L, Labrie F, Coy DH, Choh HL (1977) Stimulation of prolactin release in the rat by intraventricular injection of β-endorphin and met-enkephalin. Biochem Biophys Res Commun 75:76-82.

Elde R, Hökfelt T (1978) Distribution of hypothalamic hormones and other peptides in the brain. In: Ganong WF, Martini L (eds) Frontiers in Neuroendocrinology, Raven Press, New York, Vol. 5.

Enjalbert A, Arancibia S, Ruberg M, Priam M, Bluet-Pajot MT, Briaud B, Rotsztejn WH, Kordon C (1980) Stimulation of in vitro prolactin release by vasoactive intestinal peptide (VIP). Neuroendocrinology in press.

Enjalbert A, Moos F, Carbonell L, Priam M, Kordon C (1977a) Prolactin inhibiting activity of dopamine free subcellular fractions from rat mediobasal hypothalamus. Neuroendocrinology 24:147-161.

Enjalbert A, Priam M, Kordon C (1977b) Evidence in favor of the existence of a dopamine free prolactin inhibiting factor (PIF) in rat hypothalamic extracts. Eur J Pharmacol 41:243-244.

Enjalbert A, Ruberg M, Arancibia S, Priam M, Bauer K, Kordon C (1979a) Inhibition of in vitro prolactin secretion by histidyl-proline-diketopiperazine, a degradation product of TRH. Eur J Pharmacol 58:97-98.

Enjalbert A, Ruberg M, Arancibia S, Priam M, Kordon C (1979b) Endogenous opiates block dopamine inhibition of prolactin secretion in vitro. Nature 280:595-597.

Enjalbert A, Ruberg M, Fiore L, Arancibia S, Priam M, Kordon C (1979c) Effect of morphine on the dopamine inhibition of pituitary prolactin release in vitro. Eur J Pharmacol 53: 211-212.

Enjalbert A, Ruberg M, Fiore L, Arancibia S, Priam M, Kordon C (1979d) Independent inhibition of prolactin secretion by dopamine and gamma-aminobutyric acid in vitro. Endocrinology 105:823–826.

Ferland F, Fuxe K, Eneroth P, Gustafson JA, Skett P (1977) Effects of methionine-enekephalin on prolactin release and catecholamine levels and turnover in the median eminence. Eur J Pharmacol 43:89–90.

Gourdji D, Kerdelhue B, Tixier-Vidal A (1966) Mise en évidence d'un clone de cellules hypophysaires sécrétant de la prolactine (GH$_3$): Modification induite par l'hormone de libération de l'hormone thyrotrope (TRF). C R Acad Sci (Paris) 274:437.

Gourdji D, Bataille D, Vauclin N, Groucelle D, Rosselin G, Tixier-Vidal A (1979) Vasoactive intestinal peptide (VIP) stimulates prolactin release and cAMP production in a rat pituitary cell line (GH$_3$/B6). Additive effects of VIP and TRH on PRL relase. FEBS Lett 104:165–168.

Grandison L, Guidotti A (1979) γ-Aminobutyric acid receptor function in rat anterior: Evidence for control of prolactin release. Endocrinology 105:754–759.

Kato Y, Chihara K, Ohgo S, Iwasaki Y, Abe H, Imura H (1976) Growth hormone and prolactin release by substance P in rats. Life Sci 19:441–446.

Kato Y, Iwasaki J, Abe H, Yanaihara N, Imura H (1978) Prolactin release by vasoactive intestinal polypeptide in rats. Endocrinology 103:554–558.

Kebabian JW, Calne DB (1979) Multiple receptors for dopamine. Nature 277:93–96.

Lamberts SWJ, MacLeod RM (1978) Studies on the mechanisms of the GABA mediated inhibition of prolactin secretion. Proc Soc Exp Biol Med 158:10–13.

Locatelli V, Cocchi D, Frigerio C, Betti R, Krogsgaard-Larsen P, Racagni G, Müller EE (1979) Dual γ-aminobutyric acid control of prolactin secretion in the rat. Endocrinology 105:778–785.

Login IS, MacLeod RM (1979) Effects of opiates and DA and PRL secretion. Eur J Pharmacol 60:253–255.

MacLeod RM (1976) Regulation of prolactin secretion. In: Martini L, Ganong WF (eds) Frontiers in Neuroendocrinology. Raven Press, New York, Vol IV, pp.169–197.

MacLeod RM, Robyn C (1977) Mechanism of increased prolactin secretion by sulpiride. J Endocr 72:273–277.

Maeda K, Frohman LA (1978) Dissociation of systemic and central effects of neurotensin on the secretion of growth hormone, prolactin and thyrotropin. Endocrinology 103:1903–1909.

Meltzer HY, So R (1979) Effect of morphine, γ-endorphin and leu-enkephalin on ^{3}H-spiropiridal binding to bovine pituitary membranes. Life Sci 25:531–536.

Mioduzewski R, Grandison L, Meites J (1976) Stimulation of prolactin release in rats by GABA. Proc Soc Exp Biol Med 151:44–46.

Mueller GP, Chen HJ, Meites J (1973) In vivo stimulation of prolactin release in the rat by synthetic TRH. Proc Soc Exp Biol Med 144:613–615.

Nakano H, Fawcett CP, McCann SM (1976) Enzymatic dissociation and short term culture of isolated rat anterior pituitary cells for studies on the control of hormone secretion. Endocrinology 98:278–288.

Noel GL, Dimond RC, Wartofsky L, Earll JM, Frantz AG (1974) Studies of prolactin and FSH secretion by continuous infusion of small amounts of thyrotropin-releasing hormone (TRH). J Clin Endocrinol Metab 39:6-17.

Ojeda SR, Harms PG, McCann SM (1974) Possible role of cyclic AMP and prostaglandin E1 on the dopaminergic control of prolactin release. Endocrinology 95:1694-1703.

Ondo JG, Pass KA (1976) The effects of neurally active amino acids on prolactin secretion. Endocrinology 98:1248-1252.

Racagni G, Apud JA, Locatelli V, Cocchi D, Nistico G, Di Giorgio RM, Müller EE (1979) GABA of CNS origin in the rat anterior pituitary inhibits prolactin secretion. Nature 281:575-578.

Rivier C, Brown M, Vale W (1977) Effect of neurotensin, substance P and morphine sulfate on the secretion of prolactin and growth hormone in the rat. Endocrinology 100: 751-754.

Rivier C, Vale W (1974) In vivo stimulation of prolactin secretion in the rat by thyrotropin releasing factor, related peptides and hypothalamic extracts. Endocrinology 95:978-983.

Rivier C, Vale W, Ling N, Brown M, Guillemin R (1977) Stimulation in vivo of the secretion of prolactin and growth hormone by β-endorphin. Endocrinology 100:238-241.

Robberecht P, De Neef P, Lammens M, Deschodt-Lanckman M, Christophe JP (1978) Specific binding of vasoactive intestinal peptide to brain membranes from the guinea pig. Eur J Biochem 90:147-154.

Ruberg M, Rotsztejn WH, Arancibia S, Besson J, Enjalberg A (1978) Stimulation of prolactin release by vasoactive intestinal peptide (VIP). Eur J Pharmacol 51:319-320.

Saïd SI, Porter JC (1979) Vasoactive intestinal peptide: release into hypophyseal portal blood. Life Sci 24:227-230.

Schally AV, Dupont A, Arimura A, Takamara J, Redding TW, Shaar C (1976) Purification of a catecholamine-rich fraction with prolactin-release inhibiting factor (PIF) activity from porcine hypothalami. Acta Endocrinol 82:1-14.

Schally AV, Redding TW, Arimura A, Dupont A, Linthicum G (1977) Isolation of gamma-aminobutyric acid from pig hypothalami and demonstration of its prolactin release-inhibiting activity in vivo and in vitro. Endocrinology 100:681-691.

Schmidt MJ, Hill LE (1977) Effects of ergots on adenylate cyclase activity in the corpus striatum and pituitary. Life Sci 20:789-798.

Shaar CJ, Frederickson RCA, Dininger NB, Jackson L (1977) Enkephalin analogues and naloxone modulate the release of growth hormone and prolactin-evidence for regulation by an endogenous opioid peptide in brain. Life Sci 21:833-860.

Simantov R, Snyder S (1977) Opiate receptor binding in the pituitary gland. Brain Res. 127:178-184.

Tashjian AH, Barousky NJ, Jensen DK (1971) Thyrotropin releasing hormone: Direct evidence for stimulation of prolactin production by pituitary cells in culture. Biochem Biophys Res Commun 43:516-522.

Tappaz ML, Brownstein MJ, Kopin IJ (1977) Glutamate decarboxylase (GAD) and gamma-aminobutyric acid (GABA) in discrete nuclei of hypothalamus and substantia nigra. Brain Res. 125:109-121.

Vale W, Rivier C, Brazeau P, Guillemin R (1974) Effects of somatostatin on the secretion of thyrotropin and prolactin. Endocrinology 95:968-977.

Valverde RC, Chieffo V, Reichlin S (1972) Prolactin releasing factor in porcine and rat hypothalamic tissue. Endocrinology 91:982-992.

Vijayan E, McCann SM (1979) In vivo and in vitro effects of substance P and neurotensin on gonadotropin and prolactin release. Endocrinology 105:64-68.

Vijayan E, Samson WK, Saïd SI, McCann SM (1979) Vasoactive intestinal peptide: Evidence for a hypothalamic site of action to release growth hormone, luteinizing hormone and prolactin in conscious ovariectomized rats. Endocrinology 104:53–57.

Weiner RI, Ganong WF (1978) Role of Brain monoamines and histamine in regulation of anterior pituitary secretion. Physiol Rev 58(4):905–976.

The Role of the Central Nervous System in the Control of the Menstrual Cycle of the Rhesus Monkey

E. Knobil, Pittsburgh

The time of course of the circulating gonadotropic hormones (LH and FSH) during the menstrual cycle may be viewed as being the resultant of basal secretion interrupted, once every 28 days or so, by an abrupt discharge of these pituitary hormones, the preovulatory gonadotropin surge, that eventuates in ovulation approximately 36 h later. These secretory patterns appear to be governed by a seemingly simple control system composed of three major components: the hypothalamus, the adenohypophysis and the ovary (Knobil, 1974). The basal secretion of both LH and FSH is controlled by a classical negative feedback loop wherein ovarian estradiol-17β is the primary gonadal component. Estrogen secretion and follicular development proceed in response to basal gonadotropin secretion during the follicular phase of the menstrual cycle until serum estradiol concentrations exceed a threshold of approximately 200 pg/ml for 36 h or more. When the latter is achieved, a stimulatory or positive feedback action of estrogen on gonadotropin secretion comes into effect resulting in initiation of the preovulatory discharge of FSH and LH.

That the neural components of this control system are resident entirely within the medial basal hypothalamus (MBH) is suggested by experiments in which the hypothalamic isolation technique, devised by Halasz and co-workers for the rat (Halasz and Pupp, 1965; Halasz and Gorski, 1967), was applied to the rhesus monkey (Krey et al., 1975a). The completeness of the surgical disconnections of the MBH in female rhesus monkeys was evidenced by microscopic examination of the lesions and by various physiological criteria (Krey et al., 1975a; Krey et al., 1975b; Butler et al., 1975). The MBH "islands" produced in these animals included the median eminence and arcuate nuclei, and portions of the ventromedial nuclei and of the mammillary bodies. The preoptic area as well as the suprachiasmatic and supraoptic nuclei were excluded by the cuts. Basal FSH and LH levels were not severely altered in either intact or ovariectomized animals subjected to this procedure and the circhoral, pulsatile gonadotropin discharges characteristic of gonadectomized monkeys (Dierschke et al., 1970) remained fully evident (Krey et al., 1975a). In addition, the negative feedback inhibition of gonadotropin secretion by estradiol was easily demonstrable in these monkeys (Krey et al., 1975a). Moreover, the administration of estradiol benzoate to monkeys subjected to either complete or anterior surgical disconnection of the MBH induced gonadotropin surges indistinguishable from those produced in non-lesioned animals and, in some of the deafferented animals, normal spontaneous ovulatory menstrual cycles were observed (Krey et al., 1975a). These findings differ from those in the rat, wherein either complete or anterior deafferentation of the MBH interrupts the ovarian cycle by interfering with the preovulatory discharge of the gonadotropins. This latter species require connections from the preoptic-anterior hypothalamic area to the MBH for the transmission of a neural signal, coupled to the diurnal light-dark cycle, which initiates the preovulatory gonadotropin surge on the afternoon of proestrus (see Barraclough, 1973). This seemingly fundamental difference between the effects of MBH deafferentation in the monkey and in the rat, coupled with the report of Norman et al. (1976) that lesions in the preoptic-anterior hypothalamic area abolish the stimulatory action of estrogen on gonadotropin secretion in the rhesus monkey, raised the possibility that the surgical isolation of the monkey MBH described by Krey et al. (1975a) may not have been functionally complete. Nerve regeneration not demonstrable by ordinary histological techniques could not be ruled out nor could the transport of a neurotransmitter, or GnRH itself, to the disconnected MBH either by diffusion across the surgical scar or by way of the cerebrospinal fluid. The relatively high concentrations of GnRH reported in the region of the organum vasculosum of the lamina terminalis in the rhesus monkey (Neill et al., 1976) was of particular concern in this regard. We therefore directly addressed these possibilities by aspirating all neural tissue anterior and dorsal to the optic chiasm (Hess, 1977). Removal of the lamina terminalis, preoptic area and anterior hypothalamus and of the suprachiasmatic, as well as portions of the paraventricular, dorsal medial and ventral medial nuclei did not interfere with estrogen induced discharges of LH and FSH which were similar to those observed in animals with intact nervous systems following estradiol benzoate administration. Furthermore, we have since been unable to confirm the original report of Norman et al. (1976) that lesions in the rostral hypothalamus of the rhesus monkey block the stimulatory action of estradiol on gonadotropin release (Plant et al., 1979).

It may be concluded from the foregoing that, in the rhesus monkey, the central components of the control system which governs the basal mode of gonadotropin secretion, as well as the preovulatory surge of FSH and LH is resident within the MBH-hypophysial apparatus. The conclusion that the monkey, unlike the rat, does not require a signal from the preoptic-anterior hypothalamic area for the initiation of the preovulatory gonadotropin surge is consonant with the findings that such surges, whether spontaneous (Weick et al., 1973) or induced (Karsch et al., 1973b), are not coupled to the diurnal light-dark cycle and that neuroactive drugs such as pento-barbital, reserpine or phenoxybenzamine, which block the diurnal neural signal required for ovulation in the rat (Sawyer, 1969), have no effect on estrogen induced gonadotropin surges in the rhesus monkey (Knobil, 1974). Similarly, adult male rhesus monkeys can respond to the stimulatory action of estradiol with an LH surge (Karsch et al., 1973a), whereas similarly treated male rats, in which neonatal androgens have presumably abolished the transmision of the diurnal signal from the anterior hypothalamus to the MBH (Barraclough, 1966), cannot (Neill, 1972).

In the rhesus monkey, as in other species, the secretion of GnRH by the MBH is limiting in the control of gonadotropin secretion. Large, bilateral radiofrequency lesions in the MBH of ovariectomized rhesus monkeys, extending from the optic chiasm to the mammillary bodies and including the dorsal aspect of the median eminence, lead to a prompt decline in serum FSH and LH concentrations to immeasur-able levels and abolish the stimulatory action of estradiol on gonadotropin secretion (Plant et al., 1978a). Similarly, the iv

202

administration of antisera to synthetic GnRH to ovariectomized monkeys also results in a rapid reduction in serum gonadotropin levels which remain depressed as long as the circulating antibody titer remains elevated (McCormack et al., 1977). The rapidity of the response to the antiserum suggests that the sustained production of the releasing hormone is required for the elevated gonadotropin secretion characteristic of these animals.

That the arcuate nucleus is the primary hypothalamic structure responsible for the control of GnRH release is suggested by the finding that large radiofrequency lesions in the MBH, which spare the region of the arcuate nucleus, have little or no effect on basal gonadotropin secretion or on estrogen induced LH and FSH release, while smaller lesions restricted primarily to the region of the arcuate nucleus result in a decline of serum gonadotropins to undetectable levels as early as 48 hours after placement of the lesions (Plant et al., 1978a). Furthermore, administration of estradiol benzoate several days after placement of arcuate lesions fails to elicit a gonadotropin surge (Plant et al., 1978a).

Attempts to reestablish sustained gonadotropin secretion in animals bearing lesions of the arcuate nucleus by the continuous infusion of exogenous GnRH were unsuccessful (Plant et al., 1978a). Although impressive increases in serum gonadotropin concentrations could be observed for a day or two following initiation of the decapeptide infusion, the animals became refractory to continued treatment, serum gonadotropin returning to undetectable levels regardless of the magnitude of the continuous hypophysiotropic stimulus (Plant et al., 1978a; Nakai et al., 1978; Belchetz et al., 1978). When, however, an intermittent GnRH replacement regimen which mimicked the circhoral mode of gonadotropin secretion was instituted preoperative serum levels of LH and FSH were reestablished (Plant et al., 1978a; Belchetz et al., 1978). These unexpected observations have led us to the conclusion that the pattern of hypophysiotropic stimulation is an important new dimension in the neural control of gonadotropin secretion (Belchetz et al., 1978). In fact, we have recently demonstrated that relatively small changes in the frequency of exogenous GnRH administration to monkeys with MBH lesions profoundly influences not only the magnitude of the resulting gonadotropin response, but also the FSH:LH ratio in the circulation

(Hausler et al., 1979).   The latter phenomenon is attributable to the major differences in the metabolic clearance rates of the two glycoprotein hormones.

Using ovariectomized rhesus monkeys bearing hypothalamic lesions, which abolish gonadotropin secretion and in which pre-lesion gonadotropin levels were reestablished by unvarying intermittent administration of GnRH, we have re-explored the sites of the feedback actions of estrogen (Nakai et al., 1978; Plant et al., 1978b).   In such "hypophysiotropic clamp" preparations, which were devoid of an endogenous source of GnRH, estrogen exhibited its characteristic negative (Nakai et al., 1978; Plant et al., 1978b) and positive (Nakai et al., 1978) feedback effects thus permitting the conclusion that both these actions can be at the level of the pituitary gland. That estradiol can initiate gonadotropin surges by acting directly on the gonadotrophs has also been shown in monkeys with transected pituitary stalks (Ferin et al., 1979).

These findings are consonant with the hypothesis that GnRH may play only a permissive, albeit obligatory, role in the control of gonadotropin secretion.   We have recently tested and approved this hypothesis which predicts that in rhesus monkeys devoid of endogenous GnRH, normal ovulatory menstrual cycles should be subserved by an unvarying GnRH replacement regimen.   When such a regimen consisting of hourly pulses of the decapeptide was administered to otherwise intact monkeys bearing hypothalamic lesions, nearly all eventually exhibited normal ovulatory menstrual cycles 29 to 33 days in · duration (Knobil et al., 1980).   At the completion of the experiments these animals were ovariectomized but their serum gonadotropin levels remained undetectable, even in the face of sustained increments in circulating estrogen produced by sc injections of estradiol benzoate, suggesting that reorganization of the neural component of the control system following placement of the lesion had not taken place in the course of the study.

Our findings are consonant with the hypothesis that the ovary is the principal timer of the primate menstrual cycle and that estradiol controls gonadotropin secretion by acting directly on the pituitary gland, the intermittent release of GnRH by the hypothalamus being a permissive, but necessary, component of this control system. This conclusion has recently been reinforced by preliminary studies conducted in collaboration with M. Ferin and his colleagues, wherein experiments identical to the ones described here but performed on rhesus monkeys with transected pituitary stalks rather than hypothalamic lesions yielded essentially identical results.

There thus seems to be a major difference in the hypothalamic control of the monkey menstrual cycle on the one hand and of the rat estrous cycle on the other. In the latter, a bolus of GnRH, discharged into the pituitary portal vasculature in response to the action of estrogen on the central nervous system, is clearly necessary for the induction of the preovulatory gonadotropin surge. In the rhesus monkey, however, such an increment in hypothalamic activity is not required to initiate this phenomenon.

From all the foregoing, we have constructed a model of the neuroendocrine control system which governs gonadotropin secretion throughout the ovarian cycle of the rhesus monkey (Knobil, 1980).
It consists of a neuronal element in the region of the arcuate nucleus which, in the absence of extrahypothalamic inputs, discharges a bolus of GnRH into the hypophysial portal circulation approximately once every hour. This intermittent hypophysiotropic stimulus is required for the functional integrity of the gonadotrophs. The pattern of gonadotropin secretion throughout the menstrual cycle (basal secretion interrupted once every 28 days by a preovulatory gonadotropin surge) is not directed by alterations in GnRH secretion but by the ebb and flow of ovarian estrogen acting directly on the pituitary. The length of this cycle is determined by the duration of follicular development in response to basal gonadotropin secretion and by the preprogrammed functional lifespan of the corpus luteum (Knobil, 1973) during which follicular development is inhibited. Modulation of this system by hormones or neuronal inputs is achieved by changing the frequency of the arcuate nucleus "pulse generator".

The GnRH replacement regimen which subserves normal menstrual cycles in adult females with hypothalamic lesions (see above) can initiate normal ovulatory menstrual cycles in sexually immature monkeys (Wildt et al., 1980) suggesting that puberty is marked by the maturation of the arcuate, mechanism which underlies the circhoral discharge of GnRH.

References

Barraclough CA (1966) Modifications in the CNS regulation of reproduction after exposure of prepubertal rats to steroid hormones. V. Hormones and Development, Recent Prog Horm Res 22:503.

Barraclough CA (1973) Sex steroid regulation of reproductive neuro-endocrine processes. In: Greep RO, Ashwood EB (eds) Handbook of Physiology, Section 7: Endocrinology, vol 2, Williams and Wilkins, Baltimore.

Belchetz P, Plant TM, Nakai Y, Keogh EJ, Knobil E (1978) Hypophysial responses to continuous and intermittent delivery of hypothalamic gonadotropin releasing hormone. Science 202:631.

Butler WR, Krey LC, Espinosa-Campos J, Knobil E (1975) Surgical disconnection of the medial basal hypothalamus and pituitary function in the rhesus monkey. III. Thyroxine Secretion. Endocrinology 96:1094.

Dierschke DJ, Bhattacharya AN, Atkinson LE, Knobil E (1970) Circhoral oscillations of plasma LH levels in the ovariectomized rhesus monkey. Endocrinology 87:850.

Ferin M, Rosenblatt H, Carmel PW, Antunes JL, Vande Wiele RL (1979) Estrogen-induced gonadotropin surges in female rhesus monkeys after pituitary stalk section. Endocrinology 104:50.

Halasz B, Pupp L (1965) Hormone secretion of the anterior pituitary gland after physical interruption of all nervous pathways to the hypophysio-trophic area. Endocrinology 77:553.

Halasz B, Gorski RA (1967) Gonadotrophic hormone secretion in female rats after partial or total interruption of neural afferents to the medial basal hypothalamus. Endocrinology 80:608.

Hausler A, Wildt L, Marshall G, Plant TM, Belchetz PE, Knobil E (1979) Modulation of pituitary gonadotropin secretion by frequency of GnRH input. Fed Proc 38:1107.

Hess DL, Wilkins RH, Moossy J, Chang JL, Plant TM, McCormack JT, Nakai Y, Knobil E (1977) Estrogen-induced gonadotropin surges in decerebrated female rhesus monkeys with medial basal hypothalamic peninsulae. Endocrinology 101:1264.

Karsch FJ, Dierschke DJ, Knobil E (1973a) Sexual differentiation of pituitary function: Apparent difference between primates and rodents. Science 179:484.

Karsch FJ, Weick RF, Butler WR, Dierschke, DJ, Krey LC, Weiss G, Hotchkiss J, Yamaji T, Knobil E (1973b) Induced LH surges in the rhesus monkey: Strength-duration characteristics of the estrogen stimulus. Endocrinology 92:1740.

Knobil E (1973) On the regulation of the primate corpus luteum. Biol Reprod 8:246.

Knobil E (1974) On the control of gonadotropin secretion in the rhesus monkey. Rec Prog Hormone Res 30:1.

Knobil E (1980) The neuroendocrine control of the menstrual cycle. Rec Prog Hormone Res 36:53.

Knobil E, Plant TM, Wildt L, Belchetz PE, Marshall GR (1980) Neuro-endocrine control of the rhesus monkey menstrual cycle: Permissive role of the hypothalamic gonadotropin releasing hormone (GnRH). Science 207:1371.

Krey LC, Butler WR, Knobil E (1975a) Surgical disconnection of the medial basal hypothalamus and pituitary function in the rhesus monkey. I. Gonadotropin Secretion. Endocrinology 96:1073.

Krey LC, Lu K-H, Butler WR, Hotchkiss J, Piva F, Knobil E (1975b) Surgical disconnection of the medial basal hypothalamus and pituitary function in the rhesus monkey. II. Growth Hormone and Cortisol Secretion. Endocrinology 96:1088.

McCormack JT, Plant TM, Hess DL, Knobil E (1977) The effect of luteinizing hormone releasing hormone (LHRH) antiserum administration of gonadotropin secretion in the rhesus monkey. Endocrinology 100:663.

Nakai Y, Plant TM, Hess DL, Keogh EJ, Knobil E (1978) On the sites of the negative and positive feedback actions of estradiol in the control of gonadotropin secretion in the rhesus monkey. Endocrinology 102:1008.

Neill JD (1972) Sexual differences in the hypothalamic regulation or prolactin secretin. Endocrinology 90:1154.

Neill JD, Dailey RA, Tsou RC, Patton J, Tindall G (1976) Ovulation in the Human. Crosignani PG, Mishell DR (eds) Control of the Ovarian Cycle in the Monkey. Proceedings of the Serono Symposia, Volume 8, Academic Press Inc., London.

Norman RL, Resko JA, Spies HG (1976) The anterior hypothalamus: How it affects gonadotropin secretion in the rhesus monkey. Endocrinology 99:59.

Plant TM, Krey LC, Moossy J, McCormack JT, Hess DL, Knobil E (1978a) The arcuate nucleus and the control of gonadotropin and prolactin secretion in the female rhesus monkey (<u>Macaca</u> <u>mulatta</u>). Endocrinology 102:52.

Plant TM, Nakai Y, Belchetz P, Keogh E, Knobil E (1978b) The sites of action of estradiol and phentolamine in the inhibition of the pulsatile, circhoral discharges of LH in the rhesus monkey (<u>Macaca mulatta</u>). Endocrinology 102:1015.

Plant TM, Moossy J, Hess DL, Nakai Y, McCormack JT, Knobil E (1979) Further studies on the effects of lesions in the rostral hypothalamus on gonadotropin secretion in the female rhesus monkey (<u>Macaca mulatta</u>). Endocrinology 105:465.

Sawyer CH (1969) Regulatory mechanisms of secretion of gonadotrophic hormones. Haymaker W, Anderson E, Nauta WJH (eds) The Hypothalamus. Charles C. Thomas, Illinois.

Weick RF, Dierschke DJ, Karsch FJ, Hotchkiss J, Knobil E (1973) Periovulatory time courses of circulating gonadotropic and ovarian hormones in the rhesus monkey. Endocrinology 93:1140.

Wildt L, Marshall G, Knobil E (1980) Experimental induction of puberty in the infantile female rhesus monkey. Science 207:1373.

The Limbic System and Female Sexual Maturation

F. Döcke, Berlin

In spite of intensive studies performed mainly during the last 20 years, the physiological mechanisms underlying female sexual maturation are not yet fully elucidated. A dominant role of the central nervous system is indicated by the influence of brain lesions or tumors and of environmental stimuli on the onset of puberty in humans and animals, and by the observation that the ovary is capable of responding to gonadotropic stimulation and that the pituitary can support normal ovarian cyclicity long before puberty onset. However, it was concluded from recent investigations (Eckstein, 1976; Ojeda and Jameson, 1977; Advis et al., 1979) that age-dependent changes in ovarian steroid production and/or responsiveness to gonadotropic stimulation may also be important factors in determining the initiation of puberty.

Two experiments were performed to study the influence of the ovaries on female sexual maturation. Female rats were either ovariectomized on the first day of life and reimplanted with two ovaries under their kidney capsules at 24, 28 or 32 days of age, or ovaries of 23-day-old females were transplanted into 31-day-old recipients and, vice versa, ovaries of 35-day-old donors into 23-day-old rats. In the latter experiment, ovariectomy of the recipients was performed on the fourth day after implantation (Döcke and Dörner, 1974; Döcke et al., 1980b). None of these treatments had a significant influence on the length of the first ovarian cycle (exp. 1) and on the onset of puberty (exp. 2). Thus, the absence of ovarian hormones during an extended period of prepuberal life does not impair the maturation of the mechanisms underlying the cyclic ovarian function. Corresponding results have also been obtained in humans (Yen et al., 1972). The findings furthermore suggest that the developmental stage of the ovaries is not a decisive factor in the control of puberty onset.

It has been demonstrated repeatedly that structures of the limbic system are involved in the control of the ovarian cycle in adult female rats (for review see Sawyer, 1972; Kawakami and Terasawa, 1974; Gorski, 1974) and may also participate in the control of prepuberal gonadotropin secretion. Elwers and Critchlow (1960, 1961) reported that bilateral lesioning of the medial amygdala or interruption of the stria terminalis in 18-20-day-old female rats accelerated sexual maturation. A gonadotropin-inhibiting activity of the medial amygdala could be derived from these findings. Later studies, however, did not confirm this assumption, since puberty-delaying effects of amygdaloid lesions were found (Bloch and Ganong, 1971; Relkin, 1971; Velasco, 1972). Reinvestigating this question we obtained the following results (Döcke, 1976; Döcke et al., 1980c):

1. The onset of puberty was only advanced following bilateral lesioning of the anterior part of the medial amygdaloid nucleus (AMN). Lesions placed in adjacent sites, i.e. in the posterior part of the medial amygdaloid nucleus or in the cortical amygdaloid nucleus were ineffective in this respect.

2. In the strain of Wistar rats used, bilateral lesioning of the AMN induced precocious puberty only if performed at 20-22 days of age. Similar lesions produced in 15-day-old females resulted in a significant delay of vaginal opening and the first ovulation, and lesioning on day 26 did not influence sexual maturation.

3. In 15-day-old ovariectomized females, bilateral lesioning of the AMN suppressed completely the castration-induced elevation of the circulating LH level. In contrast, a significant increase of the LH concentration as compared to the ovariectomized controls was found in rats that had been lesioned on day 21, whereas an effect of brain damage could not be revealed in 26-day-old rats.

4. Daily s.c. injections of 0.05 μg estradiol benzoate (EB)/100 g b.w. administered to ovariectomized females from day 21 to day 26 lowered the LH concentration to the level recorded in intact rats. Bilateral lesioning of the AMN did not reduce this gonadotropin-inhibiting effect of estrogen.

5. The serum LH concentration was estimated in groups of untreated
   female rats autopsied at daily intervals from 17 to 26 days of
   age. Relatively high LH levels were found on day 17 and 18.
   Significantly lower values (p<0.001) were recorded between day
   19 and 23. After that, LH increased again significantly
   between day 24 and 26 (p<0.001).

The following conclusions may be drawn from these findings:

During the infantile period the AMN may stimulate LH and,
possibly, FSH secretion. Relkin (1971) reported that a distinct delay
of the onset of puberty resulted from bilateral lesioning of the
mediocortical amygdala in 4-day-old female rats. At about three
weeks of age, the gonadotropin-stimulating activity changes transiently to an inhibitory action that seems not to be related to the
negative estrogen feedback. The decrease in circulating plasma LH
and FSH in intact rats at this time that has also been described by
Ojeda and Ramirez (1972), Meijs-Roelofs et al. (1973), Cheng and
Johnson (1973/74), Döhler and Wuttke (1974, 1975), Eneroth et al.
(1975) and Kamberi et al. (1980) may partly be caused by this
direct central nervous inhibition, but other factors, e.g. the decline
of the estrogen-binding α-fetoprotein (Puig-Duran et al., 1979) and
an increase of progesterone secretion (Meijs-Roelofs et al., 1975) are
certainly also involved. The latter mechanisms, however, cannot
explain the renewed rise of the circulating LH levels towards the end
of the fourth week of life that was observed in the present study
and has also been recorded by Ojeda and Ramirez (1972), Cheng and
Johnson (1973/74), Döhler and Wuttke (1974, 1975) and Eneroth et al.
(1975). Possibly, both a decrease of estrogen secretion reported by
Döhler and Wuttke (1975) and Kamberi et al. (1980) and the
disappearance of the gonadotropin-inhibiting activity of the AMN may
be responsible for this phenomenon. The latter assumption is
supported by findings obtained in other species. The gonadotropic
response to neonatal ovariectomy is delayed in ewe-lambs for 4-6
weeks (Foster et al., 1975) and in monkeys castrated during infancy
to the time of puberty (Dierschke et al., 1974). According to Conte
et al. (1980), findings obtained in normal and agonadal children
lend strong support to the conclusion that a central nervous inhibitory mechanism that is independent of gonadal feedback in-

fluences and is suppressed prior to the onset of puberty, is operative in humans, too.

During the fourth week of life when the gonadotropin-inhibiting activity of the AMN vanishes, the positive estrogen feedback mechanism matures in the female rat (Ying and Greep, 1971; Caligaris et al., 1972; Puig-Duran and MacKinnon, 1978). A similar temporal relationship between the disappearance of direct central nervous inhibition of gonadotropin secretion and development of the gonadotropin-stimulating estrogen effect seems also to exist in other species, because an LH surge can first be induced by exogenous estrogen at the age of about 5 weeks in ewe-lambs (Land et al., 1970) and at the time of puberty in female monkeys (Dierschke et al., 1974) and girls (Grumbach et al., 1974). In guinea-pigs, in which a delay of the gonadotropic response to ovariectomy has not been found during the postnatal development (Donovan et al., 1975a,b), the positive estrogen feedback is operative immediately after birth (Medero and Dominguez, 1977).

In the rat, the posterior part of the medial amygdaloid nucleus may play an essential role in the maturation of the positive estrogen feedback mechanism. This assumption is based on the following findings:

1. Bilateral lesioning of the PMN at 26 or 32 days of age delayed significantly the first puberal ovulation (Döcke, 1976). Similar lesions produced on day 21 were ineffective in otherwise untreated females, but prevented the advancement of the puberal ovulation induced by lesioning of the mediobasal hypothalamus or by daily s.c. injections of 0.05 µg EB/100 g b.w. from day 5 till vaginal opening (Döcke et al., 1976).

2. Implantation of EB into the PMN induced an LH surge in 21-, 26- and 32-day-old rats and precocious ovulation when performed at 26 or 32 days of age (Döcke, 1976; Döcke et al., 1977). Since the ovarian cycle following the EB-induced ovulation was significantly prolonged, precocious puberty did not result from this treatment.

3. Superovulation caused by a single s.c. injection of 15 IU PMSG was blocked completely or to a large extent by deafferentation of the mediocortical amygdala at 23 or 27 days of age, respectively, and was also prevented by lesioning of the PMN

211

on day 27.   Both treatments were ineffective in 31- and 35-day-old females (Döcke and Moldenhauer, 1977).   Deafferentation of the amygdala was performed by bilateral transection of the stria terminalis at its origin according to the method of Colombo et al. (1975).

The findings suggest that even elevated estrogen levels in the blood produced by an increased number of maturing ovarian follicles and indicated by significantly higher uterine weight in the PMSG-treated rats (not published) cannot induce an ovulatory LH surge during the fourth week of life, if the function of the PMN is impaired. This does not apply to older prepuberal females, although spontaneous ovulation was temporarily suppressed in these animals by lesioning of the PMN.   It may be assumed that near puberty the positive estrogen feedback can be operative without participation of the medial amygdala if more than the physiological amount of estrogen is present in the blood.   During the development of this mechanism, however, a normal function of the medial amygdala is necessary for its realization indicating an essential contribution of this limbic nucleus to the maturation process.

The cortical amygdaloid nucleus (CAN), too, may be involved in the control of female sexual maturation. Implantation of EB into this region at 26 or 36 days of age induced an LH surge and, in the younger females, precocious ovulation.   As opposed to these findings, 32-day-old rats responded to this treatment with slight inhibition of LH secretion and a significant delay of the first puberal ovulation (Döcke, 1976; Döcke et al., 1977).   Furthermore, bilateral lesioning of the CAN performed on day 31 enhanced significantly the super-ovulatory response to PMSG, whereas the PMSG-induced ovulation was completely prevented by electrical stimulation of this nucleus during the critical period following the administration of the hormone. Similar effects were neither obtained in younger females nor on day 36, i.e. immediately prior to the onset of puberty (Döcke and Moldenhauer, 1977).

Taken together, the results suggest a temporary inhibitory influence of the CAN on the induction of an ovulatory LH surge by estrogen that vanishes when puberty approaches.   This activity may form an additional protective mechanism to prevent precocious ovula-tion and may at least partly be responsible for the steep fall in the super-ovulatory response to PMSG after day 28 that was first described by Zarrow and Quinn (1963) and was also found in the study quoted above.

Smith and Lawton (1972) reported that bilateral lesioning of the CAN prevented compensatory ovarian hypertrophy (COH) resulting from hemicastration in cyclic female rats. This finding could be confirmed (Bao and Döcke, 1977). If, however, similar lesions were produced in hemicastrated 28-day-old females that were autopsied on the 8th day after surgery, an effect on COH could not be revealed. Thus, the loss of the inhibitory activity of the CAN on the estrogen-induced LH peak at the time of puberty onset may be associated with the acquisition of the capacity to stimulate FSH secretion in response to lowering of the estrogen level in the blood.

Summarizing the presented findings on the influence of the mediocortical amygdala (MCA) on sexual maturation in female rats, some general conclusions may be drawn:

1. An important role of this limbic structure in the neurohormonal control of puberty can be assumed. This applies to the prepuberal inhibition of gonadotropin secretion as well as to the maturation of the gonadotropin-stimulating estrogen feedback.

2. Different nuclear regions of the MCA may be involved by variable activities and in an age-dependent manner in the control of prepuberal gonadotropin secretion. This conclusion is supported by morphological studies which demonstrated specific age-dependent alteration of neuronal cell nuclear size (Döcke and Smollich, 1978), numbers of ribosomes, and synaptogenesis (M. Wenzel, J. Wenzel, F. Döcke, in preparation) in this area. It seems that the AMN participates in the regulation of tonic gonadotropin secretion and the PMN in the maturation of the positive estrogen feedback. According to De Olmos (1974), the axonal efflux of the AMN terminates in the hypothalamic ventro-medial region and that of the PMN in the medial preoptic area. Because of the differential actions exerted in an age-dependent manner by the amygdaloid nuclei, it may no longer be justified to speak in a general way of a "puberty-inhibiting" or "puberty-advancing" activity of the MCA during female sexual maturation, and diverging results of former studies in this field may be explained by different developmental stages of the

animals employed, and/or by the investigation of different .nuclear regions.

3. High plasticity of prepuberal central nervous control of gonado-tropin secretion must be assumed. This is indicated by the oberservation that, e.g., lesions produced in the medial amyg-daloid nucleus at 21 days of age did not delay the first puberal ovulation, although damage to the tissue persisted to ages, at which similar lesioning inhibited completely the super-ovulatory response to PMSG. Compensatory mechanisms may be installed under these conditions. In adult female rats, a fourfold increase of the sensitivity of the bed nucleus of the stria terminalis to the ovulation-inducting effect of estrogen was recorded following deafferentation of the MCA (Döcke and Bao, 1978).

Riss et al. (1963) and Zarrow et al. (1969) reported that extensive or selective lesioning of the ventral hippocampus (VHPC) in immature female rats caused retardation of sexual maturation. According to Kawakami and Terasawa (1972), this effect may be due to an FSH-stimulating activity of the VHPC during prepuberal life. Reinvestigating the effect of small VHPC lesions on the onset of puberty in female rats we obtained the following results (Döcke, 1977; Döcke et al., 1980a):

1. A significant delay of vaginal opening and of the first ovulation was recorded following bilateral lesioning of the VHPC at 21, 26 or 32 days of age. A puberty-delaying effect of hippo-campal lesions produced on day 21 was also seen in rats in which precocious puberty had been induced by simultaneous, lesioning of the medial preoptic area or the hypothalamic ventro-medial-arcuate region, or by daily s.c. injections of 0.05 µg EB/100 g b.w. from day 5 till vaginal opening.

2. Irrespective of the applied treatment, the delay of sexual maturation was consistently associated with retardation of the somatic development, i.e. the body weights at the time of puberty did not differ from those recorded in the corresponding groups without damage to the VHPC. Thus, the stage of body development necessary for the occurrence of spontaneous or precocious puberty was reached at later ages in the rats with hippocampal lesions.

214

3. Both the puberty-delaying and growth-retarding effects of VHPC lesions produced on day 21 could be prevented by daily s.c. injections of 50 µg/100 g b.w. pyridostigmine from day 21 till vaginal opening, but not by the administration of 2 mg/100 g/day pargyline. These findings suggest a cholinergic mediation of stimulatory effects exerted by the hippocampus on sexual maturation and somatic development.

It has been demonstrated that the hippocampus stimulates growth hormone secretion (Martin, 1972), and that the onset of puberty is more closely related to somatic development than to age (for review see Donovan, 1974; Frisch, 1974). On the basis of these and the presented findings it may be concluded that the hippocampus is involved in the control of sexual maturation not only by way of its influence on FSH secretion, but also by its growth-stimulating activity.

As early as 1932, Hohlweg and Dohrn and Hohlweg and Junkmann postulated that an essential mechanism in the control of puberty onset in female rats is the desensitization of the hypo-thalamo-hypophyseal system to the gonadotropin-inhibiting effect of estrogen. Although several later studies (for review see Davidson, 1974) confirmed this assumption by demonstrating that the castration-induced increase of gonadotropin secretion can be inhibited by smaller doses of EB in prepuberal rats than have to be applied to postpuberal females, a significant role of this desensitization in the control of puberty onset has repeatedly been called in question (Donovan, 1974; Meijs-Roelofs et al., 1975; Ojeda et al., 1976; Advis et al., 1979). The main reason was that, in contrast to the human (Faiman and Winter, 1974), a distinct increase of circulating FSH and LH levels prior to the onset of puberty has not been found (Döhler and Wuttke, 1974; Meijs-Roelofs et al., 1975; Ojeda et al., 1976).

To reexamine this question, a series of experiments was performed in immature and postpuberal female rats on the day of the first vaginal estrus by implanting minute quantities of EB into the hypothalamic ventromedial-arcuate region of ovariectomized females and by estimating the circulating LH and FSH levels in these and in untreated intact rats at different ages (Döcke et al., 1978, 1980d).

The results obtained demonstrated that the gonadotropin-inhibiting effect of intrahypothalamically administered estrogen did not change during the fourth week of life. It decreased, however, between days 26 and 32 and showed a further distinct decline at the time of puberty. The MCA is probably not involved in this desensitization process, because bilateral transection of the stria terminalis did not influence the LH-inhibiting effect of s.c. injected EB in castrated females during the 5th week of life.

Monitoring the serum LH and FSH levels and the uterine weight in intact females at daily intervals from 25 to 36 days of age revealed relatively high concentrations of both gonadotropins between day 25 and 28. Acceleration of uterine growth around day 30 indicating increasing estrogen secretion (Advis et al., 1979) was associated with a sudden fall of circulating LH and FSH levels. After that, serum LH and to a lesser degree FSH begin again to rise in spite of a further weight gain of the uterus, so that the gonado-tropin curves, particularly that of LH, paralleled that of uterine weight for several days. Immediately before vaginal opening and the first ovulation, the FSH concentration declined as is also found in cyclic rats prior to ovulation (Butcher et al., 1974).

The findings suggest that the prepuberal hypothalamic de-sensitization to the gonadotropin-inhibiting effect of estrogen is reflected in intact rats by increasing gonadotropin concentrations in the presence of rising estrogen levels in the blood.at this time, reported by Döhler and Wuttke (1975) and Parker and Mahesh (1976).

The hypothesis is put forward that the described limbic and hypothalamic mechanisms are involved in the neurohormonal control of puberty in female rats in the following ways:

From birth through the third week of life, the MCA seems to exert a gonadotropin-stimulating activity, because lesioning of this area at 4 (Relkin, 1971) or 15 days of age delays the onset of puberty. Around day 21, this activity changes transiently to a gonadotropin-inhibiting action that may partly be responsible for the depression of gonadotropin secretion at this age. It vanishes during the fourth week of life as is indicated by the lesioning experiments and by the increase of serum LH between days 24 and 28. The gonadotropin concentrations at this time are as high as or even higher than those found during the first postpuberal ovarian cycle (Döhler and Wuttke, 1975; Döcke et al., in preparation). They therefore may be sufficient to initiate development of ovarian follicles, and the conclusion seems justified that "prepuberal ovarian cyclicity" culminating in the first puberal ovulation commences before day 30. According to Meijs-Roelofs et al. (1973) and Knudsen et al. (1974), large vesicular ovarian follicles are regularly found after this age.

The progressive follicle maturation is accompanied by gradually increasing estrogen secretion (Döhler and Wuttke, 1975; Parker and Mahesh, 1976). Because of the high sensitivity of the hypothalamus to the gonadotropin-inhibiting effect of estrogen, both serum LH and FSH are initially suppressed. Due to the hypothalamic desensitization to the feedback effect of estrogen, however, this inhibition is progressively reduced so that basal gonadotropin secretion sufficient for further stimulation of follicle development and comparable to that recorded during the first postpuberal ovarian cycle (Döhler and Wuttke, 1975; Döcke et al., in preparation) is resumed.

The second presupposition for the onset of ovarian cyclicity is the efficacy of the gonadotropin-stimulating estrogen feedback. This mechanism is installed in the female rat during the fourth week of life (Ying and Greep, 1971; Caligaris et al., 1972; Puig-Duran and MacKinnon, 1978). Probably, the medial amygdaloid nucleus plays an essential role in this process. Endogenous activation of the positive estrogen feedback, however, is delayed for one to two weeks by the sensitive negative feedback that prevents ovarian estrogen secretion from reaching the high preovulatory level. After this hindrance is removed, final maturation of the ovarian follicles associated with a sudden increase of estrogen secretion can occur. The first ovulation is then induced by intra- and extraovarian mechanisms that are comparable to those underlying cyclic ovulation in adult female rats (Döcke and Dörner, 1974; Ojeda et al., 1976; Advis et al., 1978, 1979).

At least during the second half of prepuberal development the ventral hippocampus, too, may be involved in the control of sexual maturation by means of his FSH (Kawakami and Terasawa, 1972) and growth-stimulating activities.

217

References

Advis JP, Andrews WW, Ojeda SR (1979) Changes in ovarian steroidal and prostaglandin E responsiveness to gonadotropins during the onset of puberty in the female rat. Endocrinology 104:653-658.

Advis JP, Simpkins JW, Chen HT, Meites J (1978) Relation of biogenic amines to onset of puberty in the female rat. Endocrinology 103:11-16.

Bao TN, Döcke F (1977) Different effects of amygdaloid lesions on compensatory ovarian hypertrophy in cyclic and prepubertal female rats. Endokrinologie 70:340-343.

Bloch GJ, Ganong WF (1971) Lesions of the brain and the onset of puberty in the female rat. Endocrinology 89:898-901.

Butcher RL, Collins WE, Fugo NW (1974) Plasma concentration of LH, FSH, prolactin, progesterone and estradio-17β throughout the 4-day estrous cycle of the rat. Endocrinology 94:1704-1708.

Caligaris L, Astrada JJ, Taleisnik S (1972) Influence of age on the release of luteinizing hormone induced by estrogen and progesterone in immature rats. J Endocrinol 55:97-103.

Cheng HC, Johnson DC (1973/74) Serum estrogens and gonadotropins in developing androgenized and normal female rats. Neuroendocrinology 13:357-365.

Colombo JA, Krieg RJ, Sawyer CH (1975) Limbic system involvement in the increase in plasma prolactin following cortical spreading depression in gonadotropin-treated female rats. Endocrinology 97:261-264.

Conte FA, Grumbach MM, Kaplan SL, Reiter EO (1980) Correlation of luteinizing hormone-releasing factor-induced luteinizing hormone and follicle-stimulating hormone release from infancy to 19 years with the changing pattern of gonadotropin secretion in agonadal patients: relation to the restraint of puberty. J Clin Endocrinol Metab 50:163-168.

Davidson JM (1974) Hypothalamic-pituitary regulation of puberty, evidence from animal experimentation. In: Grumbach MM, Grave GD, Mayer FE (eds) Control of the onset of puberty, John Wiley & Sons, New York, pp.79-103.

De Olmos JS (1972) The amygdaloid projection field in the rat as studied with the cupric-silver method. In: Eleftheriou BE (ed) The neurobiology of the amygdala, Plenum Press, New York-London, pp.145-204.

Dierschke DJ, Karsch FJ, Weick RF, Weiss G, Hotchkiss J, Knobil E (1974) Hypothalamic-pituitary regulation of puberty: feedback control of gonadotropin secretion in the rhesus monkey. In: Grumbach MM, Grave GD, Mayer FE (eds) Control of the onset of puberty, John Wiley & Sons, New York, pp.104-114.

Döcke F (1976) Age-dependent changes in the puberty-controlling function of the medial and cortical amygdaloid nuclei. Ann Biol anim Biochim Biophys 16:423-432.

Döcke F (1977) A possible mechanism of the puberty-delaying effect of hippocampal lesions in the female rats. Endokrinologie 69:258-261.

Döcke F, Bao TN (1978) Increased sensitivity to estrogen of the bed nucleus of the stria terminalis following deafferentation of the mediocortical amygdala: evidence for a compensatory ovulatory mechanism. Endokrinologie 72:257-264.

Döcke F, Dörner G (1974) Oestrogen and the control of gonadotrophin secretion in the immature rat. J Endocrinol 63:285-298.

Döcke F, Lange TH, Dörner G (1980a) Involvement of a cholinergic mechanism in the mediation of hippocampal influences on female sexual maturation and somatic development. Endokrinologie 75:8–12.

Döcke F, Lemke W, Okrasa R (1976) Studies on the puberty-controlling function of the mediocortical amygdala in the immature female rat. Neuroendocrinology 20:166–175.

Döcke F, Moldenhauer U (1977) Influence of the mediocortical amygdala on PMSG-induced ovulation in immature female rats. Endokrinologie 70:19–26.

Döcke F, Rohde W, Bao TN, Braun W, Dörner G (1978) Studies on the time and localization of the puberal desensitization to oestrogen in female rats. Endokrinologie 71:257–265.

Döcke R, Rohde W, Dörner G (1980b) Failure to demonstrate a significant influence of ovarian maturity on the onset of puberty in female rats. Endokrinologie (in press).

Döcke F, Rohde W, Lange TH, Dörner G (1980c) Evidence for direct central nervous inhibition of LH secretion during sexual maturation of female rats. Endokrinologie 75:1–7.

Döcke F, Rohde W, Lange TH, Geier TH, Dörner G (1980d) Further studies on the hypothalamic desensitization to estrogen in immature female rats: evidence for a possible role in the control of puberty. Endokrinologie (in press).

Döcke F, Rohde W, Moldenhauer U, Dörner G (1977) Maturation of the oestrogen-dependent LH-stimulating activity of the medio-cortical amygdala in female rats. Endokrinologie 69:262–265.

Döcke F, Smollich A (1978) Morphological differentiation of limbic nuclei during sexual maturation of female rats. Endokrinologie 72:1–8.

Döhler KD, Wuttke W (1974) Serum LH, FSH, prolactin and progesterone from birth to puberty in female and male rats. Endocrinology 94:1003–1008.

Döhler KD, Wuttke W (1975) Changes with age in levels of serum gonadotropins, prolactin, and gonadal steroids in prepubertal male and female rats. Endocrinology 97: 898–907.

Donovan BT (1974) The role of the hypothalamus in puberty. In: Swaab DF, Schadé JP (eds) Integrative hypothalamic activity, Progr in Brain Res Vol 41, Elsevier Scientific Publishing Company, Amsterdam, pp.239–252.

Donovan BT, ter Haar MB, Lockhart AN, MacKinnon PCB, Mattock JM, Peddie MJ (1975a) Changes in the concentration of luteinizing hormone in plasma during development in the guinea-pig. J Endocrinol 64:511–520.

Donovan BT, ter Haar MB, Lockhart AN, Peddie MJ (1975b) Changes in the concentration of follicle-stimulating hormone in plasma during development in the guinea-pig. J Endocrinol 64:521–528.

Eckstein B (1976) 5α-androstanediols during sexual maturation: biosynthesis by the immature rat ovary in vitro and some biological effects. Ann Biol anim Biochim Biophys 16:319–325.

Elwers M, Critchlow V (1960) Precocious ovarian stimulation following hypothalamic and amygdaloid lesions in rats. Am J Physiol 198:381–385.

Elwers M, Critchlow V (1961) Precocious ovarian stimulation following interruption of stria terminalis. Am J Physiol 201:281–284.

Eneroth P, Gustafsson J-Å, Skett P, Steinberg Å (1975) Sex-dependent prepubertal gonadotrophin surges in the rat. J Endocrinol 65:91–98.

Faiman C, Winter JSD (1974) Gonadotropins and sex hormone patterns in puberty: clinical data. In: Grumbach MM, Grave GD, Mayer FE (eds) Control of the onset of puberty, John Wiley & Sons, New York, pp.32–55.

Foster DL, Jaffe RJ, Niswender GD (1975) Sequential patterns of circulating LH and FSH in female sheep during the early postnatal period: effect of gonadectomy. Endocrinology 96:15–22.

Frisch RE (1974) Critical weight at menarche, initiation of the adolescent growth spurt, and control of puberty. In: Grumbach MM,

Grave GD, Mayer FE (eds) Control of the onset of puberty, John Wiley & Sons, New York, pp.403–423.

Gorski RA (1974) Extrahypothalamic influences on gonadotropin regulation. In: Grumbach MM, Grave GD, Mayer FE (eds) Control of the onset of puberty, John Wiley & Sons, New York, pp.182–207.

Greenstein BD, Puig-Duran E, MacKinnon PCB (1977) Measurement of the unbound oestradiol-17β fraction in sera of developing female rats by a miniature method of steady-state gel filtration. J Endocrinol 72:56P.

Grumbach MM, Roth JC, Kaplan SL, Kelch RP (1974) Hypothalamic pituitary regulation of puberty in man: evidence and concepts derived from clinical research. In: Grumbach MM, Grave GD, Mayer FE (eds) Control of the onset of puberty, John Wiley & Sons, New York, pp.115–166.

Hohlweg W, Dohrn M (1932) Über die Beziehungen zwischen Hypophysen-vorderlappen und Keimdrüsen. Klin Wochenschr 11:233–235.

Hohlweg W, Junkmann K (1932) Die hormonal-nervöse Regulierung der Funktion des Hypophysenvorderlappens. Klin Wochenschr 11:321–323.

Kamberi IA, de Vellis J, Bacleon ES, Inglish D (1980) Hormonal patterns of the hypothalamo-pituitary-gonadal axis in the rat during postnatal development and sexual maturation. Endokrinologie 75:129–140.

Kawakami M, Terasawa E (1972) Electrical stimulation of the brain on gonadotropin secretion in the female prepuberal rat. Endocrinol jap 19:335–347.

Kawakami M, Terasawa E (1974) Role of limbic forebrain structures on reproductive cycles. In: Kawakami M (ed) Biological rhythms in neuroendocrine, Igaku Shoin, Tokyo, pp.197–219.

Knudsen JF, Costoff A, Mahesh VB (1974) Correlation of serum gonado-tropins, ovarian and uterine histology in immature and prepubertal rats. Anat Rec 180:497–508.

Land RB, Thimonier J, Pelletier J (1970) Possibilité d'induction d'une décharge de LH par une injection d'oestrogène chez l'agneau femelle en fonction de l'âge. C R Acad Sci, Paris, Sér D 271:1549–1551.

Martin JB (1972) Plasma growth hormone (GH) response to hypothalamic and extrahypothalamic electrical stimulation. Endocrinology 91:107–115.

Meijs-Roelofs HMA, De Greef WJ, Uilenbroek JTHJ (1975) Plasma progesterone and its relationship to serum gonadotrophins in immature female rats. J Endocrinol 64:329–336.

Meijs-Roelofs HMA, Uilenbroek JTHJ, de Greef WJ, de Jong FH, Kramer P (1975) Gonadotrophin and steroid levels around the time of first ovulation in the rat. J Endocrinol 67:275–282.

Meijs-Roelofs HMA, Uilenbroek JTHJ, Osman P, Welschen R (1973) Serum levels of gonadotrophins and follicular growth in prepuberal rats. In: Peters H (ed) The development and maturation of the ovary and its functions. Excerpta Med Int Congr Ser, No. 267, Amsterdam, pp.3–11.

Ojeda SR, Jameson HE (1977) Developmental patterns of plasma and pituitary growth hormone (GH) in the female rat. Endocrinology 100:881–889.

Ojeda SR, Ramirez VD (1972) Plasma level of LH and FSH in maturing rats: response to hemigonadectomy. Endocrinology 90:466–472.

Ojeda SR, Wheaton JE, Jameson HE, McCann SM (1976) The onset of puberty in the female rat: changes in plasma prolactin, gonadotropins, luteinizing-hormone-releasing hormone (LHRH), and hypothalamic LHRH content. Endocrinology 98:630–638.

Parker CRJR, Mahesh VB (1976) Hormonal events surrounding the natural onset of puberty. Biol Reprod 14:347–353.

Puig-Duran E, Greenstein BD, MacKinnon PCB (1979) The effects of serum oestrogen-binding components on the unbound oestradiol-17β fraction in the serum of developing female rats and on inhibition of (^{3}H) oestradiol uptake by uterine tissue in vitro. J Reprod Fert 56:707-714.

Puing-Duran E, MacKinnon PCB (1978) Ontogeny of prolactin and luteinizing hormone responses to oestrogen and progesterone in immature rats. J Endocrinol 76:321-331.

Relkin R (1971) Relative efficacy of pinealectomy, hypothalamic and amygdaloid lesions in advancing puberty. Endocrinology 88:415-418.

Riss W, Burstein SD, Johnson RW (1963) Hippocampal or pyriform lobe damage in infancy and endocrine development of rats. Am J Physiol 204:861-866.

Sawyer CH (1972) Functions of the amygdala related to the feedback actions of gonadal steroid hormones. In: Eleftheriou BE (ed) The neurobiology of the amygdala, Plenum Press, New York, pp.745-762.

Smith SW, Lawton IE (1972) Involvement of the amygdala in the ovarian compensatory hypertrophy response. Neuroendocrinology 9:228-234.

Velasco ME (1972) Opposite effects of platinum and stainless steel lesions of the amygdala on gonadotropin secretion. Neuroendocrinology 10:301-308.

Yen SSC, Tsai CC, Vandenberg G, Rebar R (1972) Gonadotropin dynamics in patients with gonadal dysgenesis: a model for the study of gonadotropin regulation. J Clin Endocrinol Metab 35:897-904.

Ying S-Y, Greep RO (1971) Effect of age of rat and dose of a single injection of estradiol benzoate (EB) on ovulation and the facilitation of ovulation by progesterone (P). Endocrinology 89:785-790.

Zarrow MX, Naqvi RH, Denenberg VHC (1969) Androgen-induced precocious puberty in the female rat and its inhibition by hippocampal lesions. Endocrinology 84:14-19.

Zarrow MX, Quinn DL (1963) Superovulation in the immature rat following treatment with PMS alone and inhibition of PMS-induced ovulation. J Endocrinol 26:181-188.

Estrogen Facilitation of Lordosis Behavior in the Female Rat

R.A. Gorski and M. Yanase, Los Angeles

It is well established that the display of sexual behavior in the female rat is dependent upon the action of ovarian steroids upon a complex hormone responsive neural substrate. Although there are a number of components of sexual behavior in the female, the present discussion will focus on the lordosis reflex. The lordosis quotient (LQ, the number of lordosis reflexes expressed as a percentage of the number of mounts by the male) is a convenient and reliable index of sexual receptivity and thus, a useful parameter with which to evaluate steroid action on the brain. In this regard, although high rates of lordosis responding can be facilitated in the ovariectomized rat by treatment with estradiol benzoate (EB) alone, relatively prolonged injection of EB (for approximately one week) is required (Gorski, 1974; Moralí and Beyer, 1979). However, after exposure to EB for a much shorter period (see below), progesterone (P) administration will markedly facilitate the LQ that is attained four–six hours later at a time when ovariectomized females treated with EB alone are essentially non–receptive. In fact, it has been suggested that in the intact rat the facilitation of lordosis behavior by ovarian hormones involves this synergism between estrogen and P (see Gorski, 1974).

Although it is beyond the scope of this discussion, considerable progress has been made in the identification of several components of the neural substrate upon which these steroids act to facilitate lordosis behavior (Gorski, 1976; Moralí and Beyer, 1979; Sakuma and Pfaff, 1979), but our understanding of how the activity of this complex neural substrate is integrated to facilitate this behavior is severely limited. In our laboratory, however, we have studied a surgical preparation which renders the facilitation of lordosis behavior simpler, at least in terms of its hormonal requirements. The ovariectomized rat subjected to electrolytic destruction of the lateral septum attains high levels of lordosis responding following treatment with EB alone. In fact, the septal lesioned female rat is behaviorally hyperresponsive to Eb (Figure 1), but its response to exogenous P appears normal (Nance et al., 1975). Although this

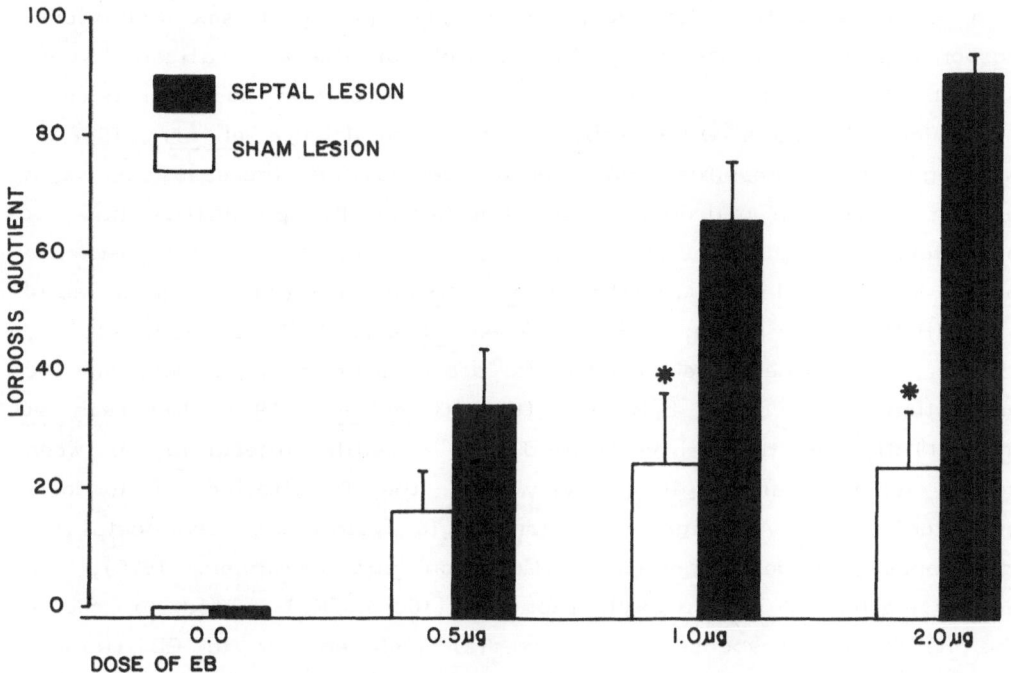

Figure 1: Mean lordosis quotient (+ standard error) of septal lesioned and sham operated ovariectomized rats primed with different doses of estradiol benzoate for three days. Behavioral tests were conducted on the fourth day. Data from Nance et al. (1975)

facilitation of the lordosis response to EB appears to be independent of adrenal P (Nance et al., 1974), this model is not simple presumably because of adaptation by intact neural systems which may exhibit functional, if not morphological, plasticity following destruction of the septum (Raisman, 1969; Loy and Melner, 1980). Nevertheless, our study of the action of EB in facilitating lordosis behavior in the septal lesioned rat has provided new information about the interaction between estrogen, aminergic activity and lordosis behavior, information which may be useful for our under-standing of the central action of estrogen also in the normal female.

Since septal lesions induce an immediate hypersensitivity to environmental stimuli, two possible explanations for the increased behavioral sensitivity to EB become apparent: the increase in LQ could be due to a generalized hypersensitivity which might render the stimuli associated with mounting more effective, or it could be due to an immediate release from tonic inhibition. Neither explana-tion appears valid, however, since the increased sex behavioral responsiveness persists after habituation of the generalized hyper-excitability and the increase in lordosis responding does not develop until four-six days after septal destruction (Nance et al., 1977). Although it is possible that septal destruction increases estrogen uptake by certain neurons, to our knowledge this possibility has not been tested. Septal lesions, however, have been reported to decrease brain serotonin levels (Heller et al., 1962) and catecholamine acti-vity (Heller and Moore, 1965; McGreer et al., 1969; Bernard et al., 1975). Since these neurochemicals presumably play a role in the regulation of lordosis behavior (Everitt et al., 1975; Meyerson et al., 1979), we have investigated the possible interaction between septal lesions, aminergic activity and the facilitation of lordosis behavior by EB. Although a serotoninergic system has been postulated to suppress lordosis behavior (Meyerson and Lewonder, 1970), the administration of 5-hydroxytryptophan (100 mg/Kg) failed to modify the heightened response of the septal lesioned rat to EB (Nance, unpublished observation). However, since serotonin may be more closely related to the behavioral action of P. (see Everitt et al., 1975), this observation is not surprising considering the observation that septal lesions facilitate the behavioral response to EB but not to P.

Since dopamine (DA) is also generally considered to be in-hibitory to lordosis behavior (Everitt et al., 1974, 1975), we administered d-amphetamine (1.0 mg/Kg), a catecholamine releaser, approximately one hour prior to behavioral testing on day four following three daily injections of 2 μg EB. This treatment elimi-nated the behavioral hyperresponsiveness to EB which had returned 24 hours later (Nance et al., 1977). Armed with this suggestion that the behavioral effectiveness of septal destruction may relate to an

224

alteration in aminergic activity, we undertook a more detailed study of the effects of three days of EB treatment on DA and norepinephrine (NE) turnover in sham-operated and septal lesioned females.

As shown in Table 1, we did not detect any effect of septal lesions or EB on NE turnover, although NE has been reported to facilitate female sexual behavior (Everitt et al., 1975). Similarly, in sham-operated rats there was no effect of EB on DA turnover, however, there was a general suppression of DA turnover in EB treated septal lesioned rats which reached statistical significance in two brain regions rich in dopaminergic terminals: the corpus striatum and the nucleus accumbens. It would appear from these results that the increased behavioral responsiveness of the septal lesioned animals could be due to an increase in the ability of EB to suppress the turnover of this behaviorally inhibitory neurotransmitter. Obviously this conclusion requires the assumption that the decreased DA turnover we observed reflects similar changes in brain regions directly involved in the regulation of lordosis behavior.

However, this simplistic interpretation appears to be contradicted by our data on the influence of EB treatment on the activity of glutamic acid decarboxylase (GAD) which is the rate limiting enzyme in the synthesis of gamma aminobutyric acid (GABA), a putative inhibitory neurotransmitter. In this case, the septal lesioned rats generally failed to respond to EB treatment, while intact animals exhibited a significant decrease in GAD activity in the region of dopaminergic cell bodies, i.e., the ventral tegmentum and substantia nigra (Table 1C). Thus, these data would at first suggest that in the case of GAD activity, it is the normal ovariectomized rat which displays hypersensitivity to EB.

However, data are available to suggest another explanation for the septal lesion effects, an explanation which takes into account the probable existence of complex interactions between central aminergic mechanisms. It is generally accepted that there exists a gabaminergic striato-nigral neuronal system which is inhibitory in nature (Kim et al., 1971; Precht and Yoshida, 1971), and similar inhibitory projections may exist for the mesolimbic dopaminergic neurons which have their cell bodies in the ventral tegmentum (Fuxe et al., 1975). Moreover, estrogen appears to reduce the efficacy of DA at the post- and/or presynaptic level (see Gordon et al., 1980). The effect of

Table 1: Effects of estradiol benzoate (EB) on catecholamine synthesis and glutamic acid decarboxylase activity in various brain areas of sham operated or septal lesioned ovariectomized rats *

	SHAM OPERATED		SEPTAL LESIONED	
	OIL	EB	OIL	EB
A. Dopamine Synthesis Rate (pmole/mg tissue/hr.)				
Striatum	23.19	20.38	25.86	13.11^a
Accumbens	17.17	16.55	16.63	11.10
Amygdala	0.64	0.81	0.55	0.22^a
B. Norepinephrine Synthesis Rate (pmole/mg tissue/hr.)				
Striatum	0.63	0.69	0.54	0.65
Accumbens	0.76	0.76	0.66	0.57
Amygdala	0.66	0.72	0.56	0.45
C. Glutamic Acid Decarboxylase Activity (nmole/mg hr.)				
Ventral Tegmentum	143±10	$101±5^{b,c}$	157±8	$162±6^b$
Substantia Nigra	375±24	$196±5^{b,c}$	437±10	$356±21^b$

* Data from Gordon et al. (1977)
a. Significantly different from that of both oil treated groups in same region based on rate constants
b. Significantly different from that of respective oil treated group
c. Significantly different from that of EB primed septal lesioned group

estrogen in reducing dopaminergic efficacy has been reported at the level of the pituitary gland in vitro (Raymond et al., 1978), circling behavior following entopeduncular lesions (Bedard et al., 1978), and the stereotyped behavior induced by apomorphine administration (Gordon et al., 1980).

On the basis of these data we have postulated the existence of a compensatory interrelationship between the dopaminergic and gaba-minergic systems. As the efficacy of DA is decreased by EB action, there may be a compensatory decrease in inhibitory GABA input on dopaminergic cell bodies. Thus we suggest that upon EB injection in the otherwise intact ovariectomized rat, DA efficacy is reduced but there is a compensatory fall in GAD activity in the regions of the DA cell bodies so that at the time of behavioral testing, the normal rat exhibits a significant decrease in GAD activity without a detectable alteration in DA activity, and the animal is essentially non-re-ceptive. The estrogen primed animal, however, can now respond to P so these changes in neurochemistry could underlie the ability of P to facilitate lordosis behavior at this time. In the septal lesioned rat, however, we propose that the compensatory response in GABA activity is altered by some unknown mechanism. Thus, upon EB administration, although DA efficacy is presumably reduced, there is no compensatory decrease in GABA input to the dopaminergic cell bodies and in the presence of this continued inhibitory input, there is a frank decrease in DA turnover, and the females are highly receptive.

If this hypothesis has any validity certain predictions can be made. Since we suggest that lordosis responding in the septal lesioned animal is high because there has been no compensatory decrease in the inhibitory gabaminergic input to dopaminergic neurons (and DA activity is significantly reduced), the local application of a GABA antagonist should increase DA activity and suppress lordosis behavior. As shown in Figure 2A, following the intranigral infusion of 5 μg picrotoxin, a GABA receptor blocker, lordosis behavior in EB-primed septal lesioned rats is acutely and transiently inhibited, as predicted.

On the other hand, if lordosis responsiveness in the intact animal primed only with EB is prevented because of a compensatory decrease in the inhibitory gabaminergic input to dopaminergic neurons, a pharmacologically induced increase in GABA activity should decrease DA and facilitate lordosis behavior. As shown in Figure 2B, this prediction was borne out when 3.0 μg hydrazino-proprionic acid, an indirect agonist of GABA since it inhibits GABA transaminase, was infused into the substantia nigra; the LQ of septum intact rats was significantly increased.

Although we attempted to identify drug induced changes in DA turnover as measured by striatal tyrosine hydroxylase activity, no significant differences were noted (McGinnis et al., 1980). However, striatal levels of homovanillic acid, one of the major metabolites of DA, were altered consistent with the model proposed. Thus, although this model is highly speculative, the data do support the view that: 1) DA turnover is modulated by a gabaminergic system; 2) EB may modulate this DA-GABA neuronal system during its facilitation of lordosis behavior; and 3) septal lesions disrupt this system.

At this point we should emphasize that the preceding behavioral and pharmacological studies on lordosis behavior were all conducted in ovariectomized rats on the fourth day after three days of priming

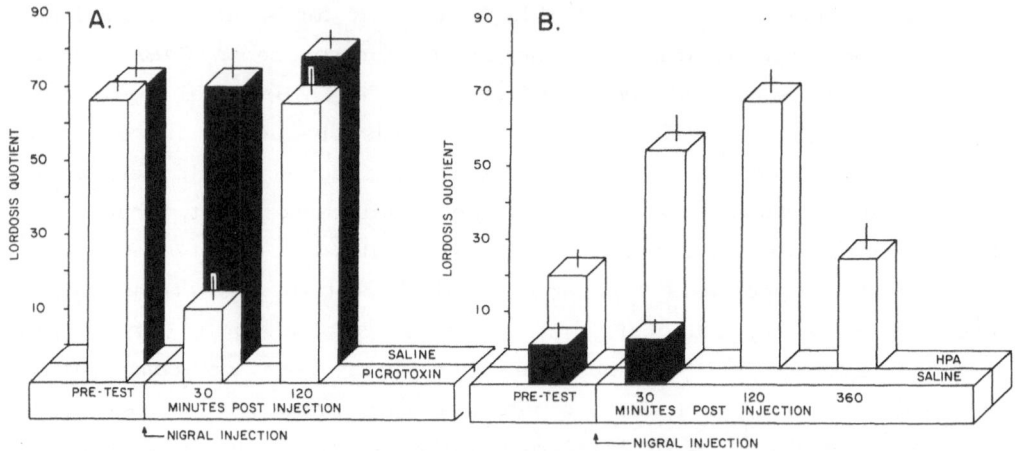

Figure 2: The influence of the intranigral infusion of drugs or saline on the mean lordosis quotient (+ standard error) of ovariectomized rats primed with 2 μg estradiol benzoate for three days. A, the influence of the infusion of 5 μg picrotoxin or saline in septal lesioned rats; B, the influence of the infusion of 3.0 μg hydrazinopropionic acid (HPA) in sham operated rats. Modified from McGinnis et al. (1980)

with EB, which is one experimental paradigm routinely used in this laboratory. However, lordosis can also be facilitated with another hormonal paradigm: a single injection of EB followed by the administration of P approximately 43 hours later with the behavioral tests conducted four-six hours later. Recently, we have used this second experimental paradigm to investigate another aspect of the possible interaction between EB, catecholamines and lordosis behavior. As shown below, we have come to the opposite conclusion: under certain conditions DA is clearly facilitatory to lordosis behavior.

In order to understand the important difference between these two paradigms, it is necessary to consider the temporal aspects of the facilitation of lordosis behavior by EB. In a study by Arai and Gorski (1968), which was recently reviewed in more modern terminology (Gorski, 1979a), we evaluated this question utilizing the anti-estrogen CN 55,945-27 (now CI-628). Although treatment with this anti-estrogen was effective in preventing behavioral facilitation by a single injection of EB, this drug had to be administered concomitantly with EB or within approximately 18 hours of steroid injection. When the anti-estrogen was given 24 hours after EB, it was not

228

effective in blocking lordosis behavior. However, in this same experiment, even though we could no longer block the behavioral action of EB after 24 hours, the response of the rat to P given 24 hours after EB was minimal. Given this information we postulated that there were at least two phases of EB action: an early phase which apparently is dependent on the uptake of estrogen, and a second or maturational phase which is independent of the continued presence of estrogen. Subsequent studies have confirmed this concept from several different approaches. There is a considerable latent period (approximately 18–24 hours) before lordosis behavior can be elicited (see McEwen et al., 1975; Feder et al., 1979; and Figure 4). Estradiol disappears from neuronal nuclei well before behavior is facilitated (McEwen et al., 1975). More recently it has been shown that estrogen induces cerebral receptors for P, and that the time course of this response is consistent with the prolonged latent period before behavior is actually facilitated (Blaustein and Feder, 1979). The latter observation, in particular, is consistent with the general-ly accepted view that the action of estrogen on the brain is mediated by genomic processes.

In the context of a complex and prolonged action of estrogen on the brain, only one early component of which may be dependent upon the actual presence of estrogen, it is clear that the preceding discussion relates to the very late phase of this process. Is there an interaction between EB and catecholamines during the early phase of estrogen action? To investigate this question we chose to use apomorphine, a DA agonist. Initially we confirmed the observation that DA is inhibitory to lordosis behavior when administered late in the course of estrogen action. Thus, the intraperitoneal injection of 1.5 or 3.0 mg apomorphine (but not less), when given 30 minutes prior to behavioral tests conducted 48 and five hours after the systemic injection of 5 µg EB and 0.5 mg P, respectively, essentially prevented lordosis behavior (Yanase and Gorski, unpublished ob-servations). Moreover, this action of apomorphine was significantly attenuated by injecting the DA receptor blockers pimozide (1.0 mg) or haloperidol (0.25 mg) two hours prior to apomorphine.

However, when apomorphine was injected simultaneously with EB, that is 48 hours prior to behavioral testing, 1.5 and 3.0 mg of this drug actually facilitated lordosis behavior (Figure 3)! An injection of 50 μg epinephrine (Epi) was similarly effective. The fact that there is a relatively narrow temporal window for this facilitatory action of these catecholamines is illustrated by the fact that apomorphine or Epi was effective in facilitating lordosis behavior only when given simultaneously with EB, or two or four hours later, but not when given two hours before, or more than six hours after EB. Although we have not yet had the opportunity to verify that these agents effectively altered central amine activity, the data clearly suggest that early in the course of estrogen action, DA as well as Epi, are facilitatory to subsequent lordosis behavior.

Since we believe that the mechanism of the behavioral facilitation by septal lesions involves the interaction between EB and aminergic activity, we have compared the possible role of pharmacological agents during the earliest phase of EB action in intact and septal lesioned ovariectomized rats. Figure 4 illustrates the

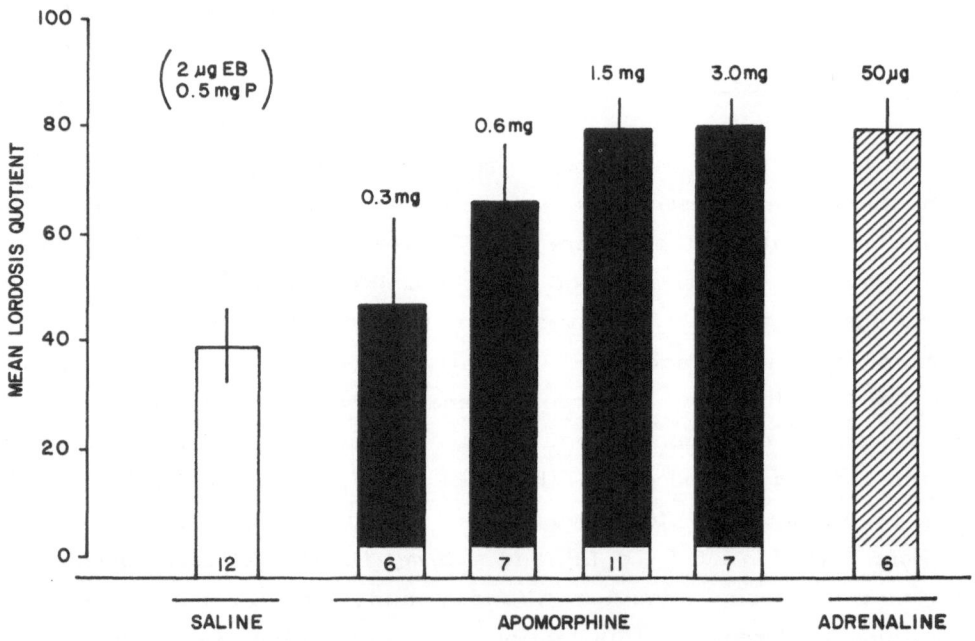

Figure 3: The facilitation of lordosis behavior produced by the administration of different doses of apomorphine or 50 μg epinephrine (adrenaline) simultaneously with the injection of 2 μg estradiol benzoate (EB). Progesterone (P; 0.5 mg) was injected 43 hours after EB and behavior tested 5 hours later. Yanase and Gorski, in preparation

difference in the time course of the facilitation of lordosis behavior in operated and control rats, the parameter we chose to investigate pharmacologically. In both groups of rats, the onset of lordosis behavior was maximal following the injection of 10 µg EB, but the septal lesioned rats clearly responded sooner.

Since we had shown that apomorphine or Epi facilitates lordosis behavior in intact rats when injected concomitantly with EB (see Figure 3), we examined the time course of the onset of lordosis responding in both sham-operated and septal lesioned rats under the same treatment regime. As shown in Figure 5, these drugs did accelerate the rate of development of the behavioral response to 5 µg EB in the intact animal. A similar effect was observed even when

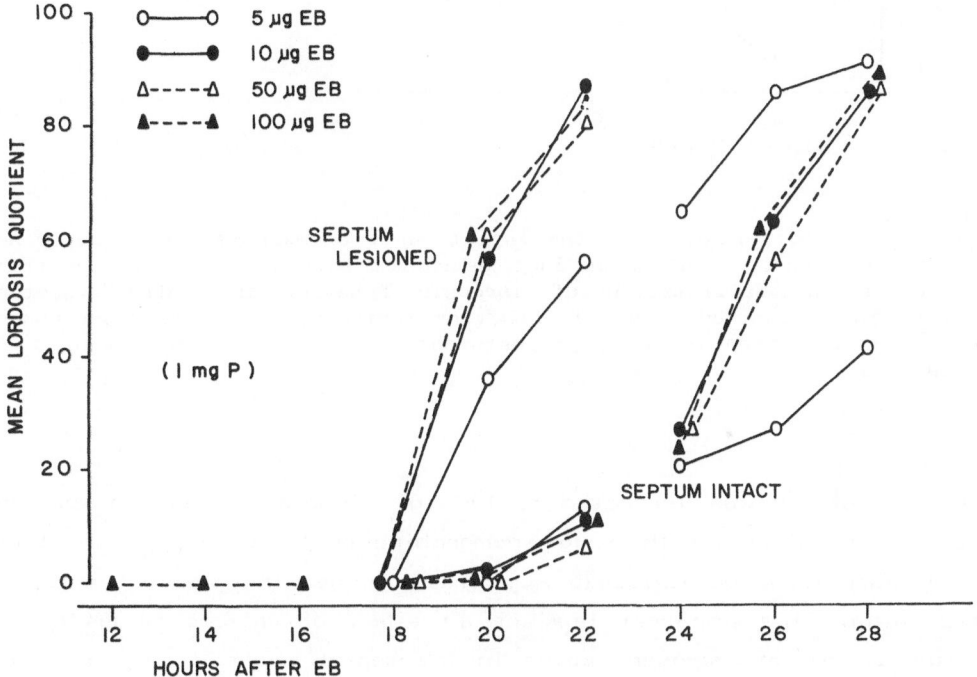

Figure 4: The influence of septal lesions on the time course of the facilitation in lordosis behavior produced by a single injection of different doses of estradiol benzoate (EB). In all cases 1 mg progesterone was administered four hours prior to behavioral testing. Yanase and Gorski, in preparation

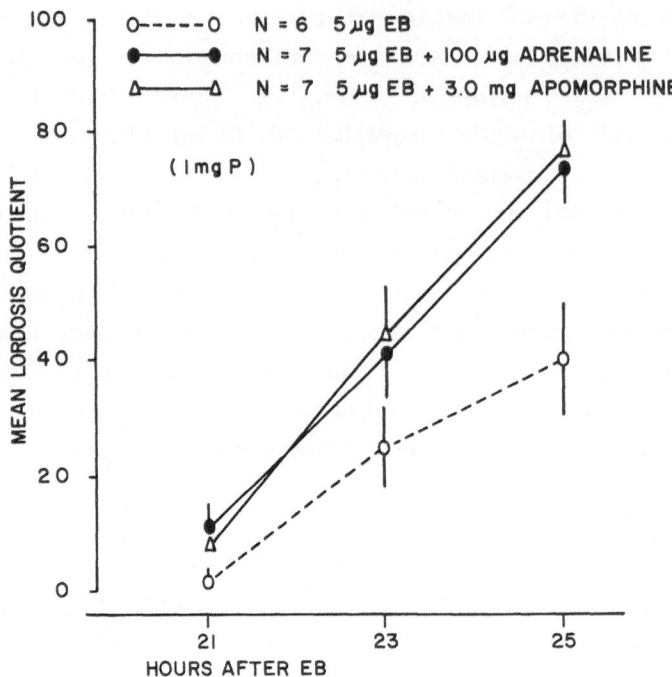

Figure 5: The influence of the injection of apomorphine or epinephrine (adrenaline) concomitant with 5 μg estradiol benzoate (EB) on the time course of the facilitation of lordosis behavior in control (septum intact) ovariectomized rats. All behavior tests were conducted four hours after the injection of 1 mg progesterone (P). Yanase and Gorski, in preparation

the dose of EB was increased to 100 μg. However, treatment of the septal lesioned rats with 3 mg apomorphine or 100 μg Epi at the time of EB administration failed to accelerate further the onset of lordosis responding. This apparent lack of an effect of catecholamines early in the course of estrogen action in the septal lesioned rat could be due to two facts: 1) catecholamines play no role in the onset of lordosis responsiveness in the septal lesioned rat, or 2) that the septal lesions alter aminergic activity such that the early phase of estrogen action is maximized.

To test these alternatives, we administered the receptor blocker, propanolol, the DA receptor blocker, pimozide, or tetra-benazine, a depletor of catecholamines, before the injection of EB.

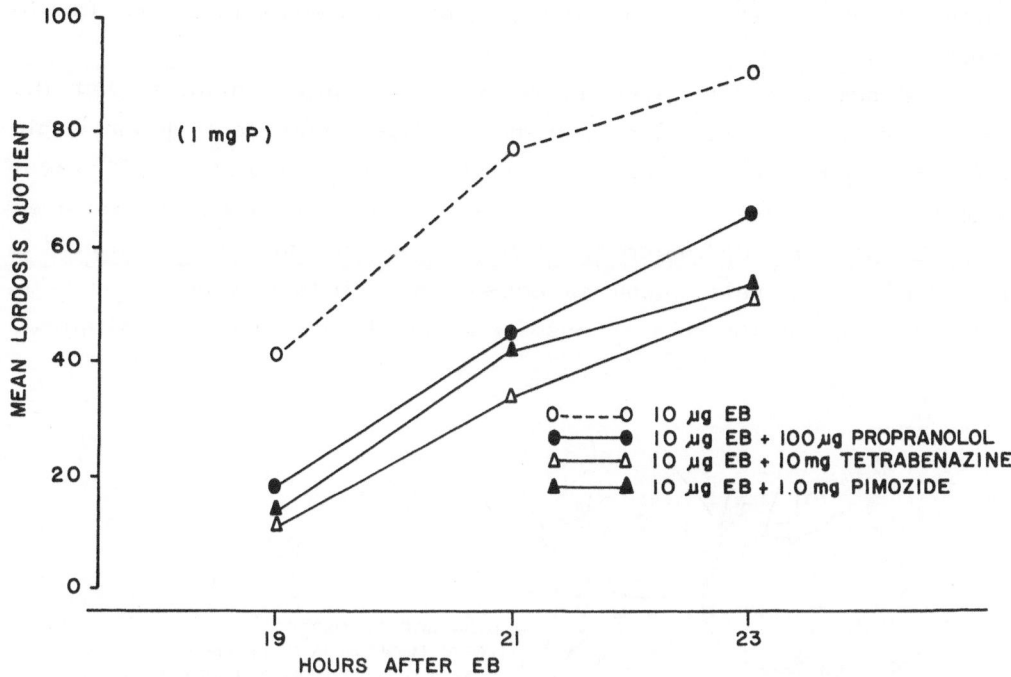

Figure 6: The influence of amine-active drugs administered prior to the injection of estradiol benzoate (EB) on the time course of the facilitation of lordosis behavior by this steroid in septal lesioned ovariectomized rats. All behavior tests were conducted four hours after the injection of 1 mg progesterone (P). Yanase and Gorski, in preparation

As shown in Figure 6, these drugs dramatically slowed the rate of onset of sexual receptivity in septal lesioned rats. These results support the view that in the septal lesioned animal, the early facilitatory action of catecholamines has been maximized as a consequence of septal destruction. In contrast, similar treatment of the septum intact rat with these same drugs was totally without effect (Yanase and Gorski, unpublished observation).

Thus, the fact that apomorphine accelerates the onset of sexual receptivity in the intact but not in the septal lesioned rat, whereas inhibitors of catecholamines delay the precocious onset of receptivity in the septal lesioned rat without any effect in the control animal, is clearly consistent with the view that septal destruction has altered aminergic activity of the remaining brain, such that the

233

early actions of EB in promoting lordosis responsiveness are facilitated.

In summary, we have presented data which suggest that the nature of the interactions between estrogen and central aminergic systems which appear to play a role in the regulation of sexual receptivity, depends upon the phase during the action of estrogen when drugs are administered. Within the first four hours after the injection of EB, catecholamines appear to facilitate lordosis behavior both in terms of its rate of onset and the final LQ that is attained.

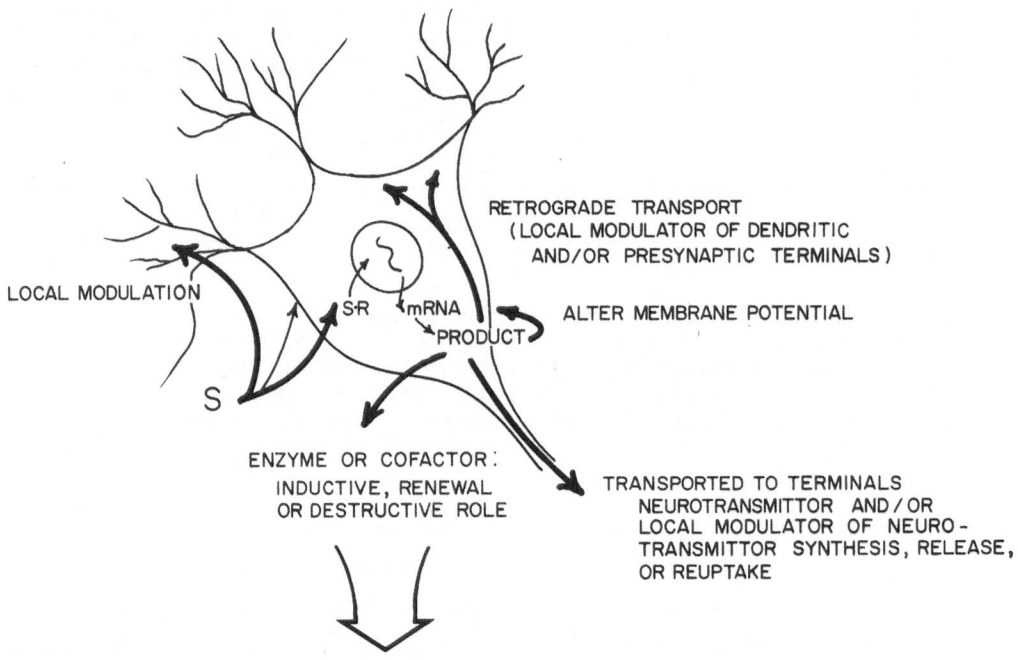

Figure 7: Highly schematic representation of possible mechanisms of action of gonadal steroid(s) in the adult brain. S-R, steroid-receptor complex. Reprinted from Gorski (1979b)

Later in the course of behavioral facilitation, at the time when P is effective, DA in particular exerts an inhibitory action on the expression of lordosis behavior. Study of the septal lesioned rat has uncovered a possible interaction between gabaminergic and dopaminergic neural systems, at least at the time of behavioral testing. Currently we have no information whether or not the gabaminergic system plays any role in the early phase of estrogen action. Study of this preparation has further shown that septal destruction clearly alters aminergic mechanisms within the surviving nervous tissue, and that these alterations may contribute to the observed behavioral hypersensitivity to estrogen.

It remains to be determined how these diverse neurochemical processes bring about the integrated response of lordosis. Figure 7 schematically represents possible modes of action of steroids on nerve cells. We may suggest that the early action of estrogen which presumably alters genomic activity could be influenced by the biogenic amines, perhaps by a membrane receptor mediated intracellular interaction with the uptake of steroid and/or the translocation of the steroid-recepetor complex into the nucleus. At this time, the catecholamines appear to be facilitatory to behavioral receptivity. Subsequently, at the time lordosis behavior can be facilitated by the action of P, at least in part because of the apparant induction of P receptors, the influence of DA is clearly inhibitory. It may be that at this time, the interaction between aminergic activity and the final neural substrate for lordosis takes place exclusively at the level of the terminals of neurons previously activated by estrogen. The present studies emphasize that future investigations of the facilitation of lordosis behavior must take time into account; clearly the interactions between aminergic systems and estrogen vary during the course of the facilitation of lordosis behavior.

Acknowledgement

The financial support of USPHS Grant HD 01182, NSF Grant BNS 78-20025 and the Ford Foundation is gratefully acknowledged.

235

References

Arai Y, Gorski RA (1968) Effect of anti-estrogen on steroid induced sexual receptivity in ovariectomized rats. Physiol and Behav 3:351-353.

Bedard P, Dankova J, Boucher R, Langelier P (1978) Effect of estrogen on apomorphine-induced circling behavior in the rat. Can J Physiol Pharmac 56:538-541.

Bernard BK, Berchek JR, Yutzey DA (1975) Alterations in brain monoaminergic functioning associated with septal lesion induced hyperreactivity. Phar Biochem Behav 3:121-126.

Blaustein JD, Feder HH (1979) Cytoplasmic progestin-receptors in guinea pig brain: Characteristics and relationship to the induction of sexual behavior. Brain Res 169:481-497.

Everitt BJ, Fuxe K, Hökfelt T, Jonsson B (1975) Pharmacological and biochemical studies on the role of monoamines in the control by hormones of sexual receptivity in the female rat. J Comp Physiol Psychol 89:556-572.

Everitt BJ, Fuxe K, Hökfelt T (1974) Inhibitory role of dopamine and 5-hydroxytryptamine in sexual behavior of female rats. Eur J Pharmac 29:187-191.

Feder HH, Landau IT, Walker WA (1979) Anatomical and biochemical substrates of the actions of estrogens and antiestrogens on brain tissues that regulate female sex behavior of rodents. In: Beyer C (ed) Endocrine control of sexual behavior. Raven Press, New York (Comprehensive endocrinology series), pp.317-340.

Fuxe K, Hökfelt T, Ljungdahl A, Agnati L, Johansson O, Perez de la Mora M (1975) Evidence for an inhibitory gabergic control of the meso-limbic dopamine neurons: Possibility of improving treatment of schizophrenia by combined treatment with neuroleptics and gabergic drugs. Med Biol 53:177-183.

Gordon JH, Nance DM, Wallis CJ, Gorski RA (1977) Effects of estrogen on dopamine turnover, glutamic acid decarboxylase activity and lordosis behavior in septal lesioned female rats. Brain Res Bull 2:341-346.

Gordon JH, Gorski RA, Borison RL, Diamond BI (1980) Postsynaptic efficacy of dopamine: Possible suppression by estrogen. Pharm Biochem Behav 12:515-518.

Gorski RA (1974) The neuroendocrine regulation of sexual behavior. In: Newton G, Riesen AH (eds) Advances in Psychobiology, Vol II. John Wiley & Sons, New York, pp.1-58.

Gorski RA (1976) The possible neural sites of hormonal facilitation of sexual behavior in the female rat. Psychoneuroendocrinology 1:371-387.

Gorski RA (1979a) The nature of hormone action in the brain. In: Hamilton TH, Clark JH, Sadler WA (eds) Ontogeny of receptors and mode of action of reproductive hormones, Raven Press, New York, pp.371-392.

Gorski RA (1979b) The neuroendocrinology of reproduction: an overview. Biol Reprod 20:111-127.

Heller A, Moore RY (1965) Effect of central nervous system lesions on brain monoamines in the rat. J Pharmac exp Ther 150:1-9.

Heller A, Harvey JA, Moore RY (1962) A demonstration of a fall in brain serotonin following central nervous system lesions in the rat. Biochem Pharmacol 11:859-866.

Kim JS, Bak IJ, Hanler R, Okada Y (1971) Role of γ-aminobutyric acid (GABA) in the extrapyramidal motor system. 2. Some evidence for the existence of a type of GABA-rich strionigral neurons. Expl Brain Res 14:95-104.

Loy R, Milner TA (1980) Sexual Dimorphism in extent of axonal sprouting in rat hippocampus. Science 208:1282-1284.

McEwen BS, Pfaff DW, Chaptal C, Luine VN (1975) Brain cell nuclear retention of H^3-estradiol doses able to promote lordosis: temporal and regional aspects. Brain Res 86:155-161.

McGinnis MY, Gordon JH, Gorski RA (1980) Influence of γ-aminobutyric acid on lordosis behavior and dopamine activity in estrogen spayed female rat. Brain Res 184:179-191.

McGreer EG, Wade JA, Terao A, Jung E (1969) Amine synthesis in various brain regions with caudate or septal lesions. Expl Neurol 24:277-284.

Meyerson BJ, Lewander T (1970) Serotonin synthesis inhibition and estrous behavior in female rats. Life Sci 9:661-671.

Meyerson BJ, Palis A, Sietnieks A (1979) Hormone-monoamine interactions and sexual behavior. In: Beyer C (ed) Endocrine control of sexual behavior, Raven Press, New York (Comprehensive endocrinology series) pp.389-404.

Moralí G, Beyer C (1979) Neuroendocrine control of mammalian estrous behavior. In: Beyer C (ed) Endocrine control of sexual behavior. Raven Press, New York (Comprehensive endocrinology series) pp.33-75.

Nance DW, Shryne J, Gorski RA (1974) Septal lesions: Effects on lordosis behavior and pattern of gonadotropin release. Horm and Behav 5:73-81.

Nance DW, Shryne J, Gorski RA (1975) Effects of septal lesions on behavioral sensitivity of female rats to gonadal hormones. Horm and Behav 6:59-64.

Nance DW, Shryne JE, Gordon JH, Gorski RA (1977) Examination of some factors that control the effects of septal lesions on lordosis behavior. Pharm Biochem Behav 6:227-234.

Precht W, Yoshida M (1971) Blockage of caudate-evoked inhibition of neurons in the substantia nigra by picrotoxin. Brain Res 32:229-233.

Raisman G (1969) Neuronal plasticity in the septal nuclei of the adult rat. Brain Res 14:24-48.

Raymond V, Beaulieu M, Labrie F, Boissier J (1978) Potent antidopaminergic activity of estradiol at the pituitary level on prolactin release. Science 200:1173-1174.

Sakuma Y, Pfaff DW (1979) Mesencephalic mechanisms for integration of female reproductive behavior in the rat. Am J Physiol 237:R285-R290.

Sex Hormone Dependent Brain Differentiation and Sexual Behavior

G. Dörner, Berlin

As early as 1938, a remarkable observation was reported by Vera Dantchakoff, which was later confirmed by Phoenix and coworkers (1959). Female guinea pigs, androgenized prenatally, exhibited increased male and decreased female behavior in adulthood. On the basis of these results, Phoenix and his coworkers distinguished an early organization period and a postpubertal activation period. Grady and Phoenix (1963) and Harris (1963) then reported that male rats orchidectomized shortly after birth showed especially strong female sexual behavior when treated with estrogen in adulthood. Similar findings were obtained in adult male rats which had been treated with anti-androgen during perinatal life (Neumann and Elger, 1966). All these observations pointed to the significance of the sex hormone level during a critical differentiation phase for the development of sexual behavior.

During the last 12 years, the following findings were obtained in our laboratories on sexual differentiation of the brain (Dörner, 1976, 1979):

1. Male rats castrated on the day of birth showed predominantly heterotypical behavior, i.e., a significant preference of sexual responsiveness to male partners, following estrogen or even androgen substitution in adulthood. In other words, genetic males exposed to an androgen deficiency during sexual differentiation of the brain, but normal or approximately normal androgen levels in adulthood were sexually excited preferentially by partners of the same sex.

2. The higher the androgen level during the differentiation

phase, the stronger was the male and the weaker the female sexual behavior during the postpubertal functional phase, irrespective of the genetic sex. Even a complete inversion of sexual behavior was observed in male and female rats following androgen deficiency in males and androgen excess in females during sex-specific brain differentiation.

3. The permanent changes of sexual behavior were associated with permanent structural and/or chemical changes in discrete brain regions controlling sexual behavior and/or gonadotropin secretion (sexual dimorphism of the brain).

4. In the male rats castrated on the day of birth, a strong positive estrogen feedback effect on LH secretion could be induced in a similar way as in normal females, but not in neonatally androgenized females. Thus, a strong positive estrogen feedback effect appears to be only evocable in adulthood if there existed a low androgen level during brain differentiation.

5. A positive estrogen feedback effect on LH release could also be elicited in homosexual men, in contrast to heterosexual and bisexual men. These findings suggest that homosexual men may possess, at least in part, a predominantly female-differentiated brain due to androgen deficiency during brain differentiation.

In view of our experimental and clinical data, the following hypothesis was deduced: An androgen deficiency occurring in genetic males during a critical period of brain organization gives rise to predominantly female differentiation of the brain. The predominantly female-differentiated brain is then activated postpubertally by an approximately normal androgen level leading to homosexual behavior.

In genetic females, the results of animal experiments obtained in various species were supported by some clinical findings which suggest that an androgen excess occurring during a critical period of brain differentiation can predispose to the development of hypo-, bi- or homosexual behavior in adult life (Dörner, 1979).

Thus in transsexual women with homosexual behavior, we could only evoke a weak or at best moderate positive estrogen feedback action on LH release as compared to the evocability of a strong estrogen feedback action found in normal heterosexual women (Dörner et al., 1976). Seyler et al. (1978a,b) then reported that the LH response to LRH after estrogen-priming also differed markedly in transsexual and homosexual women from that in heterosexual women. The LH response to LRH could not be clearly enhanced by estrogen-priming in transsexual and homosexual females, in contrast to heterosexual females.

Schwartz and Money (1976) reported on young women with adrenogenital syndrome, i.e., with an androgen excess in prenatal life, who were diagnosed and hormonally corrected from early infancy. They were delayed in establishing dating, romantic and erotic interests. Most of all, they showed a significantly increased rate of awareness of bisexuality in fantasy, with or without actual experience. These findings were also attributed to a possible delayed-action effect of excess androgenization on the foetal brain.

However, neurotransmitters – as well as sex hormones – appear to represent not only transient activators but even organizers of the brain. Thus male sexual activity was permanently decreased in neonatally pargylinized, but permanently increased in neonatally pyridostigminized rats. These permanent behavioral changes that were produced by psychotrophic drugs, which are known to affect neurotransmitter metabolism in the brain, were associated with permanent structural and biochemical changes in discrete regions of the brain. (Dörner, 1979).

According to these data, abnormal concentrations and/or turnover rates of neurotransmitters apparently produced by psychotrophic drugs during brain differentiation may act as teratogens. Similar teratogenic effects may be induced by abnormal neurotransmitter concentration and/or turnover rates produced by abnormal levels of sex hormones as well as by abnormal psychosocial influences, since both were found to affect neurotransmitter metabolism during brain differentiation. Hence, the effects of sex hormones and of the psychosocial environment on differentiation and function of the brain represent rather supplements than alternatives. Both appear to be mediated by neurotransmitter (Dörner, 1980).

However, the findings obtained in human males with Imperato-McGinley's syndrome suggest that prenatal testosterone levels may be even more important for sexual differentiation of the brain than postnatal psychosocial influences. Thus, Imperto-McGinley et al. (1977) described male pseudohermaphrodites born with ambiguity of the external genitalia. Biochemical evaluation revealed

240

normal testosterone levels, but a marked decrease in plasma di-hydrotestosterone levels due to 5α-reductase deficiency. The decrease of dihydrotestosterone in utero resulted in incomplete masculinization of the external genitalia. Thus, the affected males were born with marked ambiguity of the external genitalia, and were therefore considered and raised as girls. Psychosexual orientation, however, was unequivocally male. They considered themselves as males and had a libido directed toward females. Despite being reared as females, almost all of them even changed gender identity at the time of puberty. Hence, testosterone exposure in utero appears to be most important for the development of a male sex drive, male sexual orientation and even male gender identity.

However, prenatal psychosocial influences should also be regarded as possible etiogenetic factors in the development of sexual deviations. Thus Ingeborg Ward (1977) reported that prenatal stress in male rats demasculinized and feminized sexual behavior potentials in adult life. Since similar findings were obtained in male rats castrated on the day of birth, we have measured the plasma testosterone levels in such prenatally stressed males, i.e., in male fetuses and newborns following maternal stress between day 14 and 21 of gestation. As shown in Figure 1, the testosterone level was found to be significantly decreased, in fact, in these prenatally stressed males during prenatal and early postnatal life as compared to non-stressed control males (Stahl et al., 1978; Dörner, 1979).

Most recently, we have observed predominantly heterotypical, i.e., homosexual behavior, in prenatally stressed male rats after castration plus estrogen treatment in adulthood, whereas prenatally non-stressed but later equally treated males displayed heterosexual behavior (Götz and Dörner, in press). Hence, prenatal stress can predispose to the development of homosexual behavior in males.

In this context, it should be mentioned that in rats estrogens activate predominantly female behavior in animals with a female-differentiated brain, but predominantly male behavior in those with a male-differentiated brain. By contrast, in primates not estrogens but only androgens activate male behavior in subjects with a male-differentiated brain, whereas androgens activate – even stronger than estrogens – female behavior in subjects with a female-differentiated brain. Thus it is possible that a predominantly female-differ-

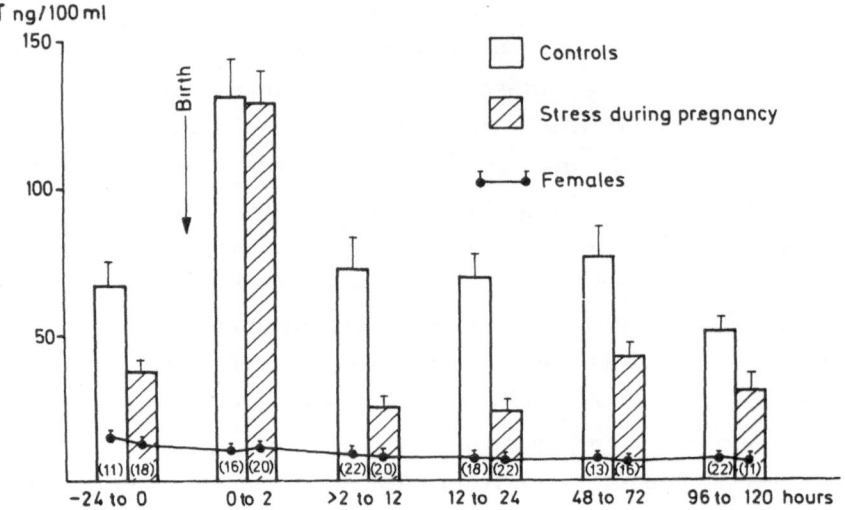

Figure 1: Plasma testosterone (T) levels of rats in pre- and early postnatal life (means ± SEM). The mother animals were stressed by restraint and illumination three times daily for 45 minutes between days 14 and 21 of gestation

entiated brain in prenatally stressed male primates may be activated in adulthood by normal endogenous testosterone levels to predominantly female-like, i.e., homosexual behavior.

In view of these data, a retrospective study was carried out to answer the question whether stressful maternal life events occurring during pregnancy may have irreversibly affected sexual differentiation of the brain in men who were born in Germany during or shortly after the stressful period of World War II. As shown in Figure 2, out of about 800 homosexual males highly significantly more homosexuals were born during the stressful war and early post-war period than in the years before or after World War II (Dörner et al., 1980). These findings suggest that stressful maternal life events, if occurring during pregnancy may represent, in fact, an etiogenetic factor for the development of sexual deviations in the male offspring.

In addition, 72 bi- or homosexual men as well as 72 hetero-sexual men of similar age were asked for maternal stressful events that may have been occurred during their prenatal life. As demonstrated in Figure 3, a highly significantly increased incidence.

242

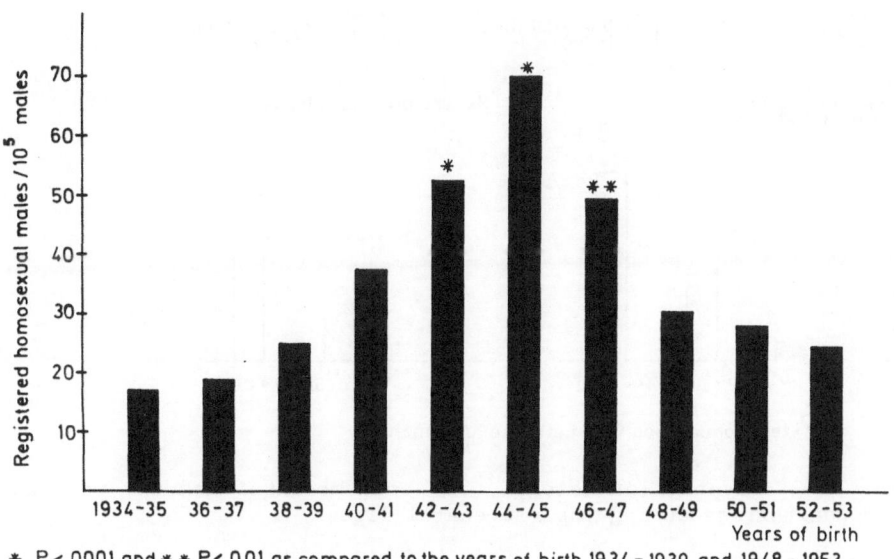

Figure 2: Relative frequency of homosexual males born in Germany (or GDR) before, during or after World War II (n = 794)

of prenatal maternal stress was found in bisexual and, in particular, in homosexual men as compared to heterosexual men (Dörner et al., in preparation). About 1/3 of the homosexual men reported to have been exposed to severe maternal stress, such as bereavement, reputation by the partner, rape or severe anxiety - and about an additional 1/3 to moderate maternal stress during their prenatal life. On the other hand, none of the heterosexual men were found to have been exposed to severe and less than 10% to moderate maternal stress during their prenatal life. These data also indicate that prenatal maternal stress may represent a risk factor for the etiogenesis of sexual deviations in later life.

References

Dantchakoff V (1938) Rôles des hormones dans les manifestations des instincts sexuals. Compt Rend Acad Sci Paris 206:945-947.
Dörner G (1976) Hormones and brain differentiation. Elsevier Scientific Publishing Company, Amsterdam-Oxford-New York.

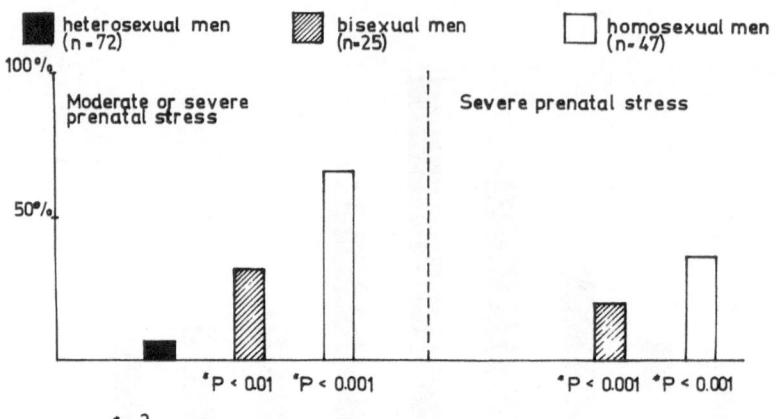

Figure 3: Percentage of hetero-, bi- or homosexual men who were exposed to maternal stress during their prenatal life

Dörner G (1979) Psychoneuroendocrine aspects of brain development and reproduction. In: Zichella L, Pancheri P (eds) Psychoneuroendocrinology in reproduction, Elsevier/North-Holland Biomedical Press, Amsterdam-Oxford, pp.43-54.

Dörner G (1980) Neurotransmitters as possible mediators of brain development. XI. International Congress of the International Society of Psychoneuroendocrinology, Florence, June 16-20, 1980, Elsevier/North-Holland Biomedical Press, Amsterdam-New York-Oxford.

Dörner G, Rohde W, Seidel K, Haas W, Schott G (1976) On the evocability of a positive oestrogen feedback action on LH secretion in transsexual men and women. Endokrinologie 67:20-25.

Dörner G, Geier TH, Ahrens L, Krell L, Münx G, Sieler H, Kittner E, Müller H (1980) Prenatal stress a possible aetiogenetic factor of homosexuality in human males. Endokrinologie, in press.

Götz F, Dörner G (1980) Homosexual behaviour in prenatally stressed male rats after castration and oestrogen treatment in adulthood. Endokrinologie, in press.

Grady KL, Phoenix CHH (1963) Hormonal determinants of mating behavior; the display of feminine behavior by adult male rats castrated neonatally. Amer Zoologist 3:482-483.

Harris GW (1963) Castration of the new-born male rat and lack of differentiation of the brain. J Physiol (London) 169:117-118.

Imperato-McGinley J, Peterson RE, Gautier T, Sturla E (1979) Male pseudohermaphroditism secondary to 5α-reductase deficiency - a model for the role of androgens in both the development of the male phenotype and the evolution of a male gender identity. J Steroid Biochem 11:637-645.

Phoenix CHH, Goy RW, Gerall AA, Young WC (1959) Organizing action of prenatally administered testosterone propionate on the tissues mediating mating behavior in the female guinea pig. Endocrinology 65:369-382.

Schwartz M, Money J (1976) Pair-bonding experience of 26 early treated adrenogenital females ages 17-27. International Congress of

Sexology, Montreal, October 28–31, 1976, Abstract No. 94.

Seyler LE Jr., Canalis E, Spare S, Reichlin S (1978a) Abnormal gonadotropin secretory responses to LRH in transsexual women after diethylstilbestrol priming. J Clin Endocrinol Metab 47:176–183.

Seyler LE Jr., Graze K, Canalis E, Spare S, Reichlin S (1978b) Abnormal gonadotropin responses to LRH during diethylstilbestrol treatment of homosexual and transsexual women. Third International Congress of Medical Sexology, Rome, October 25–28, 1978, Abstracts, p.86.

Stahl F, Götz F, Poppe I, Amendt P, Dörner G (1978) Pre- and early postnatal testosterone levels in rat and human. In: Dörner G, Kawakami M (eds) Hormones and brain development Elsevier/North-Holland Biomedical Press, Amsterdam-New York-Oxford, pp.99–109.

Ward IL (1977) Exogenous androgen activates female behavior in noncopulating, prenatally stressed male rats. J Comp Physiol Psychol 91:465–471.

Critical Evaluation of the Current Concept of Brain Differentiation – Relevance for the Primate Brain

F. Neumann and W. Elger, Berlin West and Bergkamen

It is not our intention to review the topic of hormonal brain differentiation. Some other scientists in the audience would be much more competent for doing this.

We became interested in this field around 1964/65, when we investigated the effect of a potent antiandrogen – cyproterone acetate – on male brain differentiation (Neumann und Elger, 1965; Neumann et al., 1967).

At the beginning, we would like to present a few of our own data. At that time we thought that the use of antiandrogens to study androgen-dependent differentiation processes would offer some advantages as compared with prenatal castration of male fetuses.

1. The animals are left intact. Androgen-substitution in the adult animals was not necessary. It was also not clear at that time if other hormones or substances derived from the testis, which are not affected by antiandrogens, could also influence differentiation processes of the brain.

2. It is even now under discussion, whether differentiation of certain brain centers in rodents starts only after birth or already before birth.

With the use of cyproterone acetate we were able to inhibit the androgen action at any time before and/or after birth.

3. As is known, cyproterone acetate influences very effectively somatic sexual differentiation, differentiation of the genital tract and of the external genitals, leading to the development, among other disturbances, of a vagina in males (Elger, 1966; Neumann et al., 1966, 1970). After castration and ovarian implantation in the adulthood we could very easily check by the vaginal smear pattern, whether these animals show cyclic changes or not.

Figure 1 shows an adult feminized male rat with a well developed vagina. One week following the ovarian implantation (when vaginal smears begun) most of the smears indicated a condition of estrus which generally remained for several days. Thereafter, cyclic changes were noted in some animals, but not in all of them. The findings in the smears of three feminized rats are shown in Figure 2.

By way of comparison in Figure 2 C_1 shows the cyclic changes in the vaginal epithelium of a normal castrated female rat after implantation of an ovary and C_f shows the vaginal cycle of a normal female animal. The following becomes evident: the cyclic changes in the first two feminized animals (Figure 2, Fm_1 and Fm_2) are clearly recognizable. The cycles are not as regular as in the female controls and frequently incomplete, i.e., only rarely is a distinct diestrus reached. As to the length, only a few cycles are noted that last 4 to 5 days as in normal females.

Figure 3-5 show the vaginal smear pattern of one feminized animal taken on consecutive days. This was the animal showing the most pronounced cyclic changes.

From these studies we could already conclude that ovulation did occur. Macroscopically, the ovarian transplants of feminized animals looked different, compared with the ovarian transplants of castrated normal males. This is shown in Figs. 6 and 7.

Histological examinations of the ovaries gave proof that some of the feminized animals had ovulated and old and new corpora lutea were present (see Figs. 8 and 9).

We also investigated the sexual behavior of intact feminized animals without ovarian implantation. Such animals behaved bi-sexually. They still showed male behavioral pattern, but also female behavior, when placed together with a normal male. This is in agreement with investigations performed by Dr. Dörner and his group (Dörner, 1974a). He also could induce female differentiated animals.

After ovarian implantation there was a good correlation between the cyclic state and female sexual behavior. During estrus they were mounted (Figure 10), during diestrus the animals showed defence reactions against the male (Figure 11).

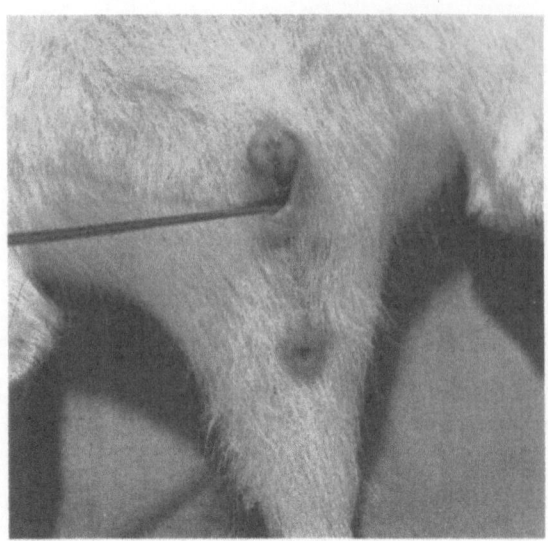

Figure 1:   External genital organs of "feminized" male rats (mother treated with 10 mg cyproterone acetate per day from the 13th to the 22nd day of gestation.   Treatment of new-born rats was continued for 3 weeks after delivery with 0.3 mg cyproterone acetate per day subcutaneously). Note the presence of a vagina

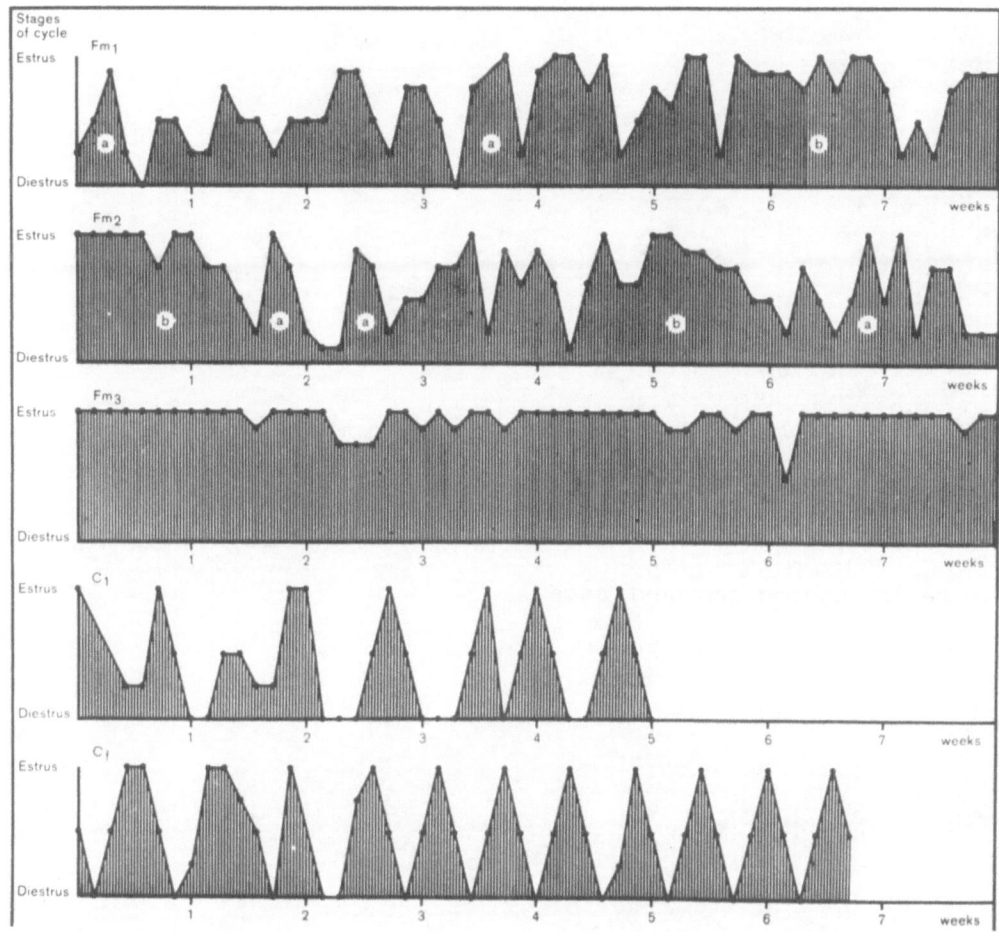

Figure 2: Cyclic changes in vaginal smears of feminized castrated male rats after implantation of ovarian tissue

Fm_1–Fm_3 = castrated feminized males with ovarian graft

C_1 = castrated female control with ovarian graft

C_f = normal female control

a = normal cycles

b = prolonged cycles

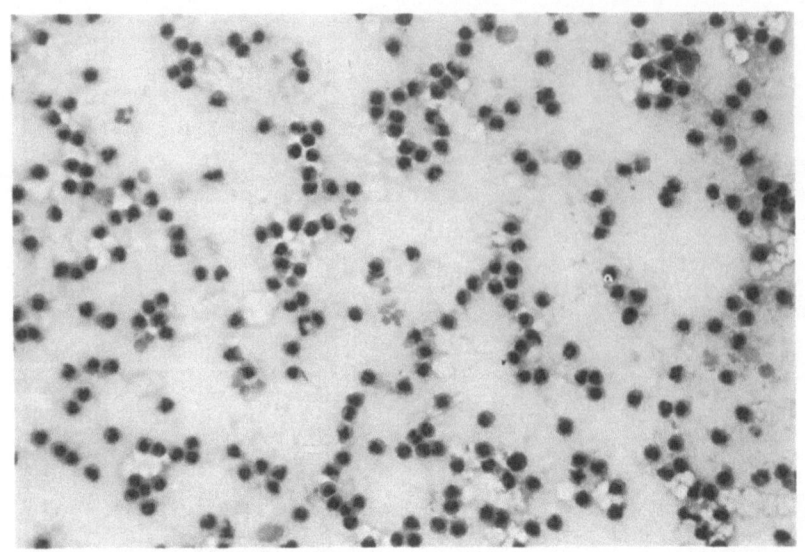

Figure 3:   Legend see next page

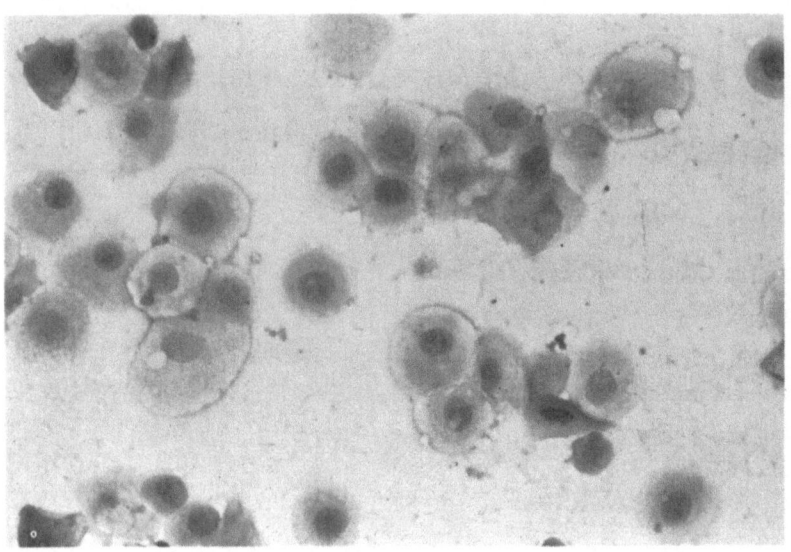

Figure 4:   Legend see next page

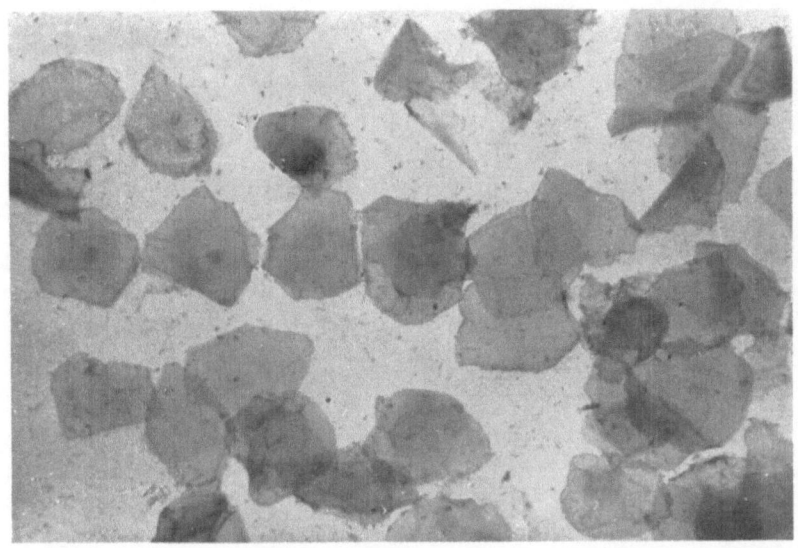

Figures 3 - 5:   Vaginal smears of a castrated feminized male rat with an ovarian graft, made on consecutive days

    Figure 3:   Diestrus,

    Figure 4:   Proestrus,

    Figure 5:   Estrus

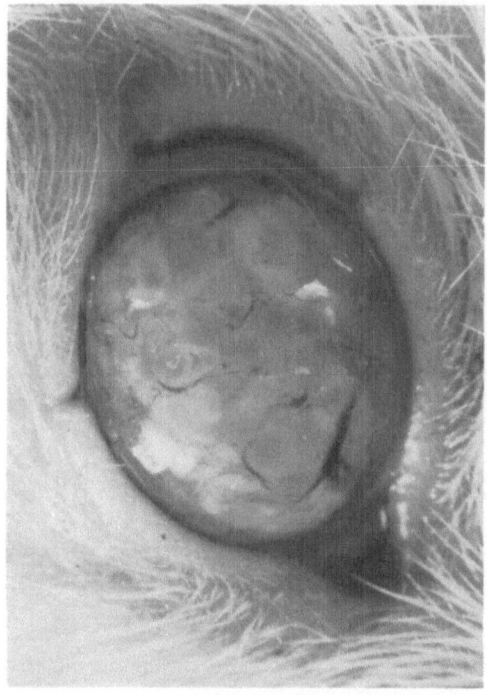

Figure 6:   Legend see next page

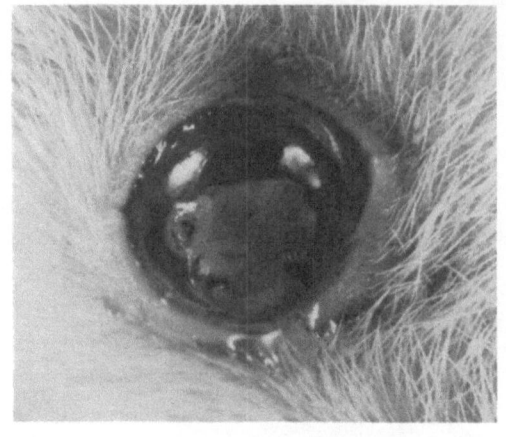

Figure 7

Figures 6 and 7: Ovarian transplants. Figure 6: Castrated male
Figure 7: Feminized male

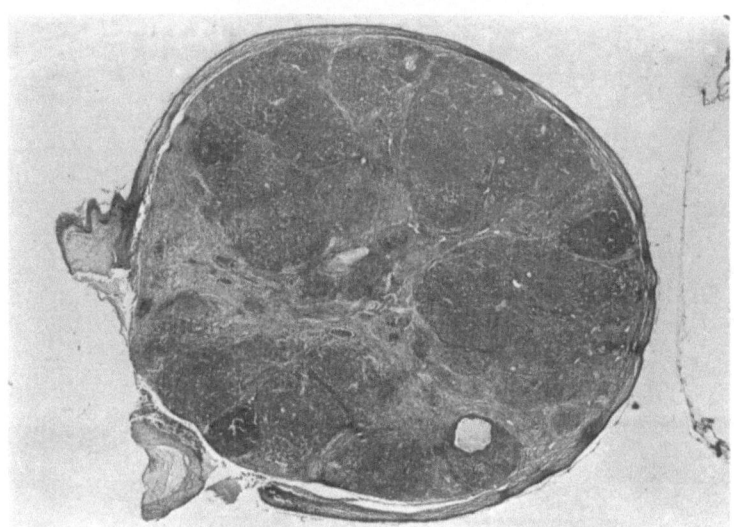

Figure 8:   Legend see next page

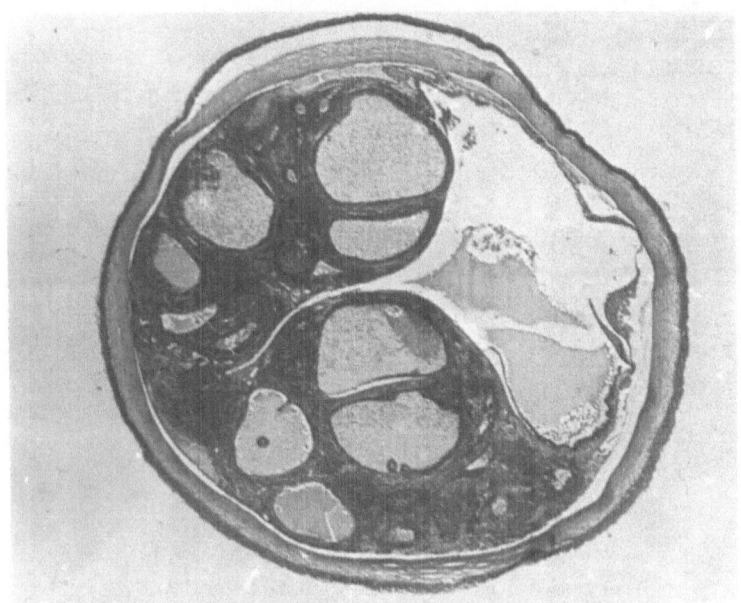

Figure 9

Figures 8 and 9: Histology of ovarian transplants

    Figure 8: Grown in a feminized male (fresh and old corpora lutea are present)

    Figure 9: Grown in a castrated male (follicles only have developed)

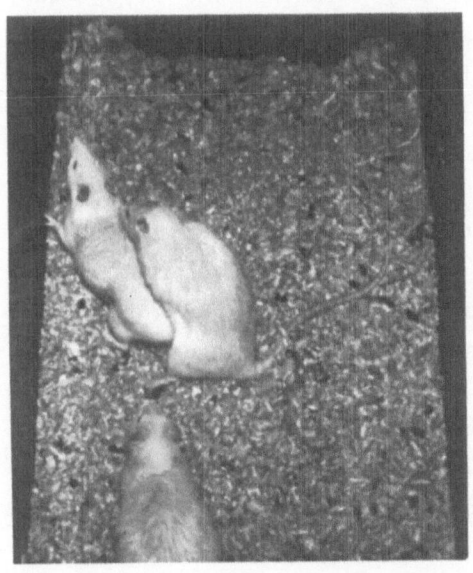

Figure 10: Legend see next page

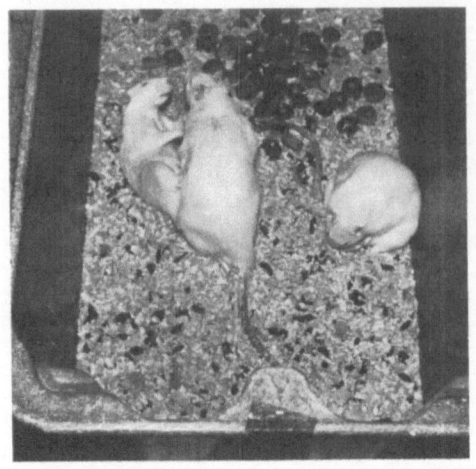

Figures 10 and 11: Mounting behavior of feminized male rats with ovarian grafts

Figure 10: Mounting attempt of the male is answered with lordosis reaction by the feminized male

Figure 11: Mounting attempt of the male is answered with defense reaction by the feminized male

Figure 11

At that time, the interpretation of these results and the results of many other research groups was very simple. It had been concluded that

1. Androgens or – as we now know – probably estrogens (for review see Brown-Grant, 1974; McEwen, 1978; McEwen et al., 1977) inhibit the development of a certain hypothalamic center, which is responsible for the cyclic release of LH.

2. Androgens or estrogens respectively establish the development of a center within the hypothalamus, which is in one way or another responsible for male sexual behavior in adulthood.

3. Without any hormonal impulse, brain differentiation occurs in the female direction. This aspect is questionable because several research groups believe now that for normal female brain differentiation estrogens are required here (for review see Döhler, 1978; Döhler et al., 1976).

In the meantime we know that in the primate and in the human, such a brain center, responsible for cyclic release in LH, does not exist. In this regard, the rat seems to be organized more complicated than the primate. This needs no further comment, because everybody is aware of the fascinating studies, done by Dr. Knobil and his group in Pittsburgh (for review see Knobil, 1974).

I will also mention another study performed at the Oregon Primate Research Center by Goy and Resko (1972). Virilized monkeys showed cyclicity and they ovulated, whereas virilized rats are

254

sterile. We cite: "Although the CNS area that mediates behavior was altered in the nine rhesus monkeys mentioned, they still appeared to release gonadotropin in a cyclic fashion. Androgenized female monkeys menstruated and had a preovulatory surge of estradiol and a functional corpus luteum".

In other experiments, performed in rats (Dörner, 1973) and also in sheep (Short, 1974) it had been shown that only animals with a female differentiated brain are able to react with LH-release after estrogen treatment, but not animals with a male type of brain differentiation.

It has then also been shown that homosexual men do also show the positive feedback reaction which does not appear in normal men (Dörner, 1974b). This was interpreted as another proof, that homosexuality is induced by hormonal disturbances during fetal live.

We will come back to this aspect later.

It was concluded that if androgens or estrogens become effective as in rodents and sheep, during the critical period of brain development certain brain centers in man also, responsible for the positive feedback reation, do not develop. This finding, in our opinion, does not agree with the results of several other groups. For instance, female virilized monkeys did not only show cyclicity, as already mentioned, they were able to a positive feedback reaction.

We cite from a paper of Resko (1977): "These observations are consistent with reports that castrated male monkeys release LH in response to estrogen treatment (Karsch et al., 1973; Steiner et al., 1974), and that prenatal androgens do not affect male monkeys as they do rats (Kidston et al., 1973; Neill, 1972) and sheep (Karsch and Foster, 1975; Short, 1974). In the latter two species, estrogens will not facilitate the release of LH in the male or the androgenized female."

Steiner et al. (1976) concluded: "The male primate contains the biochemical machinery within the hypothalamic-pituitary unit to release LH in response to estrogen."

In patients with the syndrom of testicular feminization a positive feedback is absent, theoretically those patients should have the capacity for the positive feedback reaction (Baird, 1975). In patients with gonadal agenesis it was also not possible to demonstrate a positive feedback (Mühlenstedt and Schneider, 1979).

The behavioral aspects of this problem are still under discussion concerning the relevance of animals studies for the human.

At the beginning, we and other groups postulated that several sexual deviations in humans from the so-called normal might have been induced by the absence (in males) or presence of hormones (in females) (androgens and/or estrogens) in the critical phase of fetal development. In a review paper in 1973 we wrote the following: "We know relatively little of the significance for man of the findings just described. It is reasonable to suggest that certain sexual deviations, for example transsexuality, perhaps even homosexuality, could have their cause in disturbances of the androgen balance during that phase of pregnancy in which the sexual differentiation of the brain occurs" (Hahn et al., 1973).

Some other groups even suggested prophylactically treatment to prevent homosexuality (Dörner, 1972) (the fetus would have to be treated).

We think this is a very dangerous point, because one has to consider not only the scientific aspects, but also the social ethical and even political consequences.

Do we really have good evidence to believe or do we have proof that homosexuality is hormone-induced?

1. The positive feedback reaction in homosexual men was used as a proof. But this is still questionable, as has been already mentioned before.

2. Virilized female monkeys or partially virilized girls with the adrenogenital syndrome or girls virilized because of treatment of their mothers during pregnancy with certain progestogens, never showed homosexual tendencies. These studies have been done by Ehrhardt and Money and have been discussed by Resko (1977) in a review paper (see Table 1). On the other hand, those girls have shown some other male-like behavior pattern.

3. Why should a hormonal imbalance exist at the time of brain differentiation, but not before and afterwards? If it would exist before, the somatic sexual differentiation should be also influenced.

If it would persist afterwards, the hormonal status of homosexuals should be different from normal humans and this is not

Table 1: Some behavioral characteristics of female human subjects with abnormal hormonal stimulation in fetal life

Characteristic	Syndrome[a]			Testicular[2,6] Feminization
	Progestin[1,2] induced (♀)[b]	Adreno-[2,3,4] genital (♀)	Turner[2,5] (♀ or ♂)	(♂)
Tomboyism	+↑[c]	+↑	–	–
Clothing preference	+↑	+↑	–	–
Change in childhood sexuality from genetic sex	–	–	–	–
Juvenile interest in infant care	–	+↓	–	–
Career preference over traditional marriage	+↑	+↑[d]	–	–
Homosexual tendencies	–	–	–	–

[a] Progestin-induced: Synthetic progestins administered to pregnant women to prevent abortion. Some of these compounds are also androgenic.
Adrenogenital syndrome: In this syndrome the adrenal gland is not able to biosynthesize cortisol. As a consequence, precursor substances are produced in abundance and are funneled off into the production of androgen.
Turner's syndrome: Syndrome of gonadal dysgenesis. May be either genetic males or females. In males, fetal testes do not develop, therefore sufficient androgen is not produced for differentiation.
Testicular feminization syndrome: Fetal testes produce androgen, but target tissue cannot respond to the androgen that is produced.

[b] Genetic sex of the subjects in the table.

[c] + means tendency is present and differs significantly from "normal" female controls; – means the tendency is the same as "normal" female controls. Arrow indicates the direction of the tendency: ↑ (up), ↓ (down).

[d] This characteristic was not significant in a second study (Ehrhardt and Baker, 1974).

References:
(1) Ehrhardt and Money, 1967. (2) Money and Ehrhardt, 1972. (3) Ehrhardt et al., 1968a. (4) Ehrhardt et al., 1968b. (5) Ehrhardt et al., 1970. (6) Money et al., 1968.

(From Resko, 1977)

the case. This is a question of probablility, not a scientific argument.

4. We are not familiar in this milieu, but we were told, that homosexual males do still practise male behavior and they feel like males and not like females.

The situation in the "manipulated" rat is quite different.

These are only a few questions regarding the validity of this hypothesis. We are of the opinion that this hypothesis is still only based on circumstantial evidence.

Because we do not understand too much about homosexuality, we asked Dr. Dannecker and Dr. Sigusch for a comment. They are not endocrinologists, but accepted experts in sexual research working at the University of Frankfurt/Main. We will cite a few parts from the comment we got from them:

"Homosexuality is primarily a theoretical or anthropological category. That means homosexuality is a latent behavior in the human being, which is not restricted to manifest homosexuals. If one omits such a theoretical differentiation and homosexuality is restricted only to manifest homosexuals, then motive and purpose of all research directed towards the elucidation of the etiology of homosexuality suddenly coincides with the usual discrimination of homosexuals in our society: They want to prevent any homosexual development (prophylaxis) or want to eradicate it (therapy). The manifest homosexuality should therefore be regarded as an integrated part of a personality and not as a symptom of a defect of disease which can be eradicated without destroing a personality."

We would like to close by cyting some parts of one of Goy's papers from 1970:

"As the early reports of human hermaphroditism suggested, the determination of psychosexuality may be primarily a matter of social experience. On the other hand, a growing body of evidence suggests that for the human, as for other mammals, the effectiveness of social experience is influenced in turn by the type of hormone present during an early period of embryonic, fetal or neonatal differentiation (Diamond, 1968; Money and Ehrhardt, 1968). It would be premature at this time to attempt to reconcile data and interpretations for man and animals, or to do more than suggest that the divergence between these various studies of psychosexual

258

determination has been more than slightly lessened. With the limitations of present information it is not even possible to reconcile diverse interpretations of studies restricted to experimental animals."

We think this is still the situation today. In a discussion remark, Anke Ehrhardt mentioned:

"Inborn homosexuality in man, on the other hand, may be only a question of definition. With respect to the predominance of pre- and/or postnatal causes, however, we have no evidence so far" (Ehrhardt, 1974).

It was not the intention of this contribution to prove or disprove the scientific background of this hypothesis, but we think it is too early to draw any conclusions with regard to human homosexuality from animal studies or from rather inconclusive investigations in human homosexuals, especially not from retro-spective studies as has been done by Dörner (see this volume).

References

Baird DT (1975) Abnormalities of the hypothalamic-pituitary-gonadal axis. J Endocrinol 66:13P-14P.

Brown-Grant K Recent studies on the sexual differentiation of the brain. pp.527-545.

Diamond M (1968) Genetic-endocrine interactions and human psycho-sexuality. In: Diamond M (ed) Perspectives in Reproduction and Sexual Behaviour. Indiana University Press, Bloomington, USA, pp.417-443.

Döhler K-D (1978) Is female sexual differentiation hormone-mediated? Trends in Neurosciences 1:138-140.

Döhler K-D, von zur Mühlen A, Döhler U (1976) Estrogen-gonadotropin interaction in postnatal female rats, and the induction of an-ovulatory sterility by treatment with an estrogen-antagonist. Ann Biol Anim Biochim Biophys 16:363-372.

Dörner G (1972) Sexualhormonabhängige Gehirndifferenzierung und Sexualität. Springer Verlag, Wien-New York.

Dörner G (1973) Zur Bedeutung prä- oder perinataler Umweltsbedingungen für die postnatale Regelung neuroendokriner Systeme. Endokrinologie 61:107-123.

Dörner G (ed) (1974a) Endocrinology of Sex. Differentiation and Neuro-endocrine Regulation in the Hypothalamo-Hypophysial-Gonadal-System. Proceedings of the Symposium, with International Participation, Organized by the Society for Endocrinology and Metabolic Diseases of the GDR. Johann Abrosius Barth, Leipzig.

Dörner G (1974b) Sex hormone dependent brain differentiation and sexual function. In: Dörner G (ed) Endocrinology of Sex - Differentiation and Neuroendocrine Regulation in the Hypothalamo-Hypophysial-Gonadal-System, Johann Ambrosius Barth, Leipzig, chapt.1.2., pp.30-37.

Ehrhardt AA (1974) The effects of fetal hormones in the human female on sex-related behavior and intelligence. In: Dörner G (1974) Endocrinology of Sex - Differentiation and Neuroendocrine Regulation in the Hypothalamo-Hypophysial-Gonadal-System, Johann Ambrosius Barth, Leipzig, chapt.1.8., p.79.

Ehrhardt AA, Baker SW (1974) In: Friedman RC, Richart RM and Vande Wiele RL (eds) Sex Differences in Behavior. John Wiley & Sons Inc., N.Y., p.19.

Ehrhardt AA, Epstein R, Money J (1968a) Johns Hopkins Med J 122:160.

Ehrhardt AA, Evers K, Money J (1968b) Johns Hopkins Med J 123:115.

Ehrhardt AA, Greenberg N, Money J (1970) Johns Hopkins Med J 126:237.

Ehrhardt AA, Money J (1967) J Sex Rev 3:83.

Elger W (1966) Die Rolle der fetalen Androgene in der Sexualdifferenzierung des Kaninchens und ihre Abgrenzung gegen andere hormonale und somatische Faktoren durch Anwendung eines starken Antiandrogens. Arch Anat Microsc Morphol Exp 55:657-743.

Goy RW (1970) Experimental control of psychosexuality. Phil Trans Roy Soc London, Ser B259:149-163.

Goy RW (1972) Gonadal hormones and behavior of normal and pseudohermaphroditic nonhuman female primates. Recent Progr Horm Res 28:707-733.

Hahn JD, von Hasselbach CH, Berger B, Elger W, Neumann F (1973) Sexual differentiation of the hypothalamus "prolactin inhibiting factor center" and other brain areas. Symposion on Central Mechanisms Controlling the Pituitary. In: The Endocrine Function of the Human Testis, Academic Press, Inc., New York and London, vol. 1, pp.313-341.

Karsch FJ, Dierschke DJ, Knobil E (1973) Sexual differentation of pituitary function: apparent difference between primates and rodents. Science 179:484-486.

Karsch FJ, Foster DL (1975) Sexual differentiation of the mechanism controlling the preovulatory discharge of luteinizing hormone in sheep. Endocrinology 97:373-379.

Kidston AL, Belpulsi A, Weisz J (1973) Testosterone - sterilization and "positive feedback" effect of estrogens on LH. Biol Reprod 9:77 (Abstract No. 40).

Knobil E (1974) On the control of gonadotropin secretion in the rhesus monkey. Recent Progr Horm Res 30:1-46.

McEwen BS (1978) Gonadal steroid receptors in neuroendocrine tissues. In: O'Malley BW, Birnbaumer L (eds) Receptors and Hormone Action. Academic Press, New York, San Francisco - London, vol. II, chapt. 13, pp.353-400.

McEwen BS (1980) Gonadal steroids and brain development. Biol Reprod 22:43-48.

McEwen BS, Lieberburg I, Chaptal C, Krey LC (1977) Aromatization: important for sexual differentiation of the neonatal rat brain. Hormones and Behavior 9:249-263.

Money J, Ehrhardt AA (1968) Prenatal hormone exposure: possible effects on behaviour in man. In: Michael R (ed) Endocrinology and Human Behaviour. Oxford University Press, Oxford, pp.32-48.

Money J, Ehrhardt AA (1972) Man and Woman, Boy and Girl. The Johns Hopkins University Press, Baltimore, chapt. 6, p.95.

Money J, Ehrhardt AA, Masica DN (1968) Johns Hopkins Med J 123:160.

Mühlenstedt D, Schneider HPG (1979) Sexual differentiation of the hypothalamus in gonadal agenesis and testicular feminization. Arch
Gynecol 227:97–102.

Neill JD (1972) Sexual differences in the hypothalamic regulation of
prolactin secretion. Endocrinology 90:1154–1159.

Neumann F, Elger W (1965) Proof of the activity of androgenic agents on
the differentiation of the external genitalia, the mammary gland and
the hypothalamic-pituitary system in rats. Proceedings of the IInd
Symp on Steroid Hormones "Androgens in Normal and Pathological
Conditions", Ghent 1965. Excerpta Med Found Int Congr Ser
101:168–185.

Neumann F, Elger W (1966) Permanent changes in gonadal function and
sexual behaviour as a result of early feminization of male rats by
treatment with an antiandrogenic steroid. Endokrinologie 50:209–225.

Neumann F, Elger W, Kramer M (1966) Development of a vagina in male rats
by inhibiting androgen receptors with an anti-androgen during the
critical phase of organogenesis. Endocrinology 78:628–632.

Neumann F, Hahn JD, Kramer M (1967) Hemmung von testosteroneabhängigen
Differenzierungsvorgängen der männlichen Ratte nach der Geburt. Acta
Endocrinol (Copenhagen) 54:227–240.

Neumann F, von Berswordt-Wallrabe R, Elger W, Steinbeck H, Hahn JD,
Kramer M (1970) Aspects of androgen-dependent events as studied by
antiandrogens. Laurentian Hormone Conference, Mont Tremblant/Canada
1969. Recent Progr Horm Res 26:337–410.

Resko JA (1977) Fetal hormones and development of the central nervous
system in primates. In: Thomas JA and Singhal RL (eds) Regulatory
Mechanisms Affecting Gonadal Hormone Action. Advances in Sex Hormone
Research, HM + M Medical & Scientific Publishers, Aylesburgy, Bucks,
England, vol. 3, pp.139–168.

Short RV (1974) Sexual differentiation of the brain of the sheep.
International Symposium on Sexual Endocrinology of the Perinatal
Period 32:121–142.

Steiner RA, Clifton DK, Spies HG, Resko JA (1974) Feedback control of LH
by estradiol in female, male, and female pseudohermaphroditic rhesus
monkeys. 56th Ann Meeting Endocrine Soc, Atlanta, GA, Abstract No.
280:A–195.

Steiner RA, Clifton DK, Spies HG, Resko JA (1976) Sexual differentiation
and feedback control of luteinizing hormone secretion in the rhesus
monkey. Biol Reprod 15:206–212.

261

Physiology of Somatosensory and Estrogenic Control Over the Lordosis Reflex

L.M. Kow and D.W. Pfaff, New York

During mating, when an estrous female rat is mounted by a male she becomes immobilized and displays a posture called lordosis: a prominent vertebral dorsiflexion, with elevation of the head and rump. This response by the female is an estrogen-dependent reflex. It never occurs spontaneously, but requires an appropriate stimulus. In turn, the appropriate stimulus is effective only when the female has been primed appropriately with ovarian hormone. Obviously, the reflex is reproduced by an interaction in the nervous system between the influence exerted by estrogen and the sensory input from the appropriate stimulus. The question is where and how. Our strategy to answer this question has been to identify and study the nature of the neural pathway mediating the hormone influence and that trans- mitting the requited sensory input. With this strategy, neural substrates that are both influenced by estrogen and receive the sensory input can be identified and studied to reveal the nature of the interaction.

1. Sensory Input

Sensory requirements for eliciting lordosis. Studies on the sensory requirements have been reviewed (Kow and Pfaff, 1975). Briefly, from studies using surgical and pharmacological deafferentation (Kow and Pfaff, 1976), behavioral observation (Pfaff et al., 1977), and quantitatively controlled mechanical stimulation (Kow et al., 1979a), it has been found that the skin on hindquarters, especially the flank, rump, and perineum, is the reflexogenic area, and application

262

of a touch-pressure stimulus by male rats or manually by an experimenter on this skin area is both sufficient and necessary to elicit a lordosis. Conversely, other sensory modalities, other somato-sensory submodalities, and touch-pressure cutaneous stimuli applied outside the reflexogenic area all are neither sufficient nor necessary.

In ovariectomized female rats given different doses of estrogen, the amount of pressure required to elicit a lordosis was inversely correlated with the estrogen dose given (Kow et al., 1979a). Thus, estrogen not only makes the stimulus effective in eliciting the reflex, it also reduces, quantitatively, the requirement for cutaneous input. This may be due in part to estrogen influence on the receptive field of the pudendal nerve, which innervates the skin on perineal region. It is about 30% larger in estrogen-primed than non-primed female rats (Komisaruk et al., 1972; Kow and Pfaff, 1973; Adler et al., 1977). However, this peripheral effect is not sufficient by itself to account for the induction of lordosis because 1) the effect is statistical in nature rather than all-or-none, as the behavioral effect is; 2) in rats with high estrogen doses, lordosis can still be elicited after a portion of the reflexogenic skin area was denervated by transection of pudendal nerves bilaterally (Kow and Pfaff, 1976). Therefore, we have studied interactions between estrogen influences and somatosensory input to the central nervous system.

Pathway for transmitting the sensory input. By defining the receptive fields for dorsal roots from eleventh thoracic through first sacral (Kow and Pfaff, 1975), it was clear that sensory inputs from cutaneous touch-pressure receptors in the reflexogenic area are transmitted into the spinal cord via lumbar roots. Among them, the sixth lumbar root (L_6) appears to be most important because it innervates two (rump and perineum) of the three most important skin regions. By recording single unit activity in dorsal root ganglion L_6, we studied the responses of primary sensory neurons to mechanical stimulation relevant for lordosis (Kow and Pfaff, 1979). Two types of neurons that fit the definitions for slow-adapting Type I and II receptors in cats were found to respond to cutaneous pressure stimulation. Type I units were very sensitive to touch and pressure, and were excited by an amount of pressure too small to elicit a lordosis in most cases. Furthermore, these units also were excited by hair movement stimuli that were ineffective in eliciting the reflex. In contrast, Type II neurons required more pressure. Once excited, their firing rate was increased by increments in pressure. They did not respond to hair movement. It therefore seems that the sensory inputs required for eliciting lordosis are transmitted mainly by Type II neurons. Comparisons between results from estrogen-treated and non-treated ovariectomized rats showed that all types of units present in one preparation were also present in the other, and the characteristics of each given type remained consistent regardless of hormonal condition. This lack of difference indicates that there is no lordosis-specific touch-pressure unit that functions only in the presence of estrogen influence.

Responses of lumbar spinal neurons were also studied with extracellular single unit recording technique (Kow et al., 1980). In a total of 345 units recorded, 163 responded to cutaneous pressure stimulation. Among the pressure-responsive units, 16 had response characteristics identical to that of Type I primary sensory neurons, except for larger receptive fields. One-third of pressure-sensitive units did not respond to other forms of mechanostimulation, and therefore were equivalent to Type II primary sensory neurons. However, while only excitation was observed in the peripheral neurons, spinal units could be excited, inhibited, or respond either way depending on the location stimulated. The remaining 93 pressure-responsive units also responded to hair movement and/or muscle-joint manipulation. In the absence of other stimuli, this latter group of neurons responded to pressure in the same way as the previous group did, but when other mechanostimulation was also applied the response to pressure could be altered in various ways. Obviously, responses of pressure-responsive spinal neurons are more complicated than those of primary sensory neurons. At present, it is not known how these more complicated responses are related to the elicitation of lordosis. However, it is clear that the lordosis-eliciting sensory inputs are transmitted by these peripheral and spinal neurons because they not only are pressure-responsive but also respond to the same range of pressure required to trigger lordosis (Fig. 1).

From spinal pressure-responsive neurons the lordosis-eliciting sensory inputs can be transmitted within the spinal cord to motor neurons, to supraspinal substrates, or both, to trigger the reflex.

264

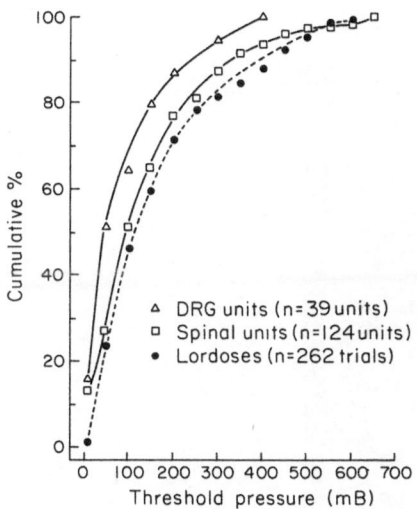

Figure 1: Comparison of pressure thresholds for eliciting lordoses (Kow et al., 1979), and evoking responses from pressure-responsive neurons in sixth lumbar dorsal root ganglion (Kow and Pfaff, 1979) and lumbosacral spinal cord (Kow et al., 1980). Lordoses were elicited by applying pressure on animal's flank, rump, and perineum, while responses from the neurons were evoked by pressure on their receptive fields. Note that the pressure thresholds for eliciting lordoses are higher than those for evoking neuronal responses. This and the close resemblance of the three curves strongly suggest that the sensory information evoked from the pressure-responsive neurons participates in triggering lordosis.

The fact that complete transection of the spinal cord at a high (T_2) or low (T_{10}) thoracic level abolished lordosis reflex (Kow et al., 1977; Kow et al., 1979b) allows but does not prove that the ascending is necessary. If it is, then the sensory inputs must be transmitted by the ascending spinal tracts located in the antero-lateral colum (ALC), for transections of all the cord except ALC (Fig. 2) at thoracic level had no effect on the performance of lordosis (Kow et al., 1977). An anatomical study of the ascending ALC fibers showed that these fibers originated in the portions of the spinal gray also occupied by spinal pressure-responsive neurons, and terminated in ventral bulbar reticular formation, mainly the lateral reticular nucleus and nucleus magnocellularis, vestibular complex, cerebellum, midbrain, and thalamus (Zemlan et al., 1978). Since lateral reticular nucleus sends its efferents to cerebellum (Brodal, 1943), and the latter was found to be unnecessary for lordosis reflex (Zemlan and Pfaff, 1975), spinal projections to these two structures could not be important for mediating lordosis-eliciting

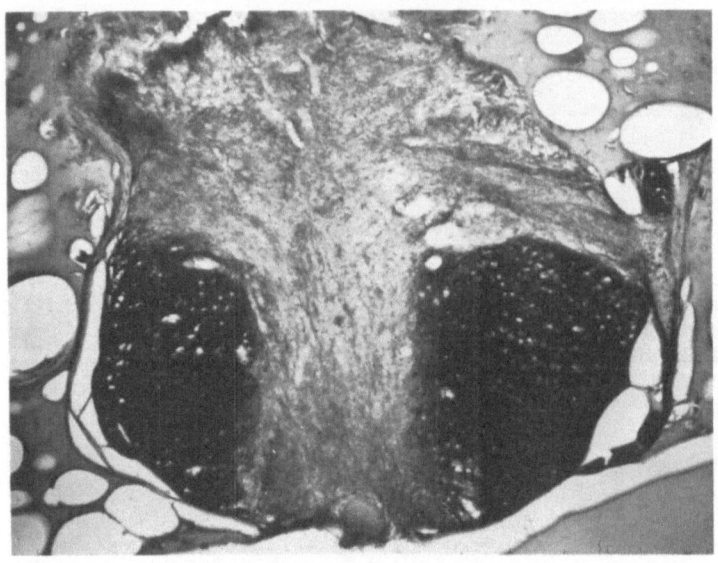

Figure 2: A coronal section through thoracic spinal cord in a rat which had been subjected to transection of the entire dorsal half of the cord plus the ventral column. The cord was embedded in albumin (the pale perforated substance surrounding the section) for orientation. The dorsal side of the cord is on top. Note the transected portion was filled with scar tissue, and the fibers in the anterolateral columns (ALC) were intact, as indicated by their dark Weil stain. This and other rats with similar spinal transection preserving only ALC showed no or little deficit in performing lordosis reflex (Kow et al., 1977; Kow and Zemlan, unpublished results)

inputs. The importance of projections to the midbrain and thalamus was also investigated. A bilateral transection of the brainstem at a pontine level, that would interrupt virtually all the ascending ALC fibers, had not effect on lordosis performance (Manogue et al., 1980). Thus, the most likely places where the lordosis-eliciting sensory inputs interact with estrogen influence are the spinal cord and/or the lower brainstem, especially the nucleus magnocellularis (or ventral portion of nucleus gigantocellularis) and vestibular complex.

2. Neural Pathways Mediating Estrogen Influence

By localizing neurons that concentrate or take up estrogen, the neural substrates that are acted upon directly by estrogen have been shown to include certain forebrain regions and mesencephalic central gray (MCG) (Pfaff and Keiner, 1973). The fact that decerebration abolished lordosis (Kow et al., 1978) indicates that the forebrain substrates are essential while MCG alone is not sufficient for mediating the lordosis-inducing effect of estrogen. The results of decerebration and the aforementioned complete spinal cord transection further show that the estrogen influence from the forebrain to lumbar spinal cord acts not through the circulatory system but through CNS pathways.

In the forebrain, the ventromedial nucleus of the hypothalamus (VMN) appears to be the only cell group that is both necessary and sufficient for the induction of lordosis by estrogen. This is indicated by: 1) cells within and around VMN concentrate estrogen (Pfaff and Keiner, 1973);   2) firing rate of VMN neurons is facilitated by estrogen (Bueno and Pfaff, 1976);   3) lordosis can be induced by implanting a minute amount of estrogen directly into VMN (Barfield and Chen, 1977; Davis et at., 1979; Rubin and Barfield, 1980);   4) lesion of VMN can abolish lordosis in hamsters (Malsbury et al., 1977) and rats (Mathews and Edwards, 1977; Pfaff and Sakuma, 1979b).   No other forebrain substrates fulfill all these criteria (cf. Introduction, Manogue et al., 1980).

A single-unit extracellular recording study (Bueno and Pfaff, 1976) has shown that VMN neurons, even after estrogen priming, fire slowly, at a rate $\lessgtr 1/\text{sec}$, and respond sluggishly or not at all to lordosis-eliciting stimuli, even though the lordosis reflex has a latency of only 161 msec (Pfaff and Lewis, 1974). In estrogen-primed female rats, electrical stimulation (Pfaff and Sakuma, 1979a) and lesion (Pfaff and Sakuma, 1979b) of VMN through chronically implanted electrodes can, respectively, facilitate and abolish lordosis, but both require long latencies, 15 minutes to one hour and 16 to 60 hours, respectively. Obviously, VMN does not participate in stimulus-by-stimulus reflex control of lordosis, but after estrogen priming must send out a tonic facilitation to the midbrain (Pfaff, 1980).

From VMN, efferent fibers descend in two routes, medial and lateral, to the midbrain and terminate mainly in the central gray (MCG) (Krieger et al., 1979). Selective brain transections that would interrupt the lateral or both groups of VMN efferents severely

267

reduced or abolished lordosis, respectively (Manogue et al., 1980). These results indicate that the tonic facilitatory estrogen influence is mediated mainly by lateral VMN efferents to MCG, and that MCG serves as a waystation for relaying the influence to the spinal cord. Indeed, in estrogen-primed female rats, electrical stimulation (Sakuma and Pfaff, 1979a) or lesion (Sakuma and Pfaff, 1979b) of MCG through chronically implanted electrodes potentiate or suppress, respectively, lordosis reflex rapidly. Furthermore, electrophysiological studies (Sakuma and Pfaff, 1980a,b) showed that some MCG neurons send efferents to nucleus gigantocellularis in the medullary reticular formation, and that these MCG neurons were facilitated by estrogen or VMN stimulation. Electrical stimulation of preoptic area that inhibited lordosis (Pfaff and Sakuma, 1979a) was also found to inhibit these MCG neurons. However, these MCG efferent neurons do not respond to the lordosis-eliciting stimulus (Sakuma and Pfaff, 1980b). Thus, despite rapid electrical stimulation or lesion effects these particular MCG neurons are obviously not responsible for stimulus-bound reflex control of lordosis either, but participate in relaying an estrogen-dependent hypothalamic signal to the lower brainstem.

Since MCG does not project directly to the spinal cord, it is obvious that at least one more waystation in the lower brainstem is necessary for relaying the estrogen influence to the cord. Anatomically, MCG has been shown to project to locus coeruleus (Russel, 1955; Sakai et al., 1977), nucleus raphe magnus (NRM), and the ventral portion of nucleus gigantocellularis (NGc) (Hamilton and Skultety, 1970; Krieger et al., 1980). Among them, only NGc and NRM are known (Zemlan et al., 1979) to give rise to descending spinal fibers through anterolateral columns, which are sufficient and essential for mediating lordosis (Kow et al., 1977). Brainstem lesion studies have shown that destruction of NRM had no effect on lordosis (Zemlan et al., 1980), while lesion in NGc affected lordosis adversely (Modianos and Pfaff, 1976, 1979; Zemlan et al., 1980). Lesions of the lateral vestibular nucleus (Modianos and Pfaff, 1979) and sub-coeruleus-pontine reticular system (Zemlan et al., 1980), that also give rise to descending ALC fibers, also had adversive effects on lordosis, but these regions do not receive projections from MCG. Thus, NGc is the only substrate that receives projection from MCG,

268

projects to the spinal cord, and, when lesioned, affects lordosis reflex. This, together with the finding that MCG neurons projecting to NGc region are facilitated by estrogen and VMN stimulation (Sakuma and Pfaff, 1980b), strongly suggests that NGc is the lower brainstem waystation for relaying estrogen influence to the spinal cord.

To study the response of NGc neurons to stimuli relevant for eliciting lordosis, bundles of fine wires (25 or 16 μ) were implanted chronically into the ventral portion of NGc to record single-unit activity. This technique allowed us to avoid using anaesthesia during recording and to observe neuronal activity and behavior simultaneously. Furthermore, the use of fine wire enabled us to follow identified units for days or even weeks, and provided an opportunity to observe the estrogen influence, which took days to develop or disappear, on the identified units. Ovariectomized rats used were given estrogen to allow lordosis. Once units were studied and identified, estrogen was withdrawn and the study continued until units were lost or the female became entirely unreceptive. Of 127 units studied, 38 were inhibited, while only 4 were facilitated by

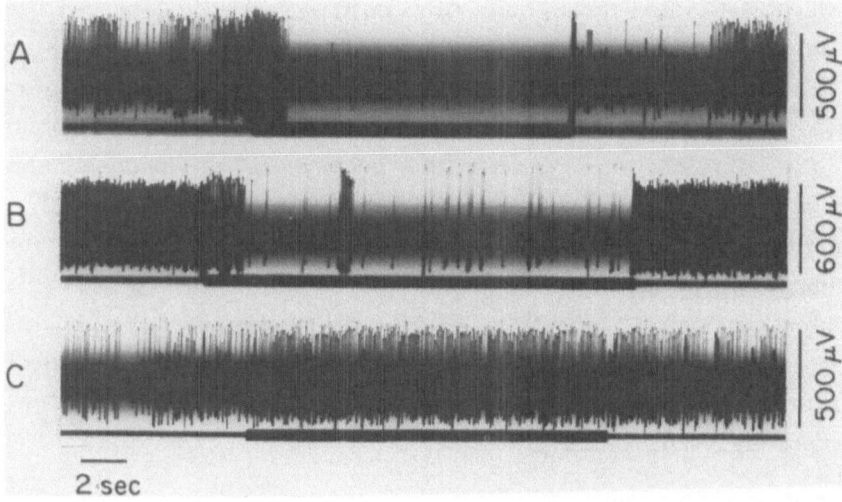

Figure 3: Examples of suppression (A), partial inhibition (B), and facilitation (C) of spontaneous unit activity by lordosis-eliciting cutaneous stimulation. Unit activity was recorded from the ventral portion of nucleus gigantocellularis in behaving female rats primed with estrogen. Widened bars below each recording indicate the application of the stimulation which elicited lordosis in all cases

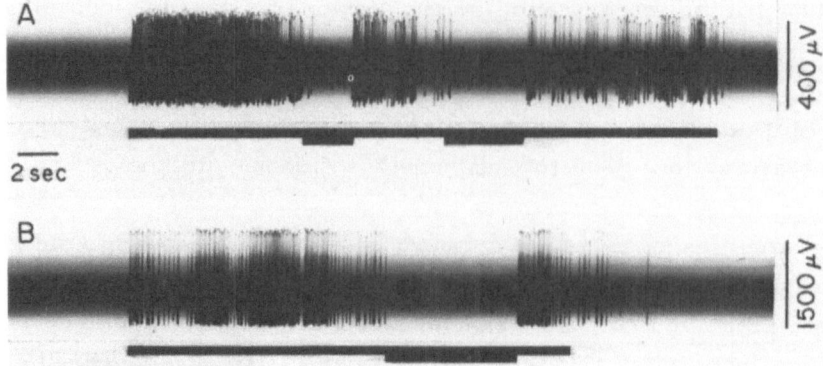

Figure 4: Effect of lordosis-eliciting cutaneous stimulation on the evoked activity of two silent neurons. Unit activity evoked by rotating the head (A, indicated by the long bar) or brushing the fur (B, long bar) was suppressed by the lordosis-eliciting cutaneous stimulation (short bars)

manual stimulation effective for eliciting lordosis. The inhibition could be exerted on spontaneous activity (Fig. 3A and 3B) and/or evoked activity (Fig. 4). The facilitatory effect was seen only on spontaneous activity (Fig. 3C). These responses were independent of estrogen influence or states of receptivity. For example, of the 35 units that were followed throughout the entire receptive-unreceptive period, 12 units (including 7 that could be antidromically activated by spinal cord stimulation) were inhibited throughout; 1 unit showed only excitatory response; and the remaining 22 units did not respond throughout. The dissociation between the occurrence of lordosis and responses to stimulation was also manifested by the observations that cellular responses could often be evoked by stimuli ineffective for eliciting lordosis. Thus, NGc neurons must participate in lordosis control not through rapid, specific, excitatory responses to lordosis-relevant stimuli, but through forebrain modulation of another aspect of NGc cellular activity, to be transmitted through reticulospinal axons to the spinal cord.

3. Summary

The simplest mechanism for lordosis behavior, as allowed by the present data, is as follows. Estrogen acts on the ventromedial nucleus of hypothalamus (VMN) to induce a tonic facilitatory output, which is relayed by neurons in mesencephalic central gray and then the medullary reticulospinal tract to the spinal cord. To trigger the lordosis reflex, sensory inputs from cutaneous touch-pressure receptors located in rump-perineal skin are required. Neural pathways exist for transmitting these inputs to motor neurons in the spinal cord and to certain supraspinal locations, but our electrophysiological studies indicate that the most likely place where these sensory inputs interact with estrogen-influenced neural activity to elicit the reflex is the spinal cord itself.

References

Adler NT, Davis PG, Komisaruk BR (1977) Variation in the size and sensitivity of a genital sensory field in relation to the estrous cycle in rats. Horm Behav 9:334-344.

Barfield RJ, Chen JJ (1977) Activation of estrous behavior in ovariectomized rats by intracerebral implants of estradiol benzoate. Endocrinology 101:1716-1725.

Brodal A (1943) The cerebellar connections of the nucleus reticularis lateralis (nucleus funiculi lateralis) in rabbit and cat. Experimental investigations. Acta Psychiat Scand 18:171-233.

Bueno J, Pfaff DW (1976) Single unit recording in hypothalamus and preoptic area of estrogen-treated and untreated ovariectomized female rats. Brain Res 101:67-78.

Davis PG, McEwen BS, Pfaff DW (1979) Localized behavioral effects of tritiated estradiol implants in the ventromedial hypothalamus of female rats. Endocrinology 104:898-903.

Hamilton BL, Skultety FM (1970) Efferent connections of the periaqueductal gray matter in the cat. J Comp Neurol 139:105-114.

Komisaruk BR, Adler NT, Hutchinson J (1972) Genital sensory field: enlargement by estrogen treatment in female rats. Science 178:1295-1298.

Kow L-M, Pfaff DW (1973) Effects of estrogen treatment on the size of receptive field and response threshold of pudendal nerve in the female rat. Neuroendocrinology 13:299-313.

Kow L-M, Pfaff DW (1975) Dorsal root recording relevant for mating reflexes in female rats: identification of receptive fields and effects of peripheral denervation. J Neurobiol 6:23-37.

Kow L-M, Pfaff DW (1976) Sensory requirements for the lordosis reflex in female rats. Brain Res 101:47-66.

Kow L-M, Pfaff DW (1977) Sensory control of reproductive behavior in female rodents. Ann N.Y. Acad Sci 290:72-97.

Kow L-M, Pfaff DW (1979) Responses of single units in the sixth lumbar dorsal root ganglion of female rats to mechanostimulation relevant for the lordosis reflex. J Neurophysiol 42:203-213.

Kow L-M, Grill HJ, Pfaff DW (1978) Elimination of lordosis in decerebrate female rats: observations from acute and chronic preparations. Physiol Behav 20:171-174.

Kow L-M, Montgomery MO, Pfaff DW (1977) Effects of spinal cord transections on lordosis reflex in female rats. Brain Res 123:75-88.

Kow L-M, Montgomery MO, Pfaff DW (1979a) Triggering of lordosis reflex in female rats with somatosensory stimulation: quantitative determination of stimulus parameters. J Neurophysiol 42:195-202.

Kow L-M, Zemlan FP, Pfaff DW (1979b) Attempts to reinstate lordosis reflex in estrogen-primed spinal female rats with monoamine agonists. Horm Behav 13:232-240.

Kow L-M, Zemlan FP, Pfaff DW (1980) Responses of lumbosacral spinal units to mechanical stimuli related to analysis of the lordosis reflex in female rats. J Neurophysiol 43:27-45.

Krieger MS, Conrad LCA, Pfaff DW (1979) An autoradiographic study of the efferent connections of the ventromedial nucleus of the hypothalamus. J Comp Neurol 183:785-816.

Krieger MS, Morrell JI, Pfaff DW (1981) Efferent connections of midbrain central gray. Manuscript in preparation.

Malsbury CW, Kow L-M, Pfaff DW (1977) Effects of medial hypothalamic lesions on the lordosis response and other behaviors in female golden hamsters. Physiol Behav 19:223-237.

Manogue KR, Kow L-M, Pfaff DW (1980) Selective brainstem transections affecting reproductive behavior of female rats: the role of hypothalamic output to the midbrain. Horm Behav, in press.

Mathews D, Edwards DA (1977) Involvement of the ventromedial and anterior hypothalamic nuclei in the hormonal induction of receptivity in the female rat. Physiol Behav 19:319-326.

Modianos DT, Pfaff DW (1976) Brain stem and cerebellar lesions in female rats. II. Lordosis reflex. Brain Res 106:47-56.

Modianos DT, Pfaff DW (1979) Medullary reticular formation lesions and lordosis reflex in female rats. Brain Res 171:334-338.

Pfaff DW (1980) Estrogens and Brain Function. Springer-Verlag, Heidelberg.

Pfaff DW, Keiner M (1973) Atlas of estradiol-concentrating cells in the central nervous system of the female rat. J Comp Neurol 151:121-158.

Pfaff DW, Lewis C (1974) Film analysis of lordosis in female rats. Horm Behav 5:317-335.

Pfaff DW, Sakuma Y (1979a) Facilitation of the lordosis reflex of female rats from the ventromedial nucleus of the hypothalamus. J Physiol 288:189-202.

Pfaff DW, Sakuma Y (1979b) Deficit in the lordosis reflex of female rats caused by lesions in the ventromedial nucleus of the hypothalamus. J Physiol 288:203-210.

Pfaff DW, Montgomery M, Lewis C (1977) Somatosensory determinants of lordosis in female rats: behavioral definition of the estrogen effect. J Comp Physiol 91:134-145.

Rubin BS, Barfield RS (1980) Priming of estrous responsiveness by implants of 17β-estradiol in the ventromedial hypothalamic nucleus of female rats. Endocrinology 106:504-509.

Russell GV (1955) The nucleus locus coeruleus (dorsolateralis tegmenti). Tex Rep Biol Med 13:939-988.

Sakai K, Touret M, Salvert D, Leger L, Jouvet M (1977) Afferent projections to the cat locus coeruleus as visualized by horseradish peroxidase technique. Brain Res 119:21-41.

Sakuma Y, Pfaff DW (1979a) Facilitation of female reproductive behavior from mesencephalic central gray in the rat. Am J Physiol 237:R278-R284.

Sakuma Y, Pfaff DW (1979b) Mesencephalic mechanisms for integration of female reproductive behavior in the rat. Am J Physiol 237:R285-R290.

Sakuma Y, Pfaff DW (1980a) Cells or origin of medullary projections in the central gray of the rat mesencephalon. J Neurophysiol, in press.

Sakuma Y, Pfaff DW (1980b) Excitability of female rat central gray cells with medullary projections: changes produced by hypothalamic stimulation and estrogen treatment. J Neurophysiol, in press.

Zemlan FP, Pfaff Dw (1975) Lordosis after cerebellar damage in female rats. Horm Behav 6:27–33.

Zemlan FP, Kow L–M, Pfaff DW (1980) Effects of brainstem lesions on lordosis and pain reflexes in female rats. Manuscript in preparation.

Zemlan FP, Kow L–M, Morrell JI, Pfaff DW (1979) Descending tracts of the lateral columns of the rat spinal cord: a study using the horseradish peroxidase and silver impregnation technique. J Anat 128:489–512.

Zemlan FP, Leonard CM, Kow L–M, Pfaff DW (1978) Ascending tracts of the lateral columns of the rat spinal cord: a study using the silver impregnation and horseradish peroxidase techniques. Exp Neurol 62:298–334.

Neural Structures Essential for the Control of Prolactin Surges in the Female Rat

M. Kawakami and J. Arita, Yokohama

Prolactin (PRL) is released from the anterior pituitary gland rapidly in response to the suckling stimulus during lactation (Amenomori et al., 1970) and to stresses, such as ether inhalation (Neill, 1970) and immobilization (Riegle and Meites, 1976; Kawakami et al., 1979). In addition, PRL surges occur spontaneously with circadian rhythms in the female rat on the day of proestrus (Kwa and Verhofstad, 1967; Niswender et al., 1969; Neill, 1970) during early pregnancy (Butcher et al., 1972) and pseudopregnancy (PSP) (Freeman et al., 1974), in the ovariectomized rat after estrogen treatment (Neill, 1972; Caligaris et al., 1974) or following uterine cervical stimulation (Smith and Neill, 1976), and in the prepuberal female rat (Kimura and Kawakami, in press). Earlier transection studies demonstrated that suckling-induced or stress-induced PRL release requires only posterior afferents to the medial basal hypothalamus (MBH) (Velasco et al., 1974; Halász et al., 1978) or posterolateral afferents as well as frontal afferents (Krulich et al., 1975; Kawakami and Higuchi, in submission), respectively. In contrast, it has been shown that the estrogen-induced PRL surge in ovariectomized rats and the induction and maintenance of PSP are dependent entirely on frontal afferents but not on posterior afferents to the MBH (Neill, 1972; Caligaris and Taleisnik, 1977; Arai, 1969; Carrer and Taleisnik, 1970), suggesting an essential role of the neural structures within or near the preoptic region in the control of the PRL surges. However, further restricted areas in the preoptic region which are essential for the surges have not been determined as yet.

Dopamine in hypophyseal portal vessels and various neurotransmitters in the brain, especially monoamines, are known to regulate the secretion of anterior pituitary hormones (Weiner and Ganong, 1978). The cell bodies of most monoaminergic neurons are located in the lower brain structures including the midbrain, pons and medulla oblongata, and their fibers ascend and terminate in the limbic-preoptic-hypothalamic system (Ungerstedt, 1971; Lindvall and Björklund, 1974). Although there is evidence suggesting that the lower brain structures are involved in the control of gonadotropin secretion, no investigation has been performed on their involvement in the control of PRL secretion.

Therefore, in the present study utilizing lesioning techniques, we attempted to determine further restricted areas in the preoptic region and the midbrain structures which are indispensable for the regulation of the afternoon surge in proestrous rats, the estrogen-induced surge in ovariectomized rats, and the nocturnal and diurnal surges in PSP rats.

1.   Neural Control of the Proestrous Surge of Prolactin

PRL surges occur spontaneously between the late afternoon and early evening of proestrus in the cycling female rat. The finding that administration of anti-estradiol serum at diestrus-2, but not at proestrus, completely abolished the proestrous PRL surge indicates that the priming action of estrogen secreted between diestrus-2 and proestrus is required for the occurrence of the proestrous surge of PRL (Neill et al., 1971). Furthermore, the experimental result that the proestrous surge of PRL was blocked by pentobarbital injected in the early afternoon of proestrus and that a normal PRL surge occurred in the late afternoon of the following day, suggests that the occurrence of the proestrous surge of PRL has a dependence on the time of day (Wuttke and Meites, 1970; Butcher et al., 1974). It was examined which part of the brain is involved in the control of the proestrous surge of PRL induced by the two events mentioned above.

Only female Wistar rats showing at least two consecutive 4-day estrous cycles were used for the experiments. Various transections were acutely made by rotating a bayonet-shaped knife in animals under ether anesthesia on the morning of the day of proestrus. In

275

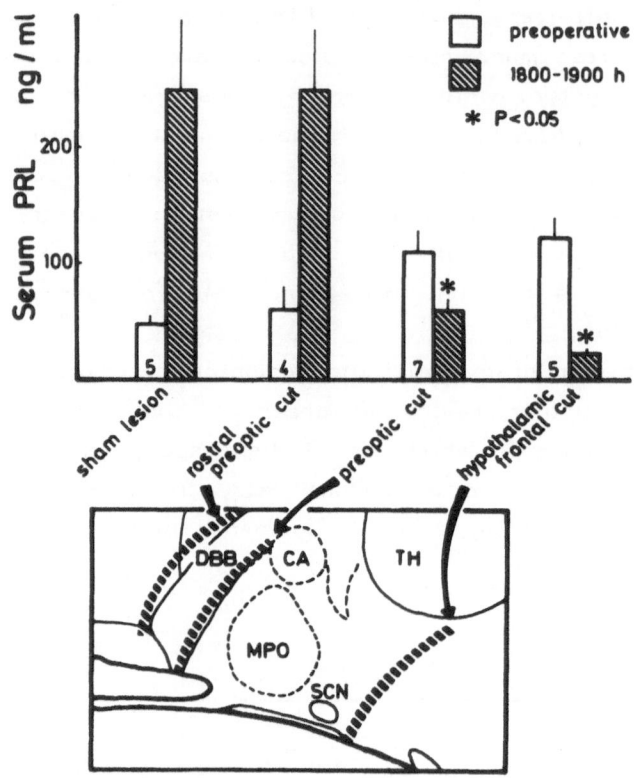

Figure 1: Effects of preoptic transections on proestrous PRL surges. Each column and vertical bar represent the mean and SEM, respectively. AC, anterior commissure; DBB, diagonal band of Broca; MPO, medial preoptic area; SCN, suprachiasmatic nucleus; TH, thalamus. Modified from Kimura and Kawakami (1978)

sham-transected animals, a PRL surge was observed in the late afternoon of proestrus and serum levels of PRL between 1800 and 1900 h were significantly higher than those in the early afternoon (P<0.05) (Fig. 1). Hypothalamic frontal deafferentation, which interrupted frontal afferents from the preoptic region to the MBH at the level immediately behind the suprachiasmatic nucleus (SCN), abolished the proestrous surge (Kimura and Kawakami, 1978). PRL levels between 1800 and 1900 h in the animals with hypothalamic frontal deafferentation were significantly lower than those in sham-transected animals (P<0.02). Preoptic deafferentation, which interrupted frontal, dorsal and lateral afferents to the preoptic region at the level caudal to the diagonal band of Broca, also blocked the proestrous PRL surge, similar to hypothalamic frontal deafferentation. When preoptic deafferentation was placed more rostrally to the level of the anterior margin of the diagonal band of Broca, a normal surge of PRL occurred, and PRL levels in the late afternoon of these animals did not differ from those of sham–transected animals (P<0.05). These results suggest that the preoptic neural structures lying rostral to the hypothalamic frontal deafferentation are essential for the control of the proestrous surge of PRL and that the preoptic structures require either or all of the neural afferents coming from the frontal, dorsal or lateral direction.

In order to transect neural fibers in the ventromedial part of the midbrain (VMM transection), a bayonet–shaped knife was lowered in the midline to the ventral surface of the neural tissue between the caudal margin of the mammillary body and the interpeduncular nucleus (Kawakami and Arita, 1980) (Fig. 2). VMM transections completely eliminated the proestrous PRL surge, which occurred in sham–transected animals with a peak at 1800 h (Fig. 3). PRL levels at 1800 h in the rats with VMM transections were significantly lower than those in sham–transected animals (P<0,05). In contrast,

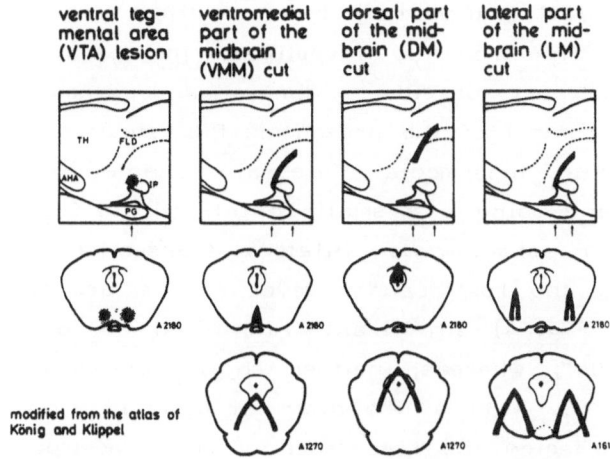

Figure 2: Schematic illustrations showing the location of lesions in the ventral tegmental area (A) and transections in the ventromedial (B)(VMM), dorsal (C)(DM) and lateral (D)(LM) parts of the midbrain. AHA, anterior hypothalamic area; FLD, fasciculus longitudinalis dorsalis; IP, interpeduncular nucleus; PG, pituitary gland. From Kawakami and Arita (1980) with permission

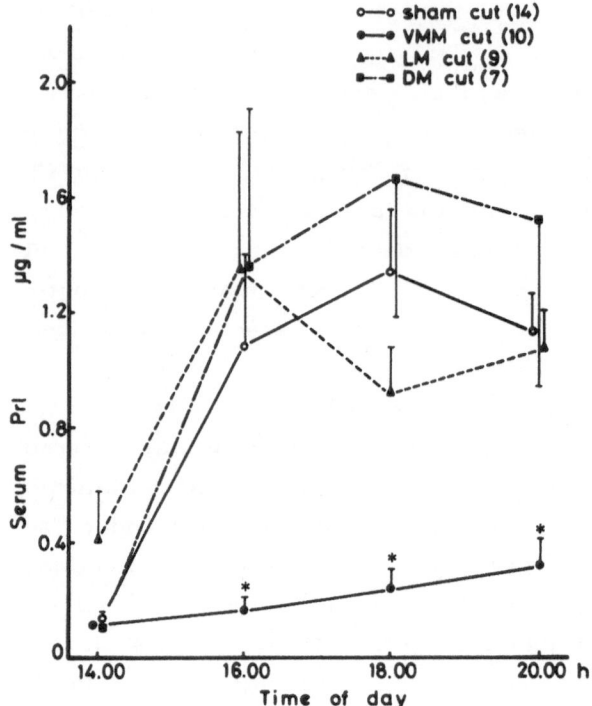

transections 2.0 mm dorsal (DM) or bilateral transections 2.0 mm lateral to VMM transections (LM transection) had no effect on the proestrous surge of PRL. In order to investigate the pathway connecting the ventromedial part of the midbrain and preoptic region, with respect to the control of the proestrous PRL surge, the lateral hypothalamus including the medial forebrain bundle, was transected in the coronal plane using a a small spatula with 1.3 mm width (Kawakami and Ando, in submission). Bilateral transections of the lateral hypothalamus at the rostrocaudal level of the arcuate nucleus (MLH transection in Fig. 4) significantly inhibited the proestrous surge of PRL (P< 0.05); whereas, neither sham transections nor bilateral transections at the level of the diagonal band of Broca (LF transection in Fig. 4) affected the occurrence of the proestrous PRL surge. Transections of the lateral hypothalamus at the level of the anterior hypothalamic area (ALH transection in Fig. 4) were also effective in abolishing the PRL surge. From these results, it is hypothesized that the neural afferents for the generation of the proestrous PRL surge ascend from the ventromedial part of the

278

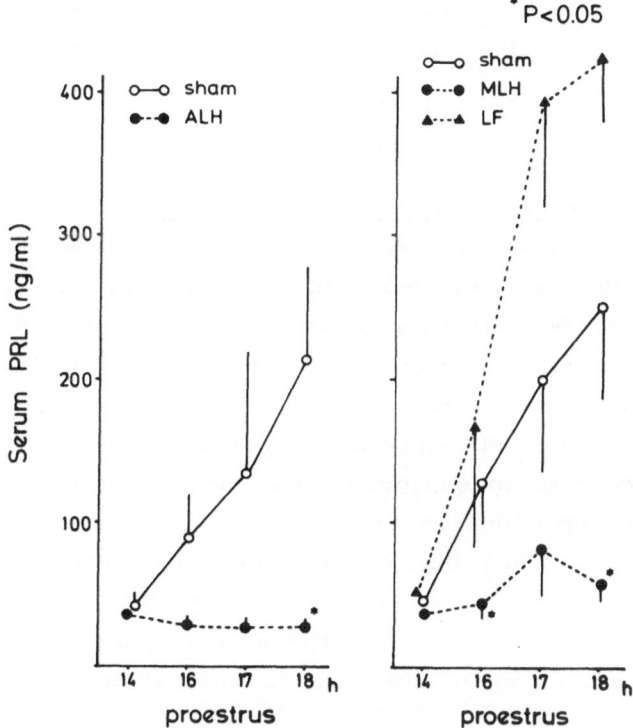

*P<0.05

Figure 4: Effects of lateral hypothalamic transection on serum PRL in proestrous rats. Bilateral transections of the lateral hypothalamus at the level of the arcuate nucleus (MLH transections), of the diagonal band of Broca (LF transections) or of the anterior hypothalamic area (ALH transections) were placed in the morning of proestrus

midbrain, not directly entering the MBH from the posterior direction, but running through the medial forebrain bundle to reach the limbin-preoptic-hypothalamic system. The neural afferents through the medial forebrain bundle may change the direction medially at the level of the preoptic region to reach the preoptic structures. It was recently demonstrated in our laboratory that some neurons in the limbic-preoptic system including the bed nucleus of the stria terminalis, lateral part of the septum and medial basal part of the suprachiasmatic area (MBSC) exhibited single unit responses to electrical stimulation of the ventromedial part of the midbrain, as measured by post-stimulus time histograms, and that percentages of neurons responding in a facilitatory manner to midbrain stimulation were higher in proestrus than in diestrus-1 (Kawakami and Ohno, unpublished data). Furthermore, it was shown that percentages of the responding neurons to midbrain stimulation were decreased by bilateral transections of the lateral hypothalamus. These electro-physiological findings strongly support our hypothesis. Of course, this hypothesis does not exclude the possibility of the involvement of the limbic inputs coming from the frontal and dorsal directions to the preoptic region.

2.   Neural Control of the Estrogen-induced Surge of Prolactin

Estrogen administration into ovariectomized rats induced a daily PRL surge in the afternoon of the following several days.   This PRL surge is known to be comparable in magnitude, duration, and timing to the proestrous surge in cycling rats (Neill, 1972; Caligaris et al., 1974). The estrogen-induced PRL surge has a common characteristic to the proestrous surge also in dependence on the time of day. The entrainment of the estrogen-induced PRL surge to light schedule has been demonstrated in the result that a phase shift of photoperiod caused a phase shift of the timing of the occurrence of the estrogen-induced surge of PRL in ovariectomized rats, and that blinded rats have PRL surges which are free running (Pieper and Gala, 1979).

First,   we   examined   the   similarity   in   the   neural   control mechanisms of the proestrous PRL surge in cycling rats and the estrogen-induced PRL surge in ovariectomized rats (Kawakami et al., 1980).   Subcutaneous injections of 50 μg estradiol benzoate into ovariectomized rats caused a marked PRL surge between 1500 and 1800 h on the third day after the injections, while at other times of the day serum PRL levels showed minimum fluctuations (Fig. 5). Hypothalamic frontal deafferentation in ovariectomized rats eliminated the estrogen-induced PRL surge observed between 1500 and 1800 h in sham-transected animals. Levels of serum PRL at 1800 h in these rats were   significantly   lower   than   those   in   sham-transected   animals ($P<0.005$) although the mean values of serum PRL in deafferented animals exhibited two small peaks occurring at 0900 and 2100 h. These results are in agreement with the results of Neill (1972).   In contrast,   Caligaris   and   Taleisnik   (1977)   reported   that   estrogen administration   into   ovariectomized   rats   with   hypothalamic   frontal deafferentation induced high PRL levels in the morning, which were comparable in magnitude to the afternoon surge in sham-deafferented animals,   and   low   levels   in   the   afternoon.   We   did   not   find   a

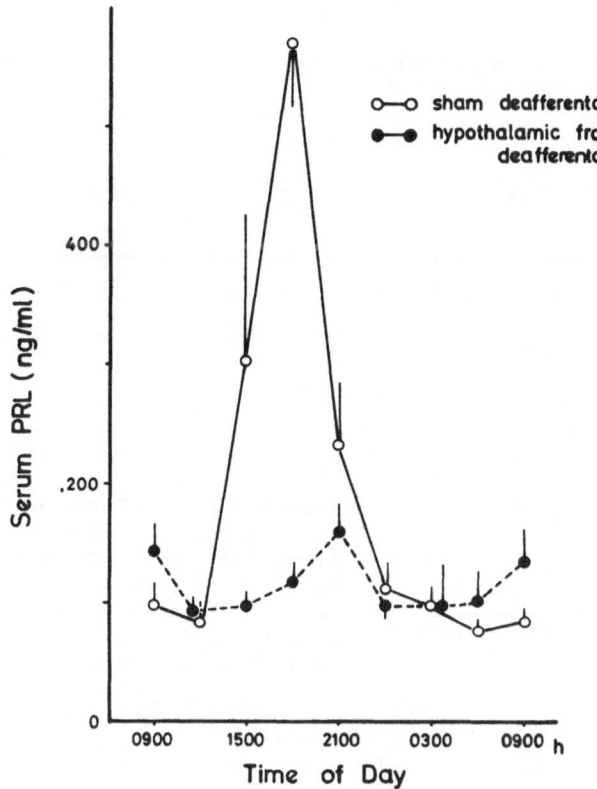

Figure 5: Effects of hypothalamic frontal deafferentation on estrogen-induced PRL surges in ovariectomized rats. The ovariectomized rats were injected sc with 50 μg estradiol benzoate 69 h before sample collection. Modified from Kawakami et al. (1980)

surge-like release of PRL in the morning as reported by Caligaris and Taleisnik, although there were slight peaks of serum PRL at 0900 h in some deafferented animals. The results in ovariectomized rats are well consistent with those in proestrous rats and both results suggest that basal secretion of PRL which is controlled by the MBH is modulated with circadian rhythms by the neural impulses from the surge centers in the preoptic region, resulting in the occurrence of the PRL surges.

On the other hand, VMM transections also abolished the PRL surge induced by estradiol benzoate injections in ovariectomized rats and serum PRL levels at 1600 h in the rats with VMM transections were significantly lower than those in sham-transected animals (P<0.02) (Fig. 6). These results in ovariectomized rats confirmed the results obtained in proestrous rats. Subramanian and Gala have demonstrated that the α-adrenergic blocker, phenoxybenzamine

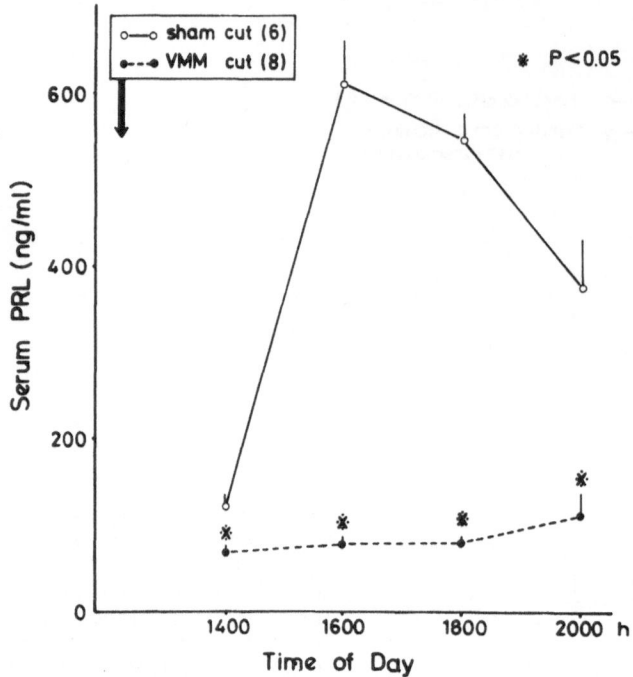

Figure 6: Effects of transections in the ventromedial part of the midbrain (VMM transection) on estrogen-induced PRL surges in ovariectomized rats

completely prevented the estrogen-induced PRL surge in ovariectomized rats. Moreover, Langelier and McCann (1977) reported that chemical lesions in the ventral noradrenergic pathway at the level of the interpeduncular nucleus by microinjections of 6-hydroxydopamine, which decreased the catecholamine fluorescence in the hypothalamus, blocked the proestrous PRL surge in cycling rats. Taken together with the present findings, it is suggested that VMM transections might interrupt ascending noradrenergic fibers in the "tegmental radiation", named by Lindvall and Björklund (1974), originating in the noradrenaline cell groups in the medulla oblongata and pons, resulting in the blockade of the proestrous surge and the estrogen-induced surge of PRL. In addition, the area of VMM transections also contains a serotoneric pathway arising from the raphe nuclei (Ungerstedt, 1971; Fuxe and Jonsson, 1974). Although it was reported that the estrogen-induced PRL surge in ovariectomized rats was prevented by the serotonergic blockers, cyprophepatidine, p-chlorophenylalanine, or methysergide (Caligaris and Taleisnik, 1974; Subramanian and Gala, 1976), further investigation will be

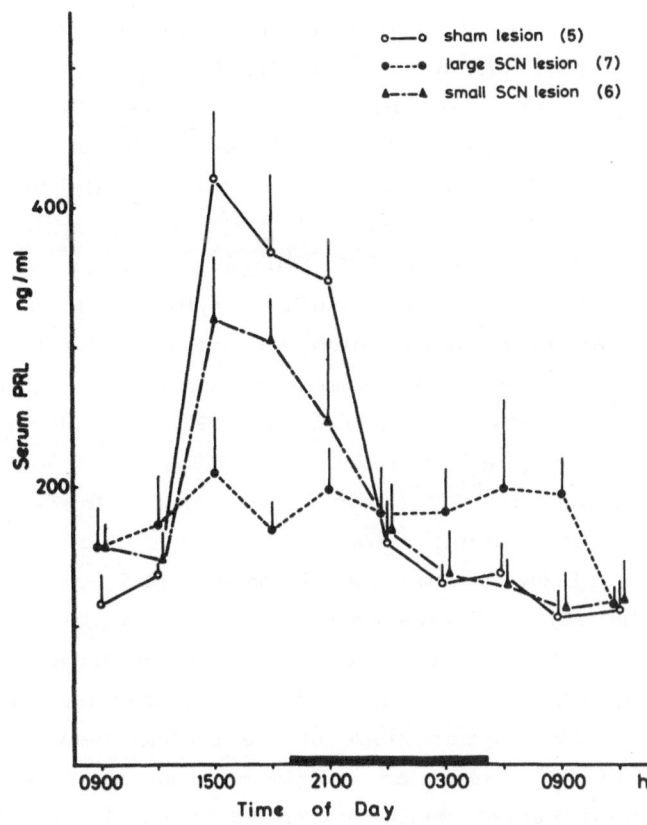

Figure 7: Effects of lesions of the supra-chiasmatic nucleus (SCN) on estrogen-induced PRL surges in ovariectomized rats. From Kawakami et al. (1980) with permission

necessary to determine whether the serotonergic pathway from the raphe nuclei is involved in the control of the proestrous surge and the estrogen-induced surge of PRL.

Second, in order to determine the exact location of the preoptic neural structures which are indispensable for the occurrence of the estrogen-induced PRL surge, small lesions were chronically placed by a platinum electrode (anodal direct current of 0.5 mA for 12 sec) in the preoptic region of ovariectomized rats, and the effects of these lesions on the estrogen-induced PRL surge were examined (Kawakami et al., 1980). Blood samples were obtained at 3-h intervals for 24 h from individual animals with an indwelling atrial cannula. In rats with large SCN lesions (destruction of more than 50% of the bilateral nuclei), pronounced surges of PRL induced by 50 μg estradiol benzoate injections were eliminated and mean values of serum PRL at 1500 h in the rats with large SCN lesions were significantly lower than those in sham-lesioned animals ($P < 0.01$) (Fig. 7). In contrast,

PRL surges comparable to those in sham-lesioned animals were observed in rats with the small lesions (destruction of ventrally or laterally adjacent structures of less than 20% of the SCN). Furthermore, most animals with large SCN lesions exhibited the pulsatile or sporadic release of PRL rather than the consistently low secretion. These results suggest that the SCN plays an essential role in the control of the estrogen-induced PRL surge. The estrogen-induced PRL surge has the attribute of a circadian rhythm mentioned above, similar to other circadian rhythms which are entrained by the light-dark cycle. It has been shown that several circadian rhythms, such as corticosterone secretion (Moore and Eichler, 1972), drinking behavior, locomotor activity (Stephan and Zucker, 1972), sleep and wakefulness (Ibuka and Kawamura, 1975), pineal serotonin N-acetyl-transferase activity (Moore and Klein, 1974) and estrous cyclicity (Barraclough et al., 1964; Brown-Grant and Raisman, 1977), were abolished by lesions of the SCN. Furthermore, it has been demon-strated that the SCN in the rat receives a direct retinohypothalamic projection (Moore and Lenn, 1972). From these findings, this neural structure is thought to be a biological clock of the central nervous system having a function of the generation and entrainment of these rhythms. The SCN may send neural impulses depending on the time of day to the MBH and to other structures in the brain for the generation of the rhythms, presumed by the electrophysiological study (Inouye and Kawamura, 1979) and the autoradiographic deoxyglucose method (Schwartz et al., 1980).

Our previous studies showed that lesions in the medial basal part of the suprachiasmatic area (MBSC), which is the periventricu-lar area lying rostrodorsal to the SCN, eliminated not only the estrogen-induced but also progesterone-induced gonadotropin surge in ovariectomized rats (Kawakami et al., 1978). The involvement of this neural structure in the control of LH surge was subsequently confirmed by other investigators (Wiegand et al., 1978; Samson and McCann, 1979). In contrast, SCN lesions abolished the estrogen-induced LH surge but not the progesterone-induced LH surge which were abolished by MBSC lesions, suggesting that the MBSC has distinct neural functions in the control of gonadotropin secretion. Therefore, the effects of MBSC lesions on the estrogen-induced PRL surge in ovariectomized rats were examined. Mean levels of serum

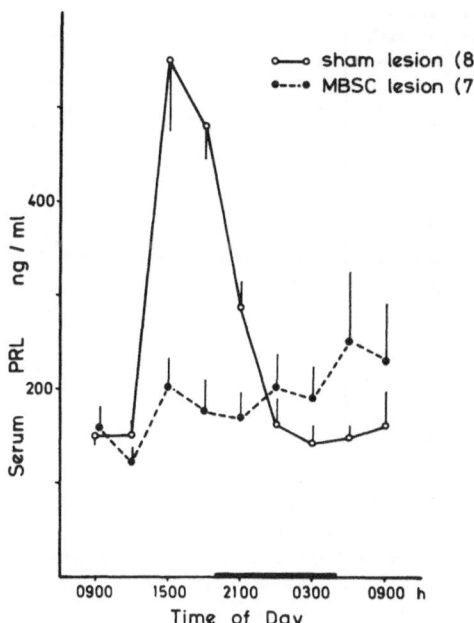

Figure 8: Effects of lesions of the medial basal part of the suprachiasmatic area (MBSC) on estrogen-induced PRL surges in ovariectomized rats

PRL of rats with MBSC lesions did not show a pronounced surge observed in sham-lesioned animals (Fig. 8). PRL values at 1500 h in MBSC-lesioned rats were significantly lower than those in sham-lesioned animals ($P < 0.01$). The effects of lesions in the MBSC and SCN on the response of PRL release to progesterone treatment were also examined. Two mg progesterone was injected into ovariectomized rats at 1200 h on the fourth day after estradiol benzoate injections. In estrogen-treated rats with sham lesions, serum PRL levels were significantly increased at 1800 h in response to progesterone injection ($P < 0.01$) (Fig. 9). PRL levels in MBSC-lesioned or SCN lesioned animals were significantly increased after progesterone injection ($P < 0.02$), and there was no statistical difference in serum PRL levels at 1800 h among sham-, MBSC- and SCN-lesioned animals. Although a difference in the neural functions between the SCN and MBSC was observed in the control of LH secretion, it was not found in the control of PRL release in response to ovarian steroids. This result suggests that, in addition to the SCN, the MBSC also consist of a surge center in the preoptic region for the generation of the estrogen-induced PRL surge in ovariectomized rats and probably of the proestrous PRL surge in cycling rats.

285

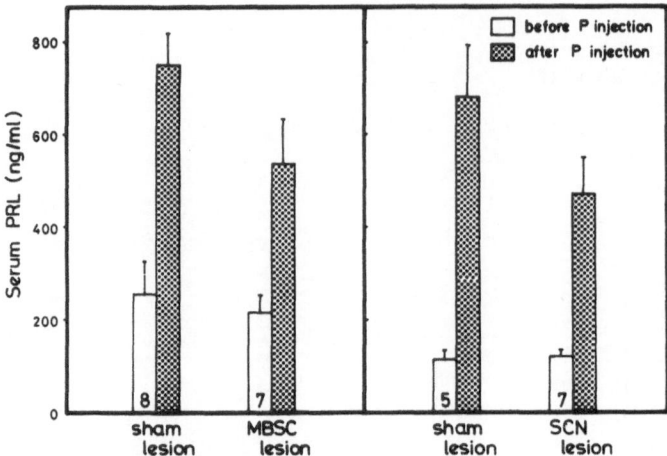

Figure 9: Effects of lesions in the MBSC and SCN on prolactin response to progesterone treatment in estrogenprimed ovariectomized rats. The ovariectomized rats were primed with 50 μg estradiol benzoate and injected with 2 mg progesterone at 1200 h on the fourth day after the estradiol benzoate injection. Blood samples were collected at 1200 and 1800 h on the fourth day

3. <u>Neural Control of the Prolactin Surge During Pseudopregnancy</u>

Stimulation of the uterine cervix induces twice daily surges during PSP. One of the daily surges is the diurnal surge occurring before lights go off, and the other is the nocturnal surge occurring before lights go one. Since the PRL surges during PSP are attenuated by ovariectomy (Freeman <u>et al.</u>, 1974; Murakami <u>et al.</u>, 1979) and cervical stimulation-induced nocturnal surges in ovariectomized rats are amplified by subcutaneous implants of progesterone (Freeman and Sterman, 1978), it is thought that progesterone secreted from the corpus luteum exerts the stimulatory feedback action on PRL release. On the other hand, it has been demonstrated that the two PRL surges in PSP rats and in ovariectomized rats with cervical stimulation occur with circadian rhythms entrained by photoperiod (Pieper and Gala, 1979; Bethea and Neill, 1979). We sought to determine the neural structures involved in the control of the diurnal and noctur-nal surges during PSP.

The uterine cervices of female rats showing regular estrous cycles were stimulated by a combination of mechanical and electrical

286

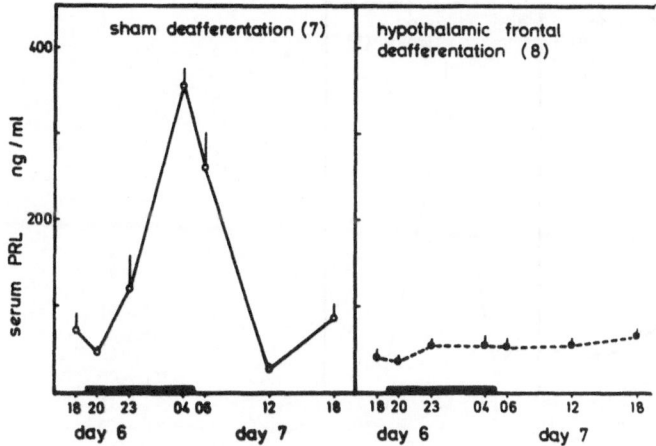

Figure 10: Effects of hypothalamic frontal deafferentation on twice daily PRL surges in pseudopregnant rats. Blood samples were collected on days 6 and 7 of pseudopregnancy

stimulation in the evening of proestrus and in the morning of estrus (day 0 of PSP). Neural transections or lesions were placed on day 1 of PSP and cannulation for blood collection was perfomed on day 2 under ether anesthesia. Blood samples were obtained at 1800, 2000 and 2300 h on day 6 and 0400, 0600, 1200 and 1800 h on day 7. Six out of 8 rats with hypothalamic frontal deafferentation showed vaginal cornification by day 5 whereas all sham-deafferented rats exhibited leucocytic smears during the period of observation. In sham-deafferented rats, pronounced nocturnal surges with peaks at 0400 h and small but significant diurnal surges with peaks at 1800 h on days 6 and 7 were observed (Fig. 10). Nadirs of serum PRL levels at 2000 h on day 6 and at 1200 h on day 7 were interposed between these nocturnal and diurnal surges. In rats with hypo-thalamic frontal deafferentation, the nocturnal surge was completely blocked (P<0.01) and the significant diurnal surge was not found at 1800 h on days 6 and 7. Arai (1969) and Carrer and Taleisnik (1970) reported that hypothalamic frontal deafferentation induced vaginal cornification and abolished the deciduoma response in PSP rats, suggesting that the frontal afferents to the MBH are required for the induction and maintenance of PSP. Freeman et al. (1974) have demonstrated that both the nocturnal and diurnal surges during

287

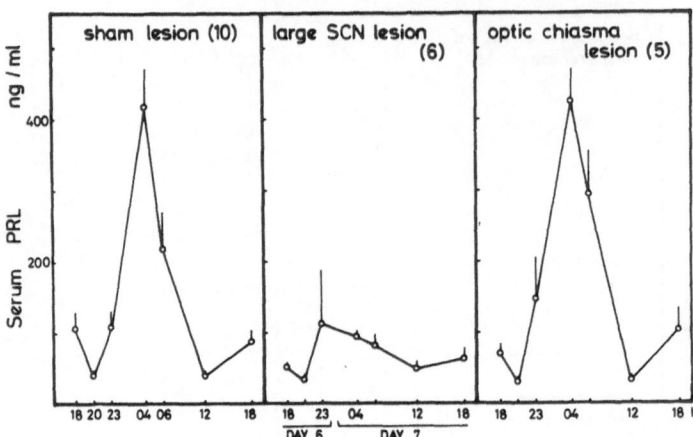

Figure 11: Effects of SCN lesions on twice daily PRL surges in pseudo-pregnant rats

PSP were abolished by hypothalamic frontal deafferentation. The present results are well consistent with those of Freeman et al. The finding that anti-PRL serum or ergocryptine administration prevented the induction and maintenance of PSP indicates that the PRL surges during PSP act on the corpus luteum as one of the luteotrophic hormones to stimulate progesterone secretion which is indispensable for the maintenance of PSP and pregnancy (McLean and Nikitovitch-Weiner, 1973; Smith et al., 1976). Consequently, it is probable that hypothalamic frontal deafferentation eliminates the twice daily surge of PRL during PSP to cause rapid luteolysis.

In order to determine the involvement of the SCN in the neural control of the PRL surges during PSP, SCN lesions were made in PSP rats. Only one out of 6 rats with large SCN lesions (destruction more than 50% of the bilateral nuclei) exhibited cornification in vaginal smears on day 4. In these SCN-lesioned rats, peak values of the nocturnal surge were attenuated to 30% of those in sham-lesioned animals (Fig. 11). For the diurnal surge, mean levels of serum PRL at 1800 h on day 6 in the SCN-lesioned rats were 50% of PRL levels at 1800 h on day 6 in sham-lesioned animals. Furthermore, serum PRL values at 1800 h on day 7 in these rats were not significantly higher compared to those at 1200 h on day 7. SCN lesions of medium size (destruction between 40% and 20% of either

288

nuclei) also diminished peak values of the nocturnal but the lesions were less effective in inhibiting the nocturnal surge than large SCN lesions. Lesions in the optic chiasma had no effect on the nocturnal and diurnal surges and the secretion pattern of serum PRL in these animals was similar to that in sham-lesioned rats. At present, why the nocturnal and diurnal surges were not suppressed by SCN lesions so completely as by hypothalamic frontal deafferentation, and why most SCN-lesioned rats exhibited leucocytic smears are unknown. It might be caused by the incompleteness of SCN lesions or the existence of other neural structures generating the PRL surges. Brown-Grant and Raisman (1977) reported that only 30% of SCN-lesioned rats which ovulated after mating became pregnant. Their results and the present results suggest that the SCN plays an important role in the control of the PRL surges during PSP. On the other hand, it has been demonstrated that rats with lesions restricted to the medial preoptic area showed repeated periods of PSP (Clemens et al., 1976; Brown-Grant et al., 1977; Freeman and Banks, 1980). Therefore, it is suggested that in the preoptic region there are facilitatory surge centers which induce the PRL surges during PSP with circadian rhythms and inhibitory systems which tonically suppress the occurrence of the PRL surges.

In order to examine the involvement of the lower brain structures in the control of the nocturnal surge during PSP, VMM, LM and DM transections were acutely placed in PSP rats. In the evening of day 5 of PSP, the transections were performed under ether anesthesia and blood samples were obtained at 2100 and 2300 h on day 5 and at 0400, 0600, 1000 and 1300 h on day 6. In sham-transected rats, marked nocturnal surges of PRL occurred with peaks between 0400 and 0600 h (Fig. 12). VMM transections, which were effective in blocking the proestrous and estrogen-induced surge of PRL, did not affect the timing and magnitude of the nocturnal surge. Neither DM transections nor LM transections also inhibited the surge. Although neural impulses of exteroceptive stimuli from the uterine cervix ascend through the spinal cord and reach the preoptic region to activate the neural centers of the neuroendocrine reflex resulting in the induction of PSP, it seems likely that the midbrain, especially ventromedial, ventrolateral and doromedial parts of the midbrain, is not involved, at least, in the maintenance of PSP.

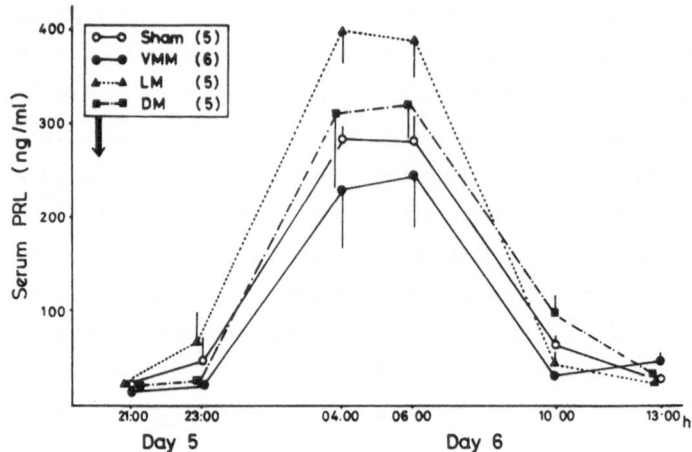

Figure 12: Effects of midbrain transections on nocturnal PRL surges in pseudopregnant rats

4. <u>Conclusion</u>

In the present study, it was indicated that the PRL surges spontaneously occurring with circadian rhythms, the proestrous surge in
cycling rats, the estrogen-induced surge in ovariectomized rats and
the diurnal and nocturnal surges in PSP rats, require the frontal
afferents from the surge centers in the preoptic region to the MBH.
The SCN, one of the surge centers, is suggested to be involved in
the control of the PRL surges as a biological clock having a function
in the generation and entrainment of the rhythms. The neural
impulses from the surge centers in the preoptic region might suppress
the activity of PRL inhibiting factor-producing neurons in the MBH,
especially arcuate dopaminergic neurons, or stimulate the activity of
PRL releasing factor-producing neurons to induce the PRL surges.
Furthermore, it was shown that the neural afferents, probably
monoaminergic afferents, from the lower brain structures to the
preoptic region are essential for the occurrence of the proestrous and
estrogen-induced surge of PRL. It is unknown and crucial to
determine whether an increase in transmission of the facilitatory
impulses from the lower brain structures to the preoptic region
occurs on the afternoon of proestrus or whether tonic discharges in
it ·is enough to maintain the neural activity of circadian rhythms
in the preoptic region.

290

Recently, numerous investigations have provided evidence suggesting that various neuropeptides participate in the physiological control of PRL secretion, and that some of them are possibly involved as PRL releasing factor. The determination of the site of actions of these neuropeptides and ovarian steroids will contribute to the understanding of the neural control of PRL secretion.

References

Amenomori Y, Chen CL, Meites J (1970) Serum prolactin levels in rats during different reproductive states. Endocrinology 86:506–510.

Arai Y (1969) Effect of hypothalamic de-afferentation on induction of pseudopregnancy by vaginal-cervical stimulation in the rat. J Reprod Fertil 19:573–575.

Barraclough CA, Yrarrazaval S, Hatton R (1964) A possible hypothalamic site of action of progesterone in the facilitation of ovulation in the rat. Endocrinology 75:838–845.

Bethea CL, Neill JD (1979) Prolactin secretion after cervical stimulation of rats maintained in constant dark or constant light. Endocrinology 104:870–876.

Brown-Grant K, Murray MAF, Raisman G, Sood MC (1977) Reproductive function in male and female rats following extra- and intra-hypothalamic lesions. Proc R Soc Lond (Biol) 198:267–278.

Brown-Grant K, Raisman G (1977) Abnormalities in reproductive function associated with the destruction of the suprachiasmatic nuclei in female rats. Proc R Soc Lond (Biol) 198:279–296.

Butcher RL, Collins WE, Fugo NW (1974) Altered secretion of gonadotropins and steroids resulting from delayed ovulation in the rat. Endocrinology 96:576–586.

Butcher RL, Fugo NW, Collins WE (1972) Semicircadian rhythm in plasma levels of prolactin during early gestation in the rat. Endocrinology 90:1125–1127.

Caligaris L, Astrada JJ, Taleisnik S (1974) Oestrogen and progesterone influence on the release of prolactin in ovariectomized rats. J Endocrinol 60:205–215.

Caligaris L, Taleisnik S (1974) Involvement of neurones containing 5-hydroxytryptamine in the mechanism of prolactin release induced by oestrogen. J Endocrinol 62:25–33.

Caligaris L, Taleisnik S (1977) Further evidence on the role of the hypothalamic afferents on the estrogen-induced prolactin release. Neuroendocrinology 23:323–329.

Carrer HF, Taleisnik S (1970) Induction and maintenance of pseudopregnancy after interruption of preoptic hypothalamic connections. Endocrinology 86:231–236.

Clemens JA, Smalstig EB, Sawyer BD (1976) Studies on the role of the preoptic area in the control of reproductive function in the rat. Endocrinology 99:728–735.

Freeman ME, Banks JA (1980) Hypothalamic sites which control the surges of prolactin secretion induced by cervical stimulation. Endocrinology 106:668–673.

Freeman ME, Smith MS, Nazian SJ, Neill JD (1974) Ovarian and hypothalamic control of the daily surges of prolactin secretion during pseudo-pregnancy in the rat. Endocrinology 94:875–882.

Freeman ME, Sterman JR (1978) Ovarian steroid modulation of prolactin surges in cervically stimulated ovariectomized rats. Endocrinology 102:1915–1920.

Fuxe K, Jonsson G (1974) Further mapping of central 5-hydroxytryptamine neurons: studies with the neurotoxic dihydroxytryptamines. Adv Biochem Psychopharmacol 10:1-

Halász B, Gerendai I, Köves K, Lukáts O, Marton J, Molnár J, Nagy G (1978) Recent data on the mechanisms controlling anterior pituitary function. In: Dörner G, Kawakami M (eds) Hormones and brain development. Elsevier/North-Holland Biomedical Press, Amsterdam, pp.399–408.

Ibuka N, Kawamura H (1975) Loss of circadian rhythm in sleep-wakefulness cycle in the rat by suprachiasmatic nucleus lesions. Brain Res 96:76–81.

Inouye ST, Kawamura H (1979) Persistence of circadian rhythmicity in a mammalian hypothalamic "island" containing the suprachiasmatic nucleus. Proc Natl Acad Sci USA 76:5962–5966.

Kawakami M, Arita J (1980) Involvement of the ventromedial part of the midbrain in the control of the proestrous surge of gonadotropins and prolactin in the rat. Neuroendocrinology 30:337–343.

Kawakami M, Arita J, Yoshioka E (1980) Loss of estrogen-induced daily surges of prolactin and gonadotropins by suprachiasmastic nucleus lesions in ovariectomized rats. Endocrinology 106:1087–1092.

Kawakami M, Higuchi T, Matsuura M (1979) Immobilization stress and prolactin secretion in male rats. Neuroendocrinology 29:262–269.

Kawakami M, Yoshioka E, Konda N, Arita J, Visessuvan S (1978) Data on the sites of stimulatory feedback action of gonadal steroids indispensable for luteinizing hormone release in the rat. Endocrinology 102:791–798.

Kimura F, Kawakami M (1978) Reanalysis of the preoptic afferents and efferents involved in the surge of LH, FSH and prolactin release in the proestrous rat. Neuroendocrinology 27:74–85.

Krulich L, Hefco E, Aschenbrenner JE (1975) Mechanism of the effects of hypothalamic deafferentation on prolactin secretion in the rat. Endocrinology 96:107–118.

Kwa HG, Verhofstad F (1967) Prolactin levels in the plasma of female rats. J Endocrinol 39:455–456.

Langelier P, McCann SM (1977) The effects of interruption of the ventral noradrenergic pathway on the proestrous discharge of prolactin in the rat. Proc Soc Exp Biol Med 154:553–557.

Lindvall O, Björklund A (1974) The organization of the ascending catecholamine neuron systems in the rat brain. Acta Physioc Scand (Suppl) 412:1–48.

McLean BK, Nikitovitch-Weiner MB (1973) Corpus luteum function in the rat: a critical period for luteal activation and the control of luteal maintenance. Endocrinology 93:316–323.

Moore RY, Eichler VB (1972) Loss of a circadian adrenal corticosterone rhythm following suprachiasmatic lesions in the rat. Brain Res 42:201–206.

Moore RY, Klein DC (1974) Visual pathways and the central neural control of a circadian rhythm in pineal serotonin N-acetyltransferase activity. Brain Res 71:17–33.

Moore RY, Lenn NJ (1972) A retinohypothalamic projection in the rat. J Comp Neurol 146:1–14.

Murakami N, Takahashi M, Suzuki Y (1979) Indispensable role of peripheral progesterone level for the occurrence of prolactin surges in pseudopregnant rats. Biol Reprod 21:263–268.

Neill JD (1970) Effect of "Stress" on serum prolactin and luteinizing hormone levels during the estrous cycle of the rat. Endocrinology 87:1192–1197.

Neill JD (1972) Sexual differences in the hypothalamic regulation of prolactin secretion. Endocrinology 90:1154–1159.

Neill JD, Freeman ME, Tillson SA (1971) Control of the proestrous surge of prolactin and luteinizing hormone secretion by estrogens in the rat. Endocrinology 89:1448–1453.

Niswender GD, Chen CL, Midgley AR, Meites J, Ellis S (1969) Radioimmunoassay for rat prolactin. Proc Soc Exp Biol Med 130:793–797.

Pieper DR, Gala RR (1979) The effect of light on the prolactin surges of pseudopregnant and ovariectomized, estrogenized rats. Biol Reprod 20:727–732.

Riegle GD, Meites J (1976) The effect of stress on serum prolactin in the female rat. Proc Soc Exp Biol Med 152:441–448.

Samson WK, McCann SM (1979) Effects of lesions in the organum vasculosum lamina terminalis on the hypothalamic distribution of luteinizing hormone-releasing hormone and gonadotropin secretion in the ovariectomized rat. Endocrinology 105:939–946.

Schwartz WJ, Davidsen LC, Smith CB (1980) In vivo metabolic activity of a putative circadian oscillator, the rat suprachiasmatic nucleus. J Comp Neurol 189:157–168.

Smith MS, McLean BK, Neill JD (1976) Prolactin: the initial luteotropic stimulus of pseudopregnancy in the rat. Endocrinology 98:1370–1377.

Smith MS, Neill JD (1976) A "critical period" for cervically-stimulated prolactin release. Endocrinology 98:324–328.

Stephan FK, Zucker I (1972) Circadian rhythms in drinking behavior and locomotor activity of rats are eliminated by hypothalamic lesions. Proc Natl Acad Sci USA 69:1583–1586.

Subramanian MG, Gala RR (1976) Further studies on the effects of adrenergic, serotonergic and cholinergic drugs on the afternoon surge of plasma prolactin in ovariectomized, estrogen-treated rats. Neuroendocrinology 22:240–249.

Ungerstedt U (1971) Stereotaxic mapping of the monoamine pathways in the rat brain. Acta Physiol Scand (Suppl) 367:1–48.

Velasco ME, Castro-Vazquez A, Rothchild I (1974) Effects of hypothalamic deafferentation on criteria of prolactin secretion during pregnancy and lactation in the rat. J Reprod Fertil 41:385–395.

Weiner RI, Ganong WF (1978) Role of brain monoamines and histamine in the regulation of anterior pituitary secretion. Physiol Rev 58:905–976.

Wiegand SJ, Terasawa E, Bridson WE (1978) Persistent estrus and blockade of progesterone-induced LH release follows lesions which do not damage the suprachiasmatic nucleus. Endocrinology 102:1645–1648.

Wuttke W, Meites J (1970) Effects of ether and pentobartital on serum prolactin and LH levels in proestrous rats. Proc Soc Exp Biol Med 135:648–652.

Electrophysiological and Morphological Properties of E$_2$-responsive Neurons

M.J. Kelly, U. Kuhnt and W. Wuttke, Pittsburgh and Göttingen

Early evidence for the influence of estrogen and progesterone on hypothalamic neurons which control pituitary gonadotropin secretion was provided by the studies of Kawakami and Sawyer (1959). They demonstrated that progesterone had a biphasic effect on the threshold (initially decreasing and then increasing) for the coitus-induced hypothalamic-rhinencephalic EEG activity in the estrogen-primed female rabbit. Single-unit recordings in the lateral hypothalamus showed increased activity with cervical probing; this activity was attenuated with large doses of progesterone (Cross and Silver, 1965). Later investigations (Lincoln and Cross, 1967; Lincoln, 1969) demonstrated that some of these effects were probably nonspecific in that they were linked to a general increase in arousal in the frontal EEG. However, Lincoln and Cross recorded from units in the preoptic, septal and anterior hypothalamus which showed a specific increase in activity after cervical probing. Furthermore, estrogen enhanced the responsiveness of preoptic units to cervical stimulation. Terasawa and Sawyer (1969) found that multiunit activity in the arcuate nucleus (ARC) increased following electrochemical stimulation of the preoptic area, a stimulus which is able to cause ovulation in the pentobarbital-anesthetized proestrous rat.

During the 4-day estrous cycle of the rat, plasma estrogen levels peak in the afternoon of proestrus (Nequin et al., 1975). Multiunit activity increases in the ARC and medial preoptic (mPOA) at this time (Kawakami et al., 1970; Wuttke, 1974). Spontaneous single-unit activity of the medial preoptic-anterior hypothalamus continuum is also highest on proestrus (Cross and Dyer, 1970; Moss and Law, 1971; Dyer et al., 1972) and lowest on estrus. These

294

"cyclic" cells apparently do not project to the medial basal hypothalamus, the presumed pathway of luteinizing hormone-releasing
hormone (LHRH) neurons, since these cyclic neurons could not be
driven antidromically by medial basal hypothalamus stimulation
(Dyer, 1973). In 1974, Wuttke made the observation that the
increased mPOA multiunit activity (and single-unit activity) in altert
freely moving rats precedes the preovulatory plasma surge of luteinizing hormone (LHRH) on proestrus.

The first studies on the effects of estrogen on single unit
activity of preoptic and hypothalamic neurons yielded ambiguous
results. The spontaneous firing frequency could increase, decrease
or not change following an intravenous (i.v.) injection of estrogen
(Yagi, 1970, 1973). Whitehead and Ruf (1974) tested 120 mPOA
neurons whose axons projected to the medial basal hypothalamus
(antidromically identified) with microelectrophoretically applied dopamine, norepinephrine and acetylcholine before and after an i.v.
injection of estrogen to ovariectomized rats. They found that
estrogen did not antagonize the actions of these putative transmitters, which led them to conclude that estrogen was acting
pre-synaptically. The spontaneous activity decreased in six of the
cells following an i.v. injection of estrogen, whereas three cells
showed a transitory increase. Bueno and Pfaff (1976) found that the
number of spontaneously active cells in the preoptic area decreased
after estrogen administration to ovariectomized rats, but there was
an increase in the number of spontaneously firing cells in the medial
basal hypothalamus. The question remained, does estrogen act
diretly on hypothalamic neurons and by what mechanism?

We attempted to answer the first question several years ago in
Dr. Robert Moss' laboratory. We utilized the microelectrophoresis
technique to apply minute quantities of an estrogen ester, 17β-
estradiol hemisuccinate, onto preoptic hypothalamic neurons of the
cycling female rat (Kelly et al., 1975, 1976). We observed both
excitatory (N=14) and inhibitory (N=40) responses but the inhibitory
effects predominated. Furthermore, these effects were extremely
rapid in onset and terminated with the iontophoretic application of
the steroid. A summary of the major findings of these studies is the
following:

(1)   17β–estradiol hemisuccinate produced a rapid inhibition (excitation) in the firing frequency of about 37% of the mPOA septal neurons tested. These changes were independent of initial firing frequency;

(2)   Four out of 18 neurons antidromically identified (AI) as having their axons projecting to the median eminence were inhibited by the microelectrophoretic application of the steroid; and

(3)   17α–estradiol hemisuccinate did not have any effect on neurons which were responsive to 17β–estradiol hemisuccinate.

At the time that we were doing these studies in the rat, Bernard Dufy and coworkers characterized the estrogen sensitivity of hypothalamic neurons with projections to the median eminence (AI neurons) in the female rabbit. Twelve out of 46 AI cells responded to an i.v. injection of estrogen with a decrease in their firing frequency (Dufy et al., 1976). This depressed activity persisted for 30–120 min. Dufy and colleagues also found that accompanying this decrease was a decrease in serum luteinizing hormone (LH) and follicle stimulating hormone (FSH) within about 40 minutes after estrogen treatment (Dufy et al., 1975). Furthermore, actinomycin D, a potent protein synthesis inhibitor, could not prevent this decrease in LH and FSH following the injection of estrogen (Dufy et al., 1976). Therefore, it appeared from these aforementioned studies that estrogen was acting directly on hypothalamic neurons to lower their firing frequency, which was temporally related to the decrease in serum LH and FSH.

To answer the question of how estrogen was acting to bring about a decrease (increase) in membrane excitability, it was necessary to perform intracellular recordings. It has been virtually impossible to obtain stable intracellular recordings in the small parvocellular neurons in vivo. Therefore, in Göttingen we developed an in vitro slice preparation for the hypothalamus to obtain long-term intracellular recordings. The slice preparation also allowed us to study whether the 17β–estradiol or its ester was causing the changes in firing frequency since we could add free steroids directly to the bathing medium.

296

1. Materials and Methods

Cycling female guinea pigs were sacrificed by a sharp blow to the neck and, six to eight sagittal hypothalamic slices of 400-450 m thickness were prepared as previously described (Kelly et al., 1979c). The slices were placed inside a recording chamber (Fig. 1), where they were kept viable for eight to ten hours by constant perfusion with artificial CSF (Kelly et al., 1980). Stimulating electrodes were placed visually in the stria terminals (ST) and the median eminence (ME) (Fig. 2). Cells which were recorded in the arcuate (ARC), ventromedial (VM) and in the cell-poor-zone (CPZ) between the ARC and the VM (Heimer and Nauta, 1969) could be driven antidromically from the ME and/or ST and orthodromically

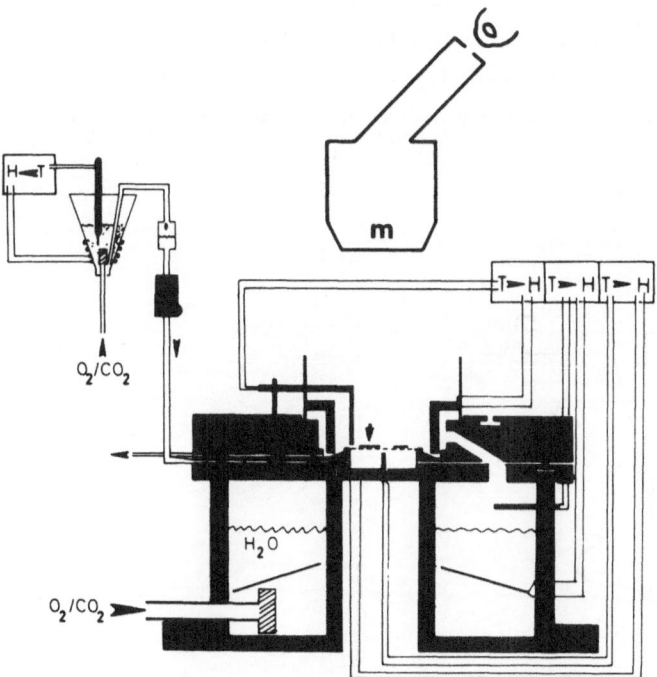

Figure 1: Schematic of slice chamber. Aerated (O_2/CO_2) medium flows from a flask containing either control medium or estrogen medium (see Material and Methods) up underneath the slice (arrow) and drains off to the side. A three-way stop-cock at the chamber reservoir inlet facilitated switching between the different media. All temperatures are controlled at 35°C. Slice is viewed from above through a stereomicroscope (m) with a fiber light source allowing the electrodes to be placed visually

from the ST and/or ME. After a recovery period of 1 1/2 hours following the removal of the guinea pig brain, intracellular recordings were made in the parvocellular neurons through single barrel micropipettes filled with 4% aqueous procion yellow (PY) solution. A bridge circuit was utilized for simultaneously passing a current and measuring the voltage across the PY pipette. The input resistance was calculated from the change in membrane potential versus the amount of current passed.

17β-estradiol (E_2) was dissolved in a separate medium reservoir at 10^{-8}M and was applied to slice by switching the inlet valve from the control medium to the E_2 medium. Estrogen was also utilized in a similar manner. More details of the procedure have been published earlier (Kelly et al., 1980).

The PY-filled electrodes afforded us the ability to label the neurons which we were recording. This intracellular fluorescent dye was pulse-injected for 10 min at tip negative currents of 0.8–1.2 nA. Following the injection the slice was fixed in 4% formalin, buffered to pH 7.35. Fluorescence microscopy was done on 30 μm cryostat sections using a Zeiss scope.

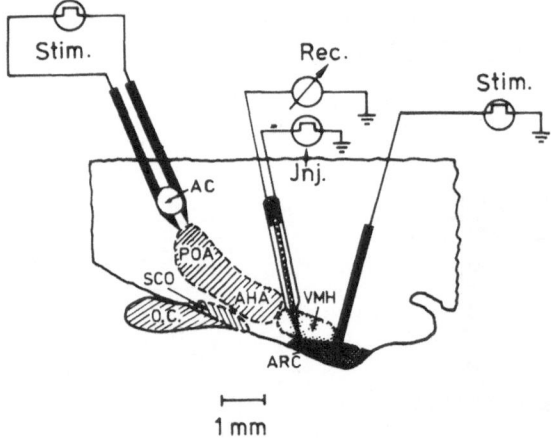

1 mm

Figure 2: Schematic of 400 μ.m thick sagittal hypothalamus slice. Stimulating electrodes (glass micropipettes filled with Wood's metal, tip diameter less than 20 μm) are placed in the stria terminalis and median eminence (ventral surface of slice). Arcuate (ARC) and ventromedial (VMH) and cell-poor-zone (CPZ) neurons are recorded through single barrel pipettes filled with PY, or theta glass micropipettes (as illustrated) AC = anterior commissure, AHA = Anterior hypothalamus, POA = preoptic, SCO = Suprachiasmatic, and OC = optic chiasm

2. Results

There were a total of eighty-five neurons recorded with an average resting membrane potential (RMP) of –35 mV. The input resistance (Rm) was found to range from 2 to 25 MΩ(N=37). Eleven of these cells were activated antidromically (AI) by ME stimulation. The antidromic latencies ranged from 1 to 20 ms (median 10 ms). A few cells (N=4) were driven orthodromically by ME stimulation. But ST stimulation resulted in orthodromic activation of more cells (ARC:N=5; CPZ:N=3; VM:N=1).

Twenty-eight neurons were tested with E_2. Eleven neurons (ARC:N=9; CPZ:N=2) were hyperpolarized from 2 to 24 mV. These membrane polarizations were found when estrogen reached concentrations in the medium reservoir of 10^{-10}M. Figures 3a and 3b exhibit DC-pen recordings from two of these neurons. Figure 3a illustrates the marked hyperpolarization which is rapidly reversed upon washing-out the E_2. The time course of the response is similar to that

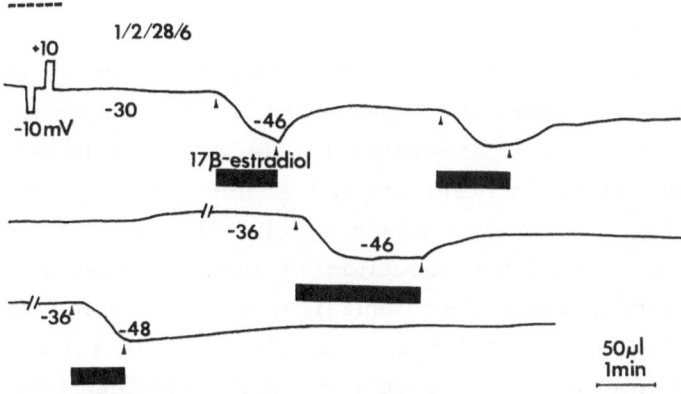

Figure 3a: Continuous script-chart recording of RMP during exposure to 17β-estradiol (E_2) in the medium (see Material and Methods). Solid bars indicate time of inflow of E_2 medium into recording chamber. Note substantial hyperpolarization of 16 mV, which occurred with concentrations of 10^{-10}M E_2 were obtained. Breaks in recording indicate passed times of 5 and 6.5 minutes respectively. Stippled line represents DC-zero reference line. Calibration mark (lower right) represents a flow rate of 50 µl/min. RMP = –30 mV. 10 mV calibration pulses are at the beginning of the record (from Kelly et al., 1980)

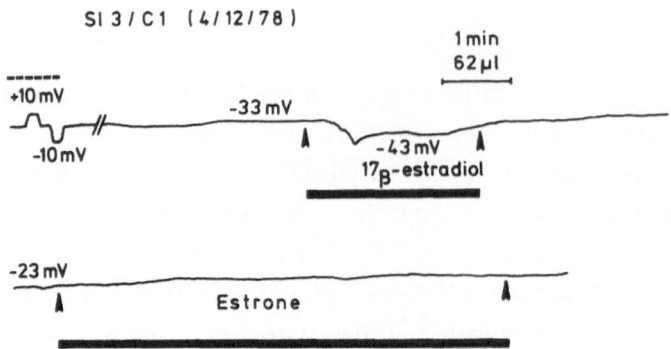

SI 3 / C1 (4/12/78)

Figure 3b: Continuous script-chart recording of RMP during exposure of ARC neuron to 17β-estradiol (upper tracing) and estrogen (lower tracing) Hyperpolarization of 10 mV by 10^{-10}M estradiol was not mimicked by higher concentrations of estrone (10^{-8}M). After application of estradiol, the cell did not return to the original resting level of -33 mV, but estradiol was still able to hyperpolarize the cell on subsequent application. Stippled line represents DC-zero reference line. Calibration mark (upper right) represents a flow rate of 62 µl/min. (from Kelly et al., 1980)

of putative transmitters applied in a perfusion system (Pittman et al., 1980). Figure 3b illustrates the specificity of this response. Estrone was not able to cause any alteration in the RMP even though it reached 100 times (10^{-8}M) the concentration. Another ARC neuron, which is not illustrated, demonstrated a reproducible hyperpolarization to 10^{-10}M E_2 and a concomitant reduction in firing frequency. The R_m was measured during the hyperpolarization and was found to decrease. Furthermore, after one hour of recording, 10^{-8}M estrone was unable to mimic any of these effects of E_2. Estrogen was applied after estrone and again was able to hyperpolarize the cell. The R_m was measured during E_2 application in two other neurons, and it did decrease in both instances.

All of the cells tested with E_2 were injected with PY. The majority of these were labeled sufficiently to make a gross morphological classification. The eleven E_2-sensitive neurons were fusiform parvocellular neurons of about 10 µm in diameter (Fig. 4). They showed very little branching of the primary dendrites and with the exception of one cell (Fig. 5), had no spine-like appendages.

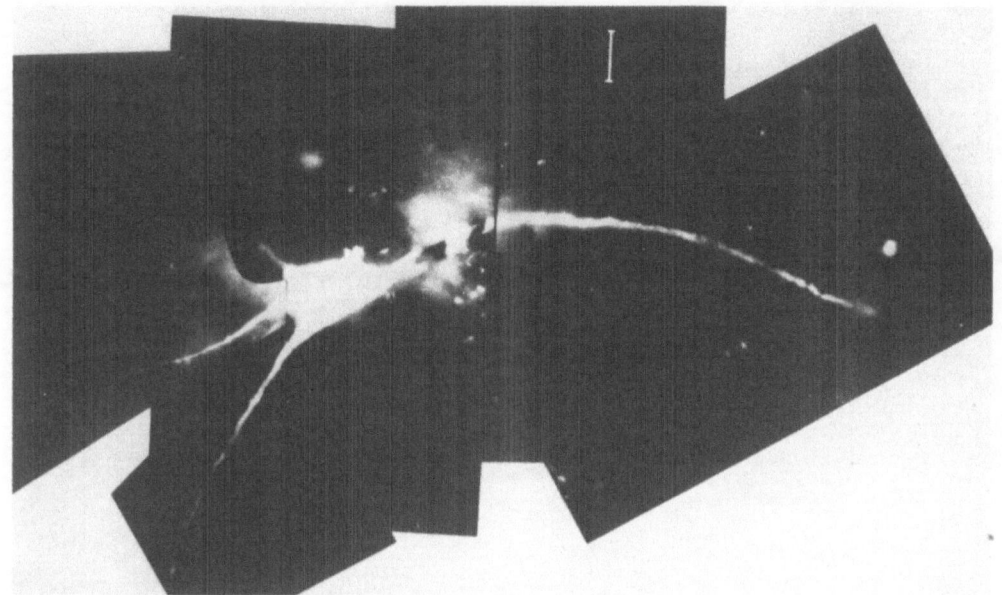

Figure 4: Montage of PY-stained ARC neuron of Fig. 3. The electrode was situated in a primary dendrite (hole surrounded by PY). The cell exhibits three primary dendrites without branches (traced for at least 200 µm) and an axon (arrow) exciting from the soma and projecting rostrally. Somal appendage (arrow head) also visable. See Fig. 6 for location. Calibration bar = 10 µm (from Kelly et al., 1980)

Three of these ARC neurons were identified antidromically, and their axons could be visualized projecting towards the ME. These cells would be considered tuberoinfundibular neurons according to Szentágothai (1964). In contrast to these simple E_2-sensitive neurons are the pyramidal-like cells with multiple dendrites with spines which did not respond to E_2 (Kelly et al., 1980). These neurons are commonly found in the VM (Millhouse, 1973, 1978) and are not as prevalent in the ARC (Szentágothai, 1964; Bodoky and Rethelyi, 1977; Kelly et al., 1977c). Figure 6 is a montage of the camera lucida drawings of most of the cells which were tested with E_2. The shaded area represents an area within 250 µm of the third ventricle which incorporates all of the labeled E_2-responsive neurons. A few neurons (N=4) in the preoptic area were tested with E_2 and were found to be unresponsive.

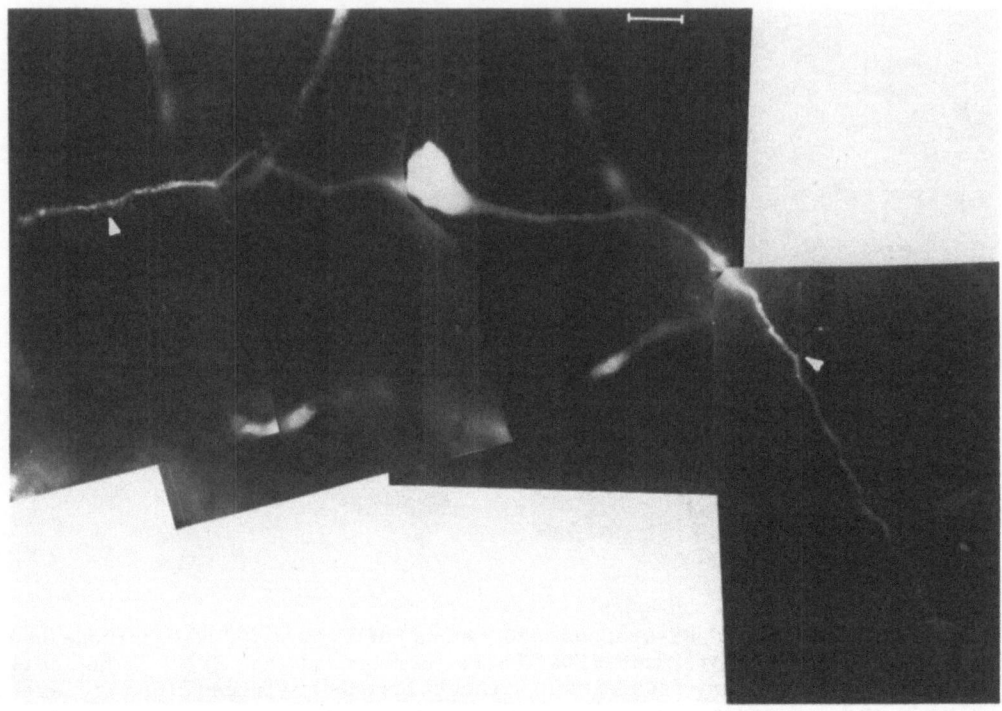

Figure 5:   Montage of another E_2-sensitive neuron.   This cell is "bipolar" exhibiting two dendrites which show no branching but do have spine-like appendages (arrowheads). An axon was not identified for this cell.   Calibration bar = 10 μm

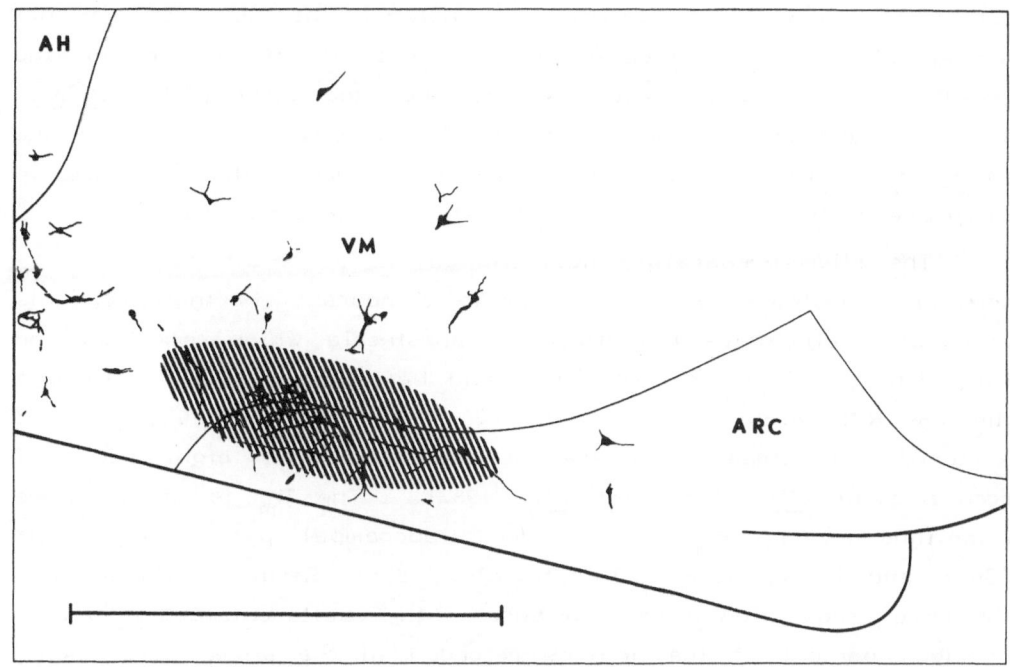

Figure 6: Parasagittal section of medial basal hypothalamus of the guinea pig with camera lucida drawings of most of the cells which were tested with estrogen and stained with PY showing their approximate location and orientation. Some of the cells were recorded in the "cell-poor-zone" between the ARC and VM nucleus. Most of the cells were located within .250 µ m in the lateral plane of the border of the third ventricle. The E_2 sensitive cells were mixed with the non-sensitive cells (shaded area) but none of the former were located in the regions as far anterior as AH (anterior hypothalamus). Calibration bar = 1 mm (modified from Kelly et al., 1980)

3. Discussion

Neuroendocrinologists have recognized for over a decade that estrogen participates in the "negative" and "positive" feedback regulation of gonadotropin-secretion at the hypothalamic-pituitary axis. This feedback pathway has been thought to involve DNA-dependent RNA transcription for the hypothalamus as well as the pituitary (McEwen and Luine, 1980). Indirect evidence comes from the early observation that tritiated estrogen is concentrated by hypothalamic neurons (Pfaff, 1968; Stumpf, 1968; Stumpf et al., 1971; Pfaff and Keiner, 1973), and that the hypothalamus contains specific nuclear receptors for estrogen (Zigmond and McEwen, 1970). However, from our earlier studies in Dallas, we concluded that estrogen was not acting solely via a nuclear-regulated event, for the latency for the effects of iontophoresed estrogen was much too short (Kelly et al., 1975). Furthermore, the inability of 17α-estradiol to change the firing frequency of these neurons was evidence that changes in membrane excitability caused by 17β-estradiol were specific.

The slice preparation has allowed us to obtain stable intra-cellular recordings for periods up to 2 hours. Furthermore, this preparation eliminates the effects of anesthesia which complicate the interpretation of the results (Dufy and Dufy-Barbe, 1979). Although the low RMP might reflect a "leaky membrane", we have sufficient evidence that these cells are healthy even after eight hours of recording in vitro (Kelly et al., 1980). The R_m is of the same magnitude as the R_m reported for hippocampal pyramidal neurons (Dodd and Kelly, 1978; Schwartzkroin, 1975). Results obtained from the slice preparation appear to agree with results obtained in vivo. Fourteen percent of the neurons recorded in the slices were driven antidromically by ME stimulation; whereas Renaud (1977) reported 15% were AI neurons from in vivo studies. Furthermore, the medial basal hypothalamic neurons (ARC, VM, CPZ) in the slice could be driven orthodromically by ST stimulation. Therefore, the slice has preserved many of the synaptic connections which have been demonstrated in vivo. This is important in classifying the cells from which we are recording.

The present data allows us to state that E_2 can specifically alter (estrone was without effect) membrane excitability presumably through ionic mechanisms. However; we have not definitely shown that estrogen is acting on the neuron from which we are recording. Unequivocal evidence will be provided when we demonstrate these same actions in a high Mg^{+2} environment, which is known to block synaptic input (Pittman et al., 1980). Additional evidence for the effects of E_2 comes from studies carried out in Dallas in which acetylcholine (Ach) and 17β-estradiol hemisuccinate were applied to preoptic neurons (Fig. 7). The application of Ach alone caused an excitation, as it did in about 60% of the cells (Kelly et al., 1977a); but when estrogen was applied simultaneously with Ach, the cell was inhibited. We interpreted these results to indicate that the steroid was acting post-synaptically. Presently, we would like to investigate

304

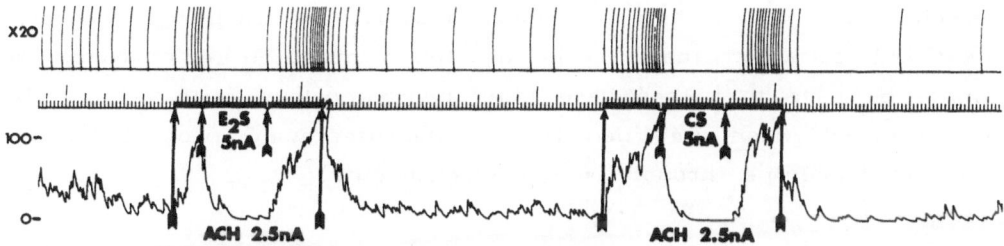

Figure 7: Extracellular recording from a medial preoptic neuron which was excited by acetylcholine (ACH) but inhibited by either 17β-estradiol hemisuccinate (E_2S) or cortisol hemisuccinate (CS) when the steroids were applied simultaneously with Ach. The arrows indicate the period for iontophoresis of the compounds. Seven out of eight mPOA neurons exhibited such a response to ACH plus E_2S. The upper trace represents standard pulses of the activity, the time base (seconds) is shown in the middle trace, and the integration of the activity is in the lower trace (modified from Kelly et al., 1977a)

the mechanism of E_2 action by looking at the specific ion conductance changes. The decrease in R_m caused by E_2 would indicate that Cl^- and/or K^+ are involved, which would be similar to γ-amino butyric acid inhibition (Krnjevic, 1974).

The spontaneous activity of hypothalamic neurons which are identified antidromically as having projections to the ME is inhibited by iontophoretically applied E_2 in the rat (Kelly et al., 1976, 1977a, 1977b) and by systemically administered E_2 in the rabbit (Dufy et al., 1976). Dufy and coworkers were able also to measure LH and FSH and to demonstrate that protein synthesis inhibitors were not able to prevent the estrogen mediated decrease in the release of the two pituitary hormones. They concluded that the reduction in electrical activity of these AI neurons is related to the "negative" feedback of E_2 on the hypothalamus. It is tempting to speculate that the hyperpolarization of AI ARC and CPZ neurons represents an inhibition of LHRH neurons or cells which are involved in LHRH release. Furthermore, E_2-sensitive neurons appeared to be the fusiform parvocellular neurons originally described by Szentágothai (1964) as the tuberoinfundibular neurons. These cells would appear to have less synaptic input from other CNS structures as deduced from the lack of spines (Palay and Chan-Palay, 1974). One could speculate therefore that these cells are under more humoral control such as "estrogen feedback". We do know that these E_2-sensitive

305

neurons are within the hypophysiotrophic area (Fig. 6), originally described by Halàsz and colleagues (1962). But although we have identified some of these cells as tuberoinfundibular neurons, we cannot be sure that these are LHRH neurosecretory cells. This will be answered when we identify the neurosecretory product in the PY-labeled neurons through immunocytochemistry.

References

Bodoky M, Rethelyi M (1977) Dendritic arborization and axon trajectory of neurons in the hypothalamic arcuate nucleus of the rat. Exp Brain Res 28:543-555.

Bueno M, Pfaff DW (1976) Single unit recordings in hypothalamus and preoptic area of estrogen-treated and untreated ovariectomized female rats. Brain Res 101:67-78.

Cross BA, Dyer RG (1970) Characterization of unit activity in hypothalamic islands with special reference to hormone effects. In: Martini L, Motta M, Fraschini F (eds) The Hypothalamus, Academic Press, New York, pp.115-122.

Cross BA, Silver IA (1965) Effect of luteal hormone on the behavior of hypothalamic neurons in pseudopregnant rats. J Endocr 31:251-263.

Dodd J, Kelly JS (1978) Is somatostatin an excitatory transmitter in the hippocampus. Nature 273:674-675.

Dufy B, Dufy-Barbe L (1979) Effects of gonadal steroids on the electrical activity of hypothalamic neurons. In: Vincent JD (ed) CNRS Collogue International sur la Biologie Cellulaire des Processes Neurosecretoires Hypothalamiques, Bordeaux, pp.207-220.

Dufy B, Dufy-Barbe L, Vincent JD (1978) Effects of protein synthesis inhibitors on the negative feedback effect of estrogen on LH release. Hormone Res 9:279-291.

Dufy B, Vincent JD, Fleury H, Du Pasquier P, Gourdji D, Tixier-Vidal A (1979) Membrane effects of thyrotropin-releasing hormone and estrogen shown by intracellular recording from pituitary cells. Science 240:509-511.

Dyer RG (1973) An electrophysiological dissection of the hypothalamic regions which regulate the pre-ovulatory secretion of luteinizing hormone in the rat. J Physiol London 234:421-422.

Dyer RG, Pritchett CJ, Cross BA (1972) Unit activity in the diencephalon of female rats during the oestrous cycle. J Endocr 53:151-160.

Halász B, Pupp L, Uhlarik S (1962) Hypophysiotrophic area in the hypothalamus. J Endocrinol 25:147-154.

Heimer L, Nauta WJ (1969) The hypothalamic distribution of the stria terminalis in the rat. Brain Res 13:284-297.

Kawakami M, Sawyer CH (1959) Neuroendocrine correlates of changes in brain activity thresholds by sex steroids and pituitary hormones. Endocrinology 65:652-668.

Kelly MJ, Dudley C, Moss RL (1975) Identification of estrogen-sensitive neurons in the preoptic-septal area of the normal cyclic female rat. Society Neurosci, 5th Ann Mtg.

Kelly MJ, Kuhnt U, Wuttke W (1979a) Effects of 17β-estradiol on hypothalamic parvocellular neurons as revealed by intracellular recordings and staining with procion yellow. The Endocrine Society, 61st Ann Mtg.

Kelly MJ, Kuhnt U, Wuttke W (1979b) Intracellular electrophysiological studies on the parvocellular neurons of the hypothalamus. Federation Proceedings 38:2557.

Kelly MJ, Kuhnt U, Wuttke W (1979c) Morphological features of physiologically identified hypothalamic neurons as revealed by intracellular marking. Exp Brain Res 34:107-116.

Kelly MJ, Kuhnt U, Wuttke W (1980) Hyperpolarization of hypothalamic neurons by 17β-estradiol and their identification through intracellular staining with procion yellow. Exp Brain Res (in press).

Kelly MJ, Moss RL, Dudley CA (1976) Differential sensitivity of preoptic septal neurons to microelectrophoresed estrogen during the estrous cycle. Brain Res 114:152-157.

Kelly MJ, Moss RL, Dudley CA (1977a) The effects of microelectrophoretically applied estrogen, cortisol and acetylcholine on medial preoptic-septal unit acitivity throughout the estrous cycle of the female rat. Exp Brain Res 30:53-64.

Kelly MJ, Moss RL, Dudley CA, Fawcett CP (1977b) The specificity of the response of preoptic septal area neurons to estrogen: 17α-estradiol versus 17β-estradiol and the response of extrahypothalamic neurons. Exp Brain Res 30:43-52.

Krnjević K (1974) Chemical nature of synaptic transmission in vertebrates. Physiol Rev 54:418-450.

Lincoln DW (1969) Responses of hypothalamic units to stimulation of the vaginal cervix: specific versus non-specific effects. J Endocr 43:683-684.

Lincoln DW, Cross BA (1967) Effect of oestrogen on the responsiveness of neurons in the hypothalamus, septum and preoptic area of rats with light-induced persistent oestrus. J Endocr 37:191-203.

McCann SM (1974) Regulation of secretion of follicle-stimulating hormone and luteinizing hormone. In: Greep RO, Astwood EB (eds) Handbook of Physiology, Section 7: Endocrinology, Vol IV. The Pituitary Gland and its Neuroendocrine Control, Part 2, American Physiological Society, Washington D.C., pp. 489-517.

McEwen BS, Luine VN (1979) Specificity, mechanisms and functional significance of steroid-receptor interactions in the brain and pituitary. In: Vincent JD (ed) CNRS Collogue International sur la Biologie Cellulaire des Processes Neurosecretoires Hypothalamiques, Bordeaux, pp.239-265.

Millhouse OE (1973) The organization of the ventromedial hypothalamic nucleus. Brain Res 55:71-87.

Millhouse OE (1978) Cytological Observations on the Ventromedial Hypothalamic Nucleus. Cell Tiss Res 191:473-491.

Moss RL, Law OT (1971) The estrous cycle: its influence on single unit activity in the forebrain. Brain Res 30:435-438.

Nequin LG, Alvarez J, Schwartz NB (1975) Steroid control of gonadotropin release. J Steroid Biochem 6:1007-1012.

Palay SL, Chan-Palay V (1977) Morphology of neurons and neuroglia. In: Bookhart JM, Mountcastle VB (eds) Handbook of Physiology, Section 1: The Nervous System, Vol. 1 Cellular Biology of Neurons, Part 1, American Physiological Society, Washington D.C., pp.5-37.

Pfaff DW (1968) Autoradiographic localization of radioactivity in rat brain after injection of tritiated sex hormones. Science 161:1355-1356.

Pfaff DW, Keiner M (1973) Atlas of estradiol-concentrating cells in the central nervous system of the female rat. J Comp Neurology 151: 121–158.

Pittman QJ, Hatton JD, Bloom FE (1980) Morphine and opiod peptides reduce paraventricular neuronal activity: Studies on the rat hypothalamic slice preparation. Proceedings National Academy Science (in press).

Renaud LP (1977) Influence of medial preoptic-anterior hypothalamic area stimulation on the excitability of mediobasal hypothalamic neurons in the rat. J Physiol 264:541–564.

Schwartzkroin PA (1975) Characteristics of CA1 neurons recorded intracellularly in the hippocamal in vitro slice preparation. Brain Res 85:423–436.

Stumpf WE (1968) Estradiol-concentrating neurons: topography in the hypothalamus by dry-mount autoradiography. Science 162:1001–1003.

Stumpf WE, Sar M, Keefer DA (1971) Atlas of estrogen target cells in rat brain. In: Stumpf WE, Grant LD (eds) Anatomical Neuroendocrinology, Krager, Basel, pp.104–133.

Szentágothai J (1964) The parvicellular neurosecretory system. In: Bargmann W, Schade JP (eds) Progress in Brain Research, Vol. 5. Lectures on the Diencephalon, Elsevier, Amsterdam, pp.135–146.

Terasawa E, Sawyer CH (1969) Changes in electrical activity in the rat hypothalamus related to electrochemical stimulation of adenohypophyseal function, Endocrinology 85:143–149.

Whitehead SA, Ruf KB (1974) Responses of antidromically identified preoptic neurons in the rat to neurotransmitters and to estrogen. Brain Res 79:185–198.

Wuttke W (1974) Preoptic unit activity and gonadotropin release. Exp Brain Res 19:205–216.

Yagi K (1973) Changes in firing rates of single preoptic and hypothalamic units following an intravenous administration of estrogen in the castrated female rat. Brain Res 53:343–352.

Yagi K (1970) Effects of estrogen on the unit activity of the rat hypothalamus. J Physiol Soc Japan 32:692–693.

Yagi K, Sawaki Y (1975) Recurrent inhibition and facilitation: demonstration in the tuberoinfudibular system and effects of strychnine and picrotoxin. Brain Res 84:155–159.

Yamada Y, Nishida E (1978) Effects of estrogen and adrenal androgen on the unit activity of the rat brain. Brain Res 142:187–190.

Zigmond RE, McEwen BS (1970) Selective retention of estradiol by cell nuclei in specific brain regions of the ovariectomized rat. J Neurochemistry 17:889–899.

Effects of Gonadal Steroids on EEG and Performance in the Human

D. Becker, M. Schwibbe and W. Wuttke, Göttingen

From neuroendocrine research it is well known that changes in the performance of behavioral tasks occur during the estrous cycle of most animals and it is also well documented that similar effects can be mimicked by treatment of castrated animals with gonadal steroids (Colwin and Sawyer, 1969; Tartellin and Gorski, 1973). An effect of gonadal steroids on both, gross electrical activity (i.e. EEG) of the brain and on single cell activity in various brain structures is also well established (Escobar, 1972; Kawakami and Sawyer, 1972). The demonstration of steroid receptive neurons in brains of all animals studied so far give the morphological substrate to these physiological findings (for details s. Stumpf and Grant, 1975).

During the menstrual cycle of women electroencephalographic as well as psychological changes are also demonstrable (Wuttke et al., 1975; Creutzfeldt et al., 1976; Becker et al., 1980). In two series of studies performed in recent years we demonstrated characteristic changes in the EEG and of a number of psychological variables in response to gonadal steroid administration which will be briefly summarized. Powerspectral analysis of the EEG and subsequent quantitation (for details s. Schwibbe and Becker, 1980) revealed that the mean alpha-frequency of the EEG is significantly accelerated during the luteal phase of the menstrual cycle when compared to the follicular phase (Fig. 1). No such effects were observed in the same subjects when they were under oral contraceptives.

The mean power spectra of the alpha range during the follicular and the luteal phase (Fig. 2) illustrates that the statistically significant acceleration of alpha-waves occurs primarily in the 11–12 Hz range.

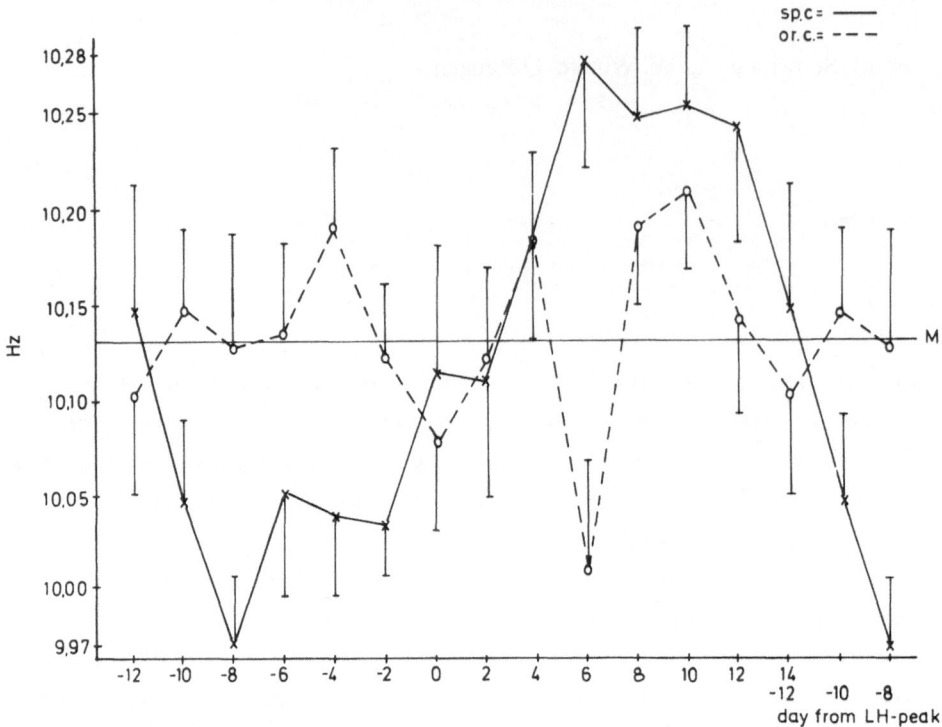

Figure 1: Mean alpha-frequency during the menstrual cycle (sp.c.) and under oral contraceptives (or.c.). Note increased alpha waves during luteal phase

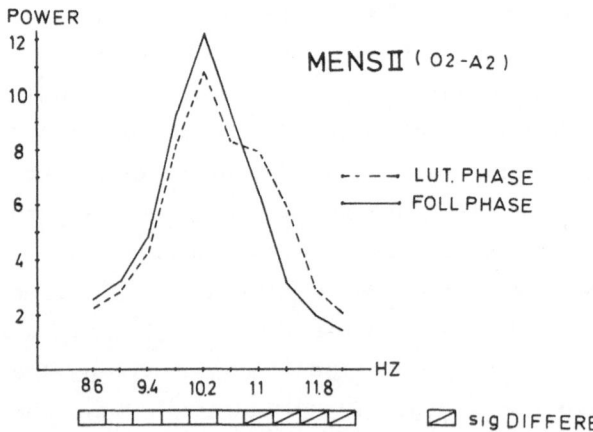

Figure 2: Power spectra of the alpha waves during luteal (lut.) and follicular (foll.) phase in women with spontaneous menstrual cycle

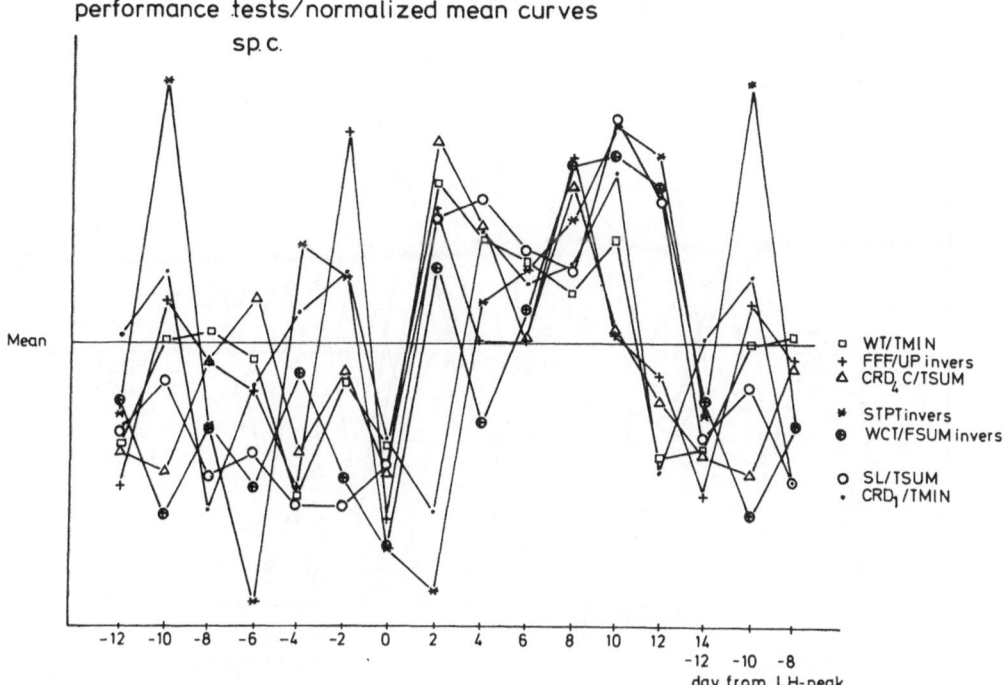

performance tests/normalized mean curves

sp.c.

Mean

- □ WT/TMIN
- + FFF/UP invers
- △ CRD₄C/TSUM
- ✳ STPT invers
- ◉ WCT/FSUM invers
- ○ SL/TSUM
- · CRD₁/TMIN

day from LH-peak

Figure 3: This figure illustrates that a number of psychological variables covary with the stage of the menstrual cycle. A downwards deflection indicates "better" performance. Note "better" performance at the periovulatory and perimenstrual period and relatively "bad" performance during luteal phase WT/TMIN = Minimal reaction time to an acoustic stimulus. FFF/UP = flicker fusion frequency as measured from low to high frequencies, $CRD_4C/TSUM$ = total time needed to react to 60 visual stimuli. STPT = personally preferred tapping frequency. WCT/FSUM = sum of incorrect reactions to a given color-tone-sequence, SL/TSUM = time needed to trace a crooked line, $CRD_1/TMIN$ = the best time needed to solve a simple arithmetic problem

From a large number of psychological variables tested (for details s. Becker et al., 1981) some proved to be significantly influenced by the stage of the menstrual cycle. As shown in Fig. 3 the most conspicuous effects can be observed at the time around preovulatory LH release (day 0) and at the perimenstrual period (day 12 and 14). The downward deflection of the curves for the different variables indicate better performance at this time. The subjects performed relatively bad during the luteal phase. The optimal performance during the periovulatory and the perimenstrual period coincides with the time of rising and falling progesterone levels and also with the time of increasing and decreasing alpha-

performance tests/normalized mean curves
       or c.

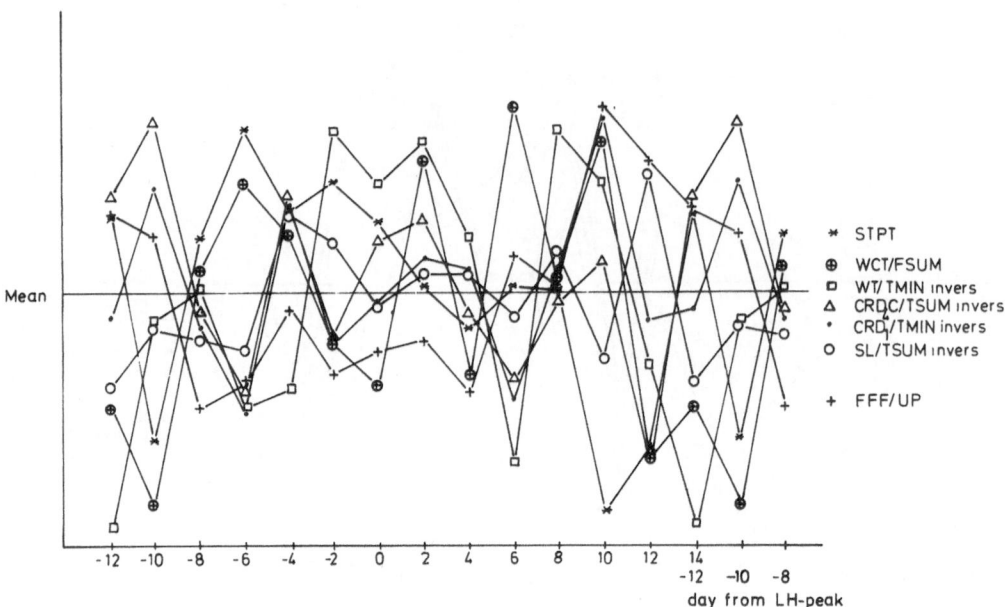

Figure 4: The same performance tests as shown in figure 3 applied to women under oral contraceptives do not change with the stage of menstrual cycle

frequencies. No cycle stage dependant changes were observed in these subjects while they received oral contraceptives (Fig. 4). These results are suggestive that at times of increasing and high progesterone levels the alpha peak frequencies are also increasing or high. Furthermore they provide the possible explanation that psychological changes occur in response to increasing or decreasing progesterone and/or alpha-frequencies.

This possibility was tested in a double blind study performed in 30 male subjects. They were treated in an unbalanced Latin-square design for one week with the following hormones: D-Norgestrel (250 mg/day), estradiol-valerate (5 mg/day), mesterolone (100 mg/day) and placebo. Between the treatment weeks one treatment-free interval of one week was introduced. Among others, the EEG was recorded and psychological performance tests were carried out during the 4th and 7th treatment days. Hormone analysis performed on bloodsamples withdrawn on these days revealed that the progestagen D-Norgestrel and the estrogen significantly reduced serum LH and FSH levels. The estrogen slightly increased serum prolactin values whereas the androgen-derivative mesterolone was ineffective in modifying serum hormone levels.

The power spectra resulting from the EEG's under the different hormone treatments are shown in Fig. 5. Mesterolon and estradiol-valerate proved to be ineffective in significantly changing the appearance of the power-spectra. The progestational compound D-Norgestrel however, shifted the mean alpha-frequencies into higher frequency-values. Hence, treatment of male subjects with the progestational compound D-Norgestrel resulted in similar effects as were normally seen during the luteal phase of spontaneously cycling female subjects.

Analysis of the psychological performance data obtained from subjects under D-Norgestrel revealed qualitatively similar results as were observed in females during the luteal phase. Hence, no sex differences in gross electrical activity and brain function as revealed by the psychological test could be demonstrated.

One interesting aspect deserves further attention. In all of our studies performed hitherto it was quite obvious that the most prominent effects on gross electrical activity of the brain and on psychological performance were observed when the subjects were under the influence of progestagens. It is inherent to these substances that they increase the basal body-temperature. This thermogenic effect causes increased temperature during the luteal phase and also in the male subjects under D-Norgestrel the sub-lingually measured temperature was elevated when compared to placebo conditions (Fig. 5). The question therefore arises whether the observed neurophysiological and psychological changes reflect a direct effect of the progestagens or represent an indirect temperature mediated effect. The latter interpretation is supported by the old qualitative results reported by Hoagland (1936) who demonstrated an acceleration of electrical brain waves in response to increased body temperature.

For this reason we looked for experimental conditions to increase the body-temperature without using progestagens. The development of a highly purified pyrogen (Galanos et al., 1979,

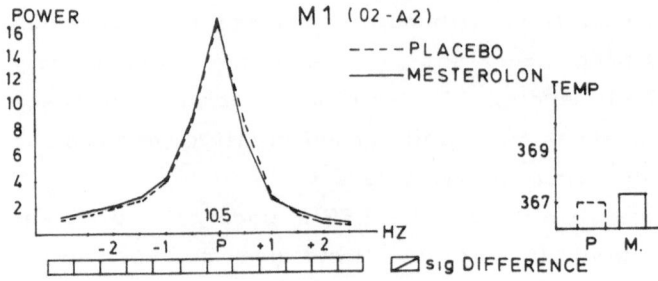

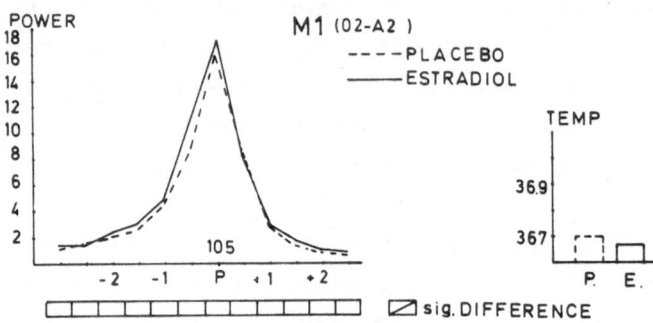

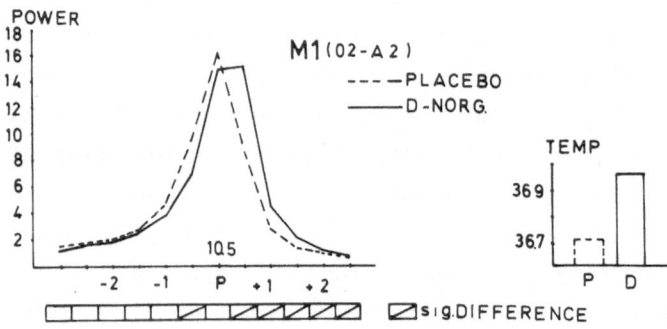

Figure 5: Power spectra of alphawaves in male subjects treated with mesterolon, estradiol-valerate, D-Norgestrel or placebo. Note the "speeding-up" effect of the progestational compound, and the increased basal body-temperature

kindly provided by Dr. O. Lüderitz, Max-Planck-Institute for Immunology, Freiburg) enabled us to investigate this problem. In this study 10 male subjects (the authors and volunteers of our laboratories) were i.v. injected with 0,03 μg Novo-Pyrexal or with placebo, using a double blind cross-over design. The effects of this treatment on body-temperature is shown in Fig. 6. Three hours

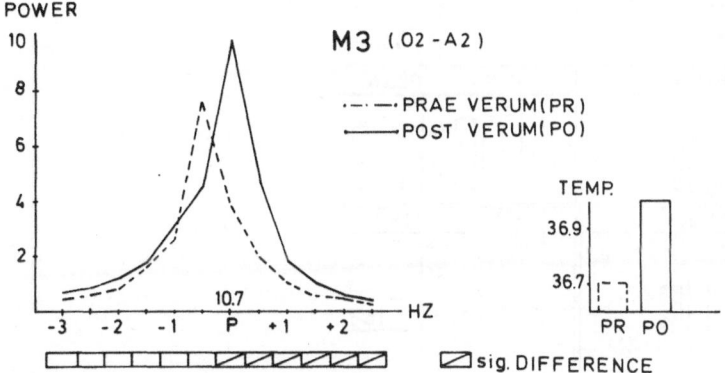

Figure 6: Power spectra of alpha waves in male subjects with normal and pyrogen-induced increased basal body-temperature. Note significantly accelerated alpha waves 3 hours after pyrogen injection (=post verum)

following Novo-Pyrexal treatment the body-temperature was significantly increased. Fig. 6 also shows that this increased body-temperature resulted in significant acceleration of alpha-waves in the EEG. The appearance of the power spectra under verum as compared to control conditions is similar to the situation observed during the luteal phase of female subjects and also to the situation found in male subjects which were under D-Norgestrel treatment. These results are suggestive that the speeding-up effect of progestagens on electrical brain waves are not direct hormone effects but rather indirectly exerted through increased body-temperature. The feedback action of D-Norgestrel on pituitary LH and FSH release was not mimicked by just increasing the body-temperature. Many of the psychological variables analyzed sofar were also influenced by elevated body-temperature in a similar manner as observed under D-Norgestrel treatment. Although analysis of all psychological data is not yet completed it is obvious that the ability to calculate simple arithmetic problems (Pauli 1) and to memorize results of these calculations for a short time (Pauli 2) is better (Fig. 7) at higher basal temperature. Under these conditions reaction time to a color-tone sequence is shorter (Fig. 7) and the time needed to trace a crooked line with a pen (Schoppe-line tracing) is shorter. In this test the subjects with increased body-temperature (i.e. under D-Norgestrel or under the pyrogen) made more errors.

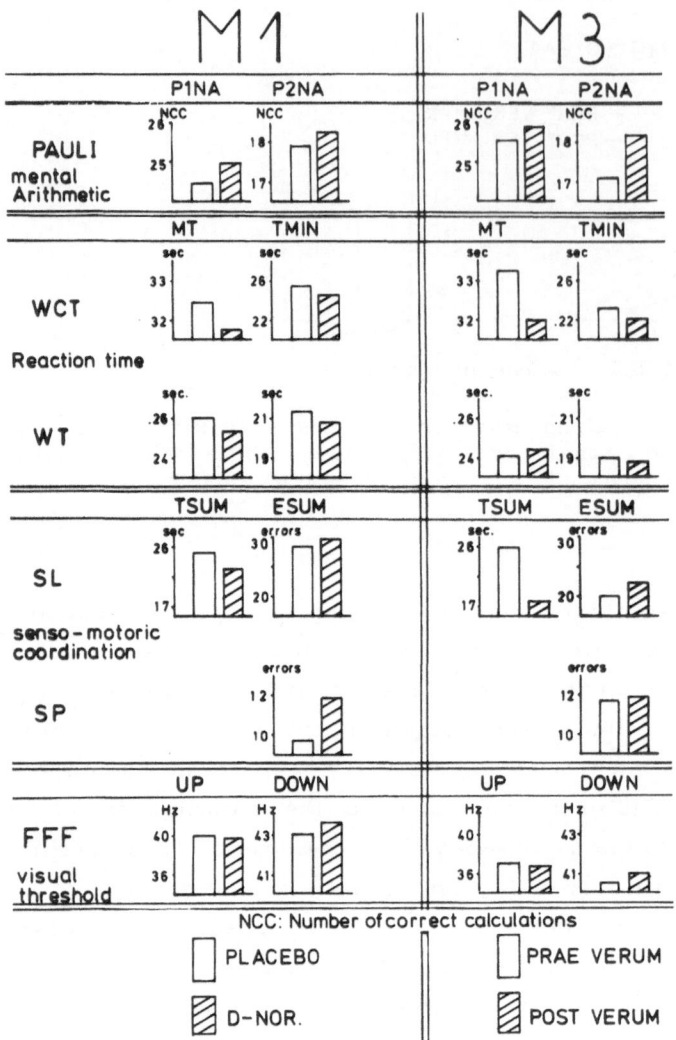

Figure 7: Comparison of D-Norgestrel-mediated (M1) with temperature-mediated (M3) effects on psychological performance. Note that effects are qualitatively always the same

These results are suggestive that some of the electrophysiological and psychotropic actions of progestagens can be mimicked by increased body-temperature. They do not allow the conclusion that all psychopharmacological effects of progestagens are indirectly exerted through increased body-temperature but in future experiments the temperature factor should always be considered.

References

Becker D, Creutzfeldt OD, Schwibbe M, Wuttke W (1980) Electro-physiological and psychological changes induced by steroid hormones in men and women. Suppl Arch Psychiatr Belg, in press.

Becker D, Creutzfeldt OD, Schwibbe M, Wuttke W Changes of physiological, EEG and psychological parameters during the menstrual cycle and under oral contraceptives. Submitted to Psychoneuroendocrinology.

Creutzfeldt OD, Arnold P-M, Becker B, Langenstein S, Tirsch W, Wilhelm H, Wuttke W (1976) EEG changes during spontaneous and controlled menstrual cycles and their correlation with psychological performance. EEG clin Neurophysiol 40:113-131.

Colvin GB, Sawyer CH (1969) Induction of running activity by intra-cerebral implants of estrogen in ovariectomized rats. Neuro-endocrinology 4:309-320.

Escobar LO (1972) Cortical evoked potentials in normal and ovariectomized rats. Acta med phill 8:104-109.

Galanos C, Lüderitz O, Westphal O (1979) Preparation and properties of a standardized lipopoly sacharide from Salmonella abortus equi (Novo-Pyrexal) Zbl Bkt Hyg 243:226-244.

Hoagland H (1936) Electrical brain waves and temperature. Science 84:139-140.

Kawakami M, Sawyer CH (1967) Effects of sex hormones and antifertility steroids on brain thresholds in the rabbit. Endocrinology 80:857-871.

Schwibbe M, Becker D (1980) Intersituativer und interindividueller Vergleich von Faktorstrukturen power-spektral-analysierter EEGs. In: Kubicki ST, Herrmann WM, Laudahn G (eds) Faktoranalyse und EEG-Frequenzbänder. Springer, Berlin.

Stumpf UE, Grant LD (1975) Anatomical Neuroendocrinology. Karger, Basel.

Tartellin MF, Gorski RA (1973) The effects of ovarian steroids and water intake and body weight in the female rat. Acta Endocrinol 72:551-568.

Wuttke W, Arnold P, Becker B, Creutzfeldt O, Langenstein S, Tiersch W (1975) Circulating hormones, EEG and performance in psychological tests of women with and without oral contraceptives. Psychoneuroendocrinology 1:141-151.

Concluding Remarks on Gonadal Steroids and Brain Function

C.H. Sawyer, Los Angeles

We have heard so many excellent presentations of different topics over the past two days that it would be quite impossible to comment on all of them in a brief talk entitled "Concluding Remarks". Rather I should like to emphasize a few items which I feel have a particular bearing on the subject of interactions between gonadal steroids and brain function. These include feedback circuits, steroid receptors, neurotransmitters, various levels of brain function and hypothalamo–pituitary mechanisms, subjects which were already widely discussed at the time of my Harris Memorial Lecture six years ago (Sawyer, 1975).

At that time Knobil's laboratory had already reported that the completely deafferented hypothalamus could maintain reproductive cyclicity and ovulation in the monkey (Knobil, 1974), and we compared deafferentation levels in the monkey with those in the rat in which the integrity of preoptico–hypothalamic pathways was required to maintain cyclicity and ovulation. In more recent brilliant research summarized in this symposium and reviewed in his recent Laurentian Hormone Conference presentation, Knobil (1980) has all but eliminated the brain as a site of estrogen's feedback action in facilitating an ovulatory surge of LH in the monkey. All that is required of the basal hypothalamus is the periodic discharge of GnRH pulses into the hypophysial portal system, for which an intravenous pump or "hypothalamic prosthesis" can be substituted in animals with arcuate nucleus lesions or infundibular stalk sections. Consecutive hourly pulsatile infusions of GnRH can maintain ovarian function and menstrual cycles in monkeys with isolated pituitaries and even start ovarian cyclicity in a prepubertal female. Knobil suggests that in the intact monkey progesterone may block the initiation of gonado-

318

tropin surges by acting on the central nervous system, but that its modulating action in advancing estrogen-induced gonadotropin surges is exerted at the level of the pituitary gland, estrogen's target organ.

A new development in neuroendocrine phenomena, discussed in this symposium by McEwen, is the induction of progestin receptors by estrogen in monkey and rat brains, recently observed in his laboratory (MacLusky et al., 1980) and in the guinea pig by Blaustein and Feder (1980). In the monkey estrogen fails to raise the level of progestin receptors in the preoptic area as it does in the other two species. Blaustein and Feder have reported that in the guinea pig the facilitation of estrous behavior by progesterone parallels the elevation of progestin receptors in the brain and that anestrus ensues as the receptor levels drop or are "down regulated" by progesterone as described here by McEwen.

The guinea pig maintains a long pseudopregnancy estrous cycle less bound by circadian rhythms than the short cycles of the rat and hamster, and as in the monkey the guinea pig cycle continues after complete hypothalamic deafferentation (Butler and Donovan, 1971; Terasawa and Wiegend, 1978). Also as in the ovariectomized monkey, the OVX guinea pig responds to exogenous estrogen with an LH surge that is not inhibited by barbiturate anesthesia. However, Terasawa et al. (1980) have recently shown that a smaller priming dose of estrogen followed some time later by progesterone will trigger an LH surge which can be blocked with either phenobarbital or repeated injections of pentobarbital. This implies a CNS site of progesterone action in the guinea pig, and essentially identical results have been more recently described in the monkey by Terasawa and Noonan (1980). Still more recently she and her colleagues (Noonan et al., 1980) have described the induction of precocious menarche in the monkey by posterior hypothalamic lesions. These findings suggest that the monkey brain may influence pituitary-ovarian function by something more than the "permissive action of GnRH" suggested by Knobil (1980).

The sites of stimulatory feedback action of estrogen and progesterone in triggering surges of gonadotropins and prolactin in the rat have been subjects of detailed investigation by Kawakami et al. (1978 a,b). Primary sites are the pituitary gland and the hypothalamus.   Employing electrolytic lesions, stereotaxic brain surgery and intracerebral implants of the steroids in OVX rats, they have observed that extrahypothalamic stimulatory feedback effects of estradiol on serum LH are exerted on limbic structures including the bed nucleus of the stria terminalis, the lateral septum and the preoptic suprachiasmatic area.   The main sites of stimulatory feed-back action of progesterone on LH release appear to be located in the diagonal band of Broca, the preoptic suprachiasmatic area and the anterior hypothalamus.   With minor discrepancies the steroids act on the same areas to stimulate FSH secretion (Kawakami et al., 1978b).   With respect to their synergistic actions on pituitary-ovarian function and sex behavior, expressed as biphasic stimulatory and inhibitory feedback influences, the effects of sequential estrogen and progesterone administration on thresholds of brain EEG activity in the rabbit should not be forgotten (Kawakami and Sawyer, 1959, 1967; Sawyer et al., 1966).   Later single unit recording and microiontophoresis studies in the laboratories of Kawakami and Moss and Kelly were reviewed by Sawyer (1975). More recently Kelly et al. (1976) reported that the response of preoptic neurons to microelectro-phoresed 17β E$_2$S shifted from excitation on diestrus 1 to inhibition on diestrus 2, proestrus and estrus.   In this symposium Kelly has extended his approach to intracellular recording of the effects of estrogen on the membranes of hypothalamic parvocellular neurons, and the methodology, developed in Wuttke's laboratory, looks very promising.   The estrogen-induced facilitation of neural transmission from the ventromedial hypothalamic nucleus (VMH) to the midbrain central grey parallel with the promotion of lordotic behavior, describ-ed by Pfaff in this symposium, is a very exciting new development. So, too, is the activation of lordosis by electrical stimulation of VMH or lesion of the preoptic area as well as the anatomical analysis of the participating neural pathways.

The possible involvement of a noradrenergic mechanism in brain-pituitary-ovarian function has been recognized for many years since it was shown that reflex ovulation in the rabbit could be blocked with rapid postcoital injections of the anti-adrenergic agent Dibenamine (Sawyer et al., 1947) and that ovulation could be induced with intraventricular infusions of norepinephrine (Sawyer, 1952).   Intraventricular norepinephrine (NE) was effective in inducing ovulation only in the estrous or estrogen-primed rabbit, and its ovulatory stimulus could be blocked not only by specific receptor-blocking drugs but also by the anesthetic pentobarbital, suggesting a central site of action (Sawyer, 1952; Sawyer and Radford, 1978). Anti-adrenergic agents and barbiturates were also found to be effective in blocking the ovulatory proestrous LH surge in the cyclically ovulating rat (Everett et al., 1949, 1950).

During the past 30 years the concept of interactions between gonadal steroids and central noradrenergic neurotransmission in controlling the ovulatory surge of LH and sex behavior in the rat and rabbit has been strengthened by a tremendous amount of data from many disciplines, and the evidence is far too vast to be reviewed here. Ever since the early experiments of Everett (reviewed in 1960) the estrogen-progesterone model has been widely employed in such studies, especially in the rat. A surge of LH release was stimulated by intraventricular NE in the OVX-estrogen-progesterone-primed rat (Krieg and Sawyer, 1976) and ovulation in the persistent estrous rat (Tima and Flerkó, 1974). The progesterone-induced LH surge in the OVX-estrogen-primed rat was blocked by diethyldithio-carbamate (DDC), which inhibits NE synthesis, and restored by treatment with dihydroxyphenylserine (DOPS), which bypasses the DDC inhibition and restores NE directly (Kalra et al., 1972; Kalra and McCann, 1974). Brain NE was released into the jugular vein on the afternoon of natural proestrus and prior to the LH surge in response to progesterone in the estrogen-primed OVX rat (Nagle and Rosner, 1976, 1980). Estrogen and progesterone priming reversed the effect of intraventricular injection of NE in the OVX rat from inhibition of the pulsatile surge to the stimulation of an LH surge resembling that of proestrus (Gallo, 1980). The proestrous or estrogen-progesterone-induced LH surge was blocked in acute experiments by destroying the ventral noradrenergic bundle with 6-hydroxydopamine (6-OHDA) (Martinovic and McCann, 1977). An elevated NE turnover has been demonstrated in the anterior hypothalamus-preoptic area on the afternoon of proestrus or the estrogen-progesterone-LH surge by Munaro (1977) and Simpkins et al. (1979) and most convincingly in the medial preoptic area by Honma and Wuttke (1980). Changes in the rate of hypothalamic catecholamine turnover can influence reproductive senescence (Meites, this volume) and the facilitation of lordosis behavior (Gorski, this volume).

These data all suggest a close relationship between hypothalamic noradrenergic synapses and the ovulatory surge of pituitary gonadotropin. However, the importance of this relationship has been questioned by recent findings. Nicholson et al. (1978) reported that the ventral noradrenergic bundle could be destroyed by injecting 6-OHDA into the ventral pons in mature female rats without prolonged effects on estrous cycles, in spite of a 60 - 75% drop in median eminence NE. The ovulatory LH surge had not recovered to normal peak levels by the second proestrus after 6-OHDA injections into the ventral noradrenergic bundle (Hancke and Wuttke, 1979). Nevertheless, Clifton and Sawyer (1979) observed independently that transection of midbrain noradrenergic pathways are consistent with complete ovulation and an undiminished proestrous LH surge in rats lacking 85% of their hypothalamic NE 40 - 50 days after stereotaxic surgery (Fig. 1). In these rats treatment with DDC, which almost completely blocks the proestrous LH surge and ovulation in intact rats while inhibiting their NE synthesis, is quite ineffective in blocking ovulation. Furthermore, the potent α-receptor blocker phenoxybenzamine (Fig. 2) also fails in the complete-cut OVX-

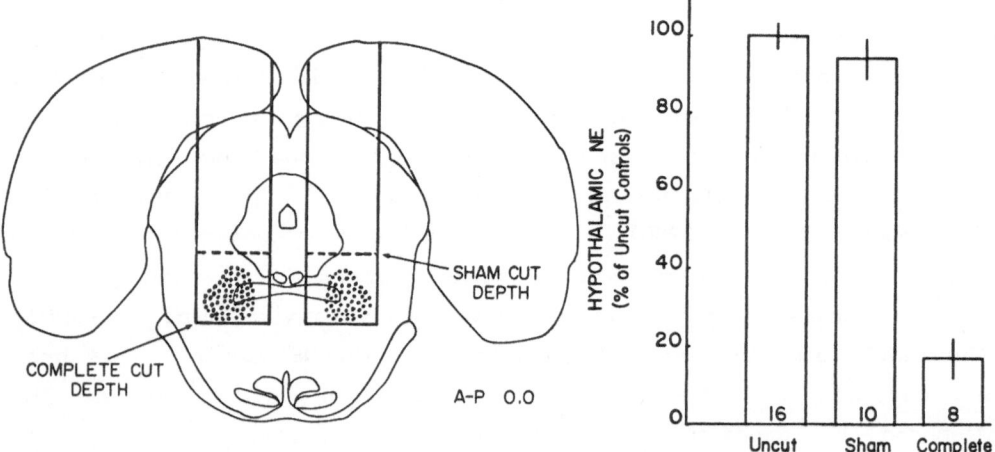

Figure 1: Diagram of coronal section illustrating the extent of sham and complete transections in the mesencephalon and the effects of the cuts on hypothalamic NE. Stippled area indicates the location of the ascending noradrenergic pathway. From Clifton and Sawyer (1979) courtesy of Neuroendocrinology

322

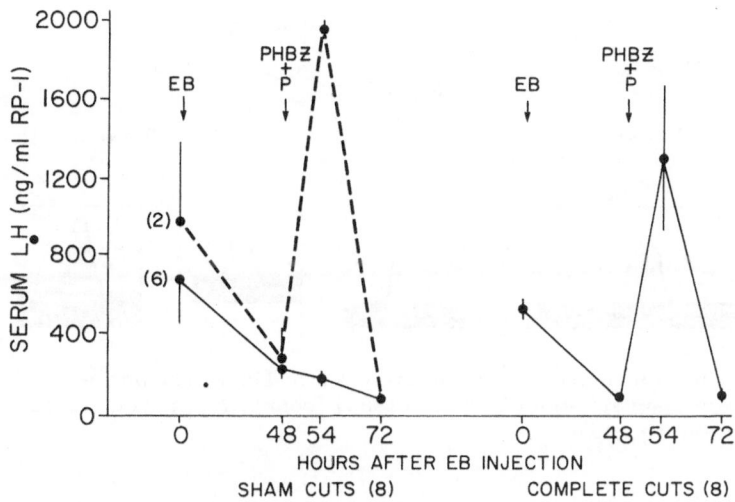

Figure 2: Effects of phenoxybenzamine on estrogen-progesterone-induced LH release in long-term ovariectomized "sham cut" and "complete cut" rats. Phenoxybenzamine (PHBZ; 20 mg/kg i.p.) and progesterone (P; 2 mg s.c.) were administered 48 h after estradiol benzoate (EB; 5 µg s.c.). Blood samples were taken just before each treatment. Dashed line represents data from 2 sham-cut animals in which the surge was not blocked by phenoxybenzamine. From Clifton and Sawyer (1980) courtesy of Endocrinology

estrogen-primed rat to block the progesterone-induced LH surge (Clifton and Sawyer, 1980). Similarly, in female rabbits copulation-induced LH release and ovulation still occur after intraventricular 6-OHDA has destroyed 85% of the hypothalamic NE (Rabii et al., 1980), and preliminary results indicate that phenoxybenzamine is ineffective in blocking the ovulatory reflex in such rabbits (Sawyer et al., unpublished results).

A hypothetical model of how hypothalamic noradrenergic inputs interact with the gonadal-steroid-induced LH surge mechanism in the rat is shown in Fig. 3 (Sawyer and Clifton, 1980). On the right are possible modes of recovery following chronic loss of the NE input. Simplified schematic diagrams of the model with intact NE fibers are seen at the top left and with severed NE pathways on the top right. Below are estimates of membrane potential under various conditions. The relative contributions of the different inputs to the total depolarization are coded the same as in the top diagrams. TP is the threshold potential and RP the resting potential. Far left—mem-

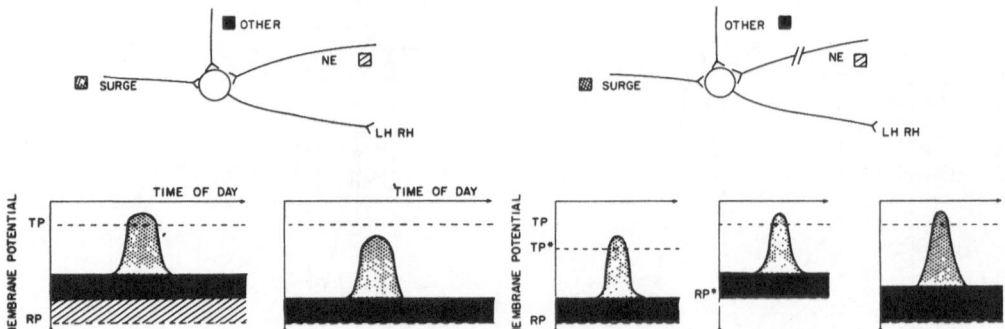

Figure 3: Model of noradrenergic interaction with LHRH neuron and LH surge in the rat. From Sawyer and Clifton (1980) courtesy of Federation Proceedings. Explanation in text

brane potential of neurosecretory LH-RH neuron on the afternoon of proestrus or in the progesterone-treated estrogen-primed animal. Next-membrane potential following acute inhibition of noradrenergic input, e.g., via phenoxybenzamine, acute lesion or DDC treatment. Next-membrane potentials after chronic development of nonspecific supersensitivity as follows: a lowering of the threshold potential, TP*, a modification of the resting potential, RP*, and an increased response to surge and other inputs.

In a way, modulation may be considered a pervasive theme in this symposium. It would appear that gonadal steroids, brain peptides and aminergic neurotransmitters are all modulators of brain-pituitary-gonadal function and sex behavior without, in most cases, being absolutely mandatory to the processes. Modulation involves changing thresholds of central nervous activity as first suggested many years ago in "Hormones and Behavior" by Frank Beach (1948). The responsiveness of CNS neurons to either electrical stimulation or treatment with monoamines may be completely reversed with appropriate hormonal treatment such as estrogen after long-term ovariectomy. One of the methods by which estrogen modulates is to influence the production of specific receptors, e.g., induction of progestin receptors. According to a very recent study by Hruska and Silberberg (1980) estrogen also increases the number of dopamine receptors in the rat striatum via a pituitary-dependent mechanism, and one wonders whether the steroid might similarly raise the level

324

of the NE receptors recently demonstrated in the medial basal
hypothalamus and median eminence by Young and Kuhar (1980). In
a modulatory sense NE can trigger patterns of nervous activity
conducive to an ovulatory surge of LH in the proestrous rat or the
estrous rabbit. Is this due to an estrogen-induced elevation in NE
receptors? There are suggestions that the monoaminergic receptors
may become supersensitive when their synaptic pathways are destroyed and/or that much more of the transmitter may ordinarily be
present than is needed to modulate the neuroendocrine effects. The
rapid adaptation of the brain to the loss of an important aminergic
input exemplifies its remarkable plasticity in the regulation of
neuroendocrine phenomena. An understanding of the mechanisms
underlying this central nervous plasticity must remain a major goal
in neuroendocrine research.

Acknowledgements

Research in the author's laboratory has been supported by grants from NIH
(NS01162) and the Ford Foundation.

References

Beach FA (1948) Hormones and behavior, Hoeber, New York.
Blaustein JD, Feder HH (1980) Nuclear progestin receptors in guinea pig
    brain measured by an in vitro exchange assay after hormonal treat-
    ments that affect lordosis. Endocrinology 106:1061-1069.
Butler JEM, Donovan BT (1971) The effect of surgical isolation of the
    hypothalamus upon reproductive function in the female guinea pig. J
    Endocr 50:507-514.
Clifton DK, Sawyer CH (1979) LH release and ovulation in the rat
    following depletion of hypothalamic norepinephrine: Chronic vs acute
    effects. Neuroendocrinology 28:442-449.
Clifton DK, Sawyer CH (1980) Positive and negative feedback effects of
    ovarian steroids on luteinizing hormone release in ovariectomized
    rats following chronic depletion of hypothalamic norepinephrine.
    Endocrinology 106:1099-1102.
Everett JW (1960) The mammalian female reproductive cycle and its
    controlling mechanisms. In: Young WC (ed) Sex and internal secre-
    tions, 3rd ed, vol 1, Williams and Wilkins, Baltimore, pp.497-555.
Everett JW, Sawyer CH, Markee JE (1949) A neurogenic timing factor in
    control of the ovulatory discharge of luteinizing hormone in the
    cyclic rat. Endocrinology 44:234-250.
Everett JW, Sawyer CH (1950) A 24-hour periodicity in the "LH-release
    apparatus" of female rats, disclosed by barbiturate sedation. Endo-
    crinology 47:198-218.

Gallo RV (1980) Neuroendocrine regulation of pulsatile luteinizing hormone release in the rat. Neuroendocrinology 30:122–131.

Hancke JL, Wuttke W (1979) Effects of chemical lesion of the ventral noradrenergic bundle or of the medial preoptic area on preovulatory LH release in rats. Exp Brain Res 35:127–134.

Honma K, Wuttke W (1980) Norepinephrine and dopamine turnover rates in the medial preoptic area and the mediobasal hypothalamus of the rat brain after various endocrinological manipulations. Endocrinology 106:1848–1853.

Hruska RE, Silbergeld EK (1980) Increased dopamine receptor sensitivity after estrogen treatment using the rat rotation model. Science 208:1466–1468.

Kalra PS, Kalra SP, Krulich L, Fawcett CP, McCann SM (1972) Involvement of norepinephrine in transmission of the stimulatory influence of progesterone on gonadotropin release. Endocrinology 90:1168–1176.

Kalra SP, McCann SM (1974) Effects of drugs modifying catecholamine synthesis on plasma LH and ovulation in the rat. Neuroendocrinology 15:79–91.

Kawakami M, Sawyer CH (1959) Neuroendocrine correlates of changes in brain activity thresholds by sex steroids and pituitary hormones. Endocrinology 65:652–668.

Kawakami M, Sawyer CH (1967) Effects of sex hormones and antifertility steroids on brain threshold in the rabbit. Endocrinology 80:857–871.

Kawakami M, Yoshioka E, Konda N, Arita J, Visessuvan S (1978a) Data on the sites of stimulatory feedback action of gonadal steroids indispensable for luteinizing hormone release in the rat. Endocrinology 102:791–798.

Kawakami M, Arita J, Yoshioka E, Visessuvan S, Akema T (1978b) Data on the sites of the stimulatory feedback action of gonadal steroids indispensable for follicle-stimulating hormone release in the rat. Endocrinology 103:752–759.

Kelly MJ, Moss RL, Dudley CA (1976) Differential sensitivity of preoptic-septal neurons to microelectrophoresed estrogen during the estrous cycle. Brain Res 114:152–157.

Knobil E (1974) On the control of gonadotropin secretion in the rhesus monkey. Recent Progr Hormone Res 30:1–46.

Knobil E (1980) Neuroendocrine control of the menstrual cycle. Recent Progr Hormone Res 36:53–88.

Krieg R, Sawyer CH (1976) Effect of intraventricular catecholamines on luteinizing hormone release in ovariectomized-steroid-primed rats. Endocrinology 99:411–419.

MacLusky NJ, Liederburg I, Krey LC, McEwen BS (1980) Progestin receptors in the brain and pituitary of the bonnet monkey (Macaca radiata): Differences between the monkey and the rat in the distribution of progestin receptors. Endocrinology 106:185–191.

MacLusky NJ, McEwen BS (1980) Progestin receptors in the rat brain: distribution and properties of ·cytoplasmic progestin-binding sites. Endocrinology 106:192–202.

Martinovic JV, McCann SM (1977) Effects of lesions in the ventral noradrenergic tract produced by microinjection of 6-hydroxydopamine on gonadotropin release in the rat. Endocrinology 100:1206–1213.

Munaro NI (1977) The effect of ovarian steroids on hypothalamic norepinephrine neuronal activity. Acta Endocrinol 86:235–242.

Nagle CA, Rosner JM (1976) Plasma norepinephrine during the rat estrous cycle and after progesterone treatment to the ovariectomized estrogen-primed rat. Neuroendocrinology 22:89–96.

Nagle CA, Rosner JM (1980) Rat brain norepinephrine release during progesterone-induced LH secretion. Neuroendocrinology 30:33-37.

Nicholson G, Greeley G, Humm J, Youngblood W, Kizer JS (1978) Lack of effect of noradrenergic denervation of the hypothalamus and medial preoptic area on the feedback regulation of gonadotropin secretion and the estrous cycle of the rat. Endocrinology 103:559-566.

Noonan JJ, Nass TE, Terasawa E (1980) Lesions of the posterior hypothalamus induce precocious menarche in the female rhesus monkey. Program 62nd Annual Meeting, The Endocrine Society, Abstr 125, p.106.

Rabii J, Ehlers C, Clifton D, Sawyer CH (1980) Effects of intraventricular infusions of 6-hydroxydopamine (6-OHDA) on pituitary LH release and ovulation in the rabbit. Neuroendocrinology 30:362-368.

Sawyer CH (1952) Stimulation of ovulation in the rabbit by the intraventricular injection of epinephrine or norepinephrine. Anat Rec 112:385.

Sawyer CH (1975) Some recent developments in brain-pituitary-ovarian physiology. Neuroendocrinology 17:97-124.

Sawyer CH, Clifton DK (1980) Aminergic innervation of the hypothalamus. Fed Proc, in press.

Sawyer CH, Kawakami M, Kanematsu S (1966) Neuroendocrine aspects of reproduction. In: Endocrines and the central nervous system. Assoc Res Nerv Ment Dis 43:59-85.

Sawyer CH, Markee JE, Hollinshead WH (1947) Inhibition of ovulation in the rabbit by the adrenergic-blocking agent dibenamine. Endocrinology 41:395-402.

Sawyer CH, Radford HM (1978) Effects of intraventricular injections of norepinephrine on brain-pituitary-ovarian function in the rabbit. Brain Res 146:83-93.

Simpkins JW, Huang HH, Advis JP, Meites J (1979) Changes in hypothalamic NE and DA turnover resulting from steroid-induced LH and prolactin surges in ovariectomized rats. Biol Reprod 20:625-630.

Terasawa E, Wiegand SJ (1978) Effects of hypothalamic deafferentation on ovulation and estrous cyclicity in the female guinea pig. Neuroendocrinology 26:229-248.

Terasawa E, King MK, Wiegand SJ, Bridson WE, Goy RW (1979) Barbiturate anesthesia blocks the positive feedback effect of progesterone, but not of estrogen, cn luteinizing hormone release in ovariectomized guinea pigs. Endocrinology 104:687-692.

Terasawa E, Noonan JJ (1980) Pentobarbital anesthesia blocks the progesterone-induced luteinizing hormone release in ovariectomized monkey. Program of the 6th International Congress of Endocrinology, Abstr. No 833.

Tima L, Flerkó B (1974) Ovulation induced by norepinephrine in rats made anovulatory by various experimental procedures. Neuroendocrinology 15:346-354.

Young WS, Kuhar MJ (1980) Noradrenergic 1 and 2 receptors: light microscopic autoradiograph localization. Proc Natl Acad Sci USA 77:1696-1700.

Abstracts of Poster Presentations

Effect of Low Doses of Continuously Administered Catecholestrogens on Peripheral and Central Target Organs

P. Ball, U. Gethmann and G. Emons, Lübeck

Catecholestrogens, especially 2-hydroxyestrogens have been known to constitue quantitatively the most important metabolic products of primary estrogens. Recently, the importance of another class of catecholestrogens, the 4-hydroxyestrogens, was forwarded (for review see Ball and Knuppen, 1980). On incubation of radioactive precursors both classes are not only formed in the liver but also in the pituitary, and hypothalamus of rat and man. Moreover, their endogenous occurrence in significant quantities has been demonstrated in urine, plasma and tissue.

4-Hydroxyestrogens show considerable binding to cytoplasmatic and nuclear receptors, whereas the reported receptor affinities for 2-hydroxyestrogens are comparatively low (Martucci and Fishman, 1979). Accordingly, 4-hydroxyestrogens exhibit a clear-cut influence on different estrogen dependent processes as e.g. premature ovulation in the PMS treated immature rat and on sexual behaviour in the ovariectomized adult rat. 2-Hydroxyestrogens show no such effect. On the other hand, they are supposed to influence the gonadotrophin release. This biological action is, however, until now, only poorly understood.

The following study was undertaken to further assess the biological activity of 4-hydroxyestradiol (4-OHE$_2$) and 2-hydroxyestradiol (2-OHE$_2$) after long term administration. To this end osmotic minipumps containing low doses of either 4-OHE$_2$ or 2-OHE$_2$ were implanted s.c. for 152 h to immature male and female rats. At the end of the test period (17.00 day 6) the animals were killed and the uterine weight, the vaginal opening, the gonadotrophin serum levels and the gonadal weight were monitored.

331

Table: Effect of Catecholestrogens on Uterine Weight, Vaginal Opening, Gonadotrophins and Gonadal Weight. The steroids dissolved in ethanol/acetic acid/propylene glycol/ascorbic acid were infused s.c. by osmotic minipumps at a rate of $0.1\,\mu g/h$ over 6 1/3 days. 8 groups of 10 immature rats, each, were used. The figures represent the mean $\pm$ standard deviation (S.E.)

	Parameter	No Steroid		2-OHE$_2$		4-OHE$_2$		Estradiol	
Female Rats	Uterine Weight (mg)	44	15	55	17	140	27	180	55
	Vaginal Opening	2		1		10		10	
	LH (ng/ml)	51	13	77	48	62	35	47	19
	FSH (ng/ml)	440	72	350	130	440	66	390	80
	Body Weight Inc. (g)	31		28		24		21	
Male Rats	LH (ng/ml)	39	10	67	38	43	15	35	9
	FSH (ng/ml)	770	100	900	170	620	190	460	70
	Gonadal Weight (mg)	740	20	750	30	520	80	360	20
	Body Weight Inc. (g)	40		37		35		30	

The following results were obtained (Table):

1. A significant increase in the uterine weight and a consistent vaginal opening were observed after 4-OHE$_2$ treatment.

2. LH-levels increased after 2-OHE$_2$ but not after 4-OHE$_2$; the increase was, however, not significant.

3. FSH-levels and gonadal weights were lowered by 4-OHE$_2$ treatment in male rats only; 2-OHE$_2$ had no effect on FSH-levels in both sexes.

4. In no instance an antiestrogenic effect of either catecholestrogen was observed.

It is concluded that 4-hydroxyestrogens have no role in LH-release, but a significant importance on uterine growth, whereas 2-hydroyestrogens may increase LH-levels but are nearly ineffective with respect to peripheral parameters.

Ball P, Knuppen R (1980) Acta Endocrinol 93, Suppl. 232:1-127.
Martucci CH, Fishman J (1979) Endocrinology 105:1288-1292.

LHRH Changes Concomitant with Catecholamine Turnover Rates in Discrete Hypothalamic Nuclei and Median Eminence: Effects of Ovariectomy, Estradiol (E$_2$) and Progesterone (P$_4$) Therapy and Phenobarbital Treatment

C.A. Barraclough, P.M. Wise and N. Rance, Baltimore

The present studies examined changes which occur in LHRH concentrations and in catecholamine (CA) turnover rates in discrete microdissected hypothalamic nuclei during proestrus or diestrus day 1 and after phenobarbital blockade of proestrous gonadotropin surges. Concomitant measurements of plasma E$_2$, P$_4$, LH, FSH and prolactin were made in these cyclic rats. The specific regions microdissected were: suprachiasmatic preoptic nucleus (SPN), medial preoptic nucleus (MPN), suprachiasmatic nucleus (SCN), anterior hypothalamic nucleus (AHN), retrochiasmatic area (RCA), arcuate nucleus (AN) and median eminence (ME). During proestrus, LHRH concentrations increased between 0900 and 1200 h (Prior to gonadotropin surges which begin between 1300 – 1500 h) and decreased between 1200 and 1500 h (during LH, FSH surges) and remained low at 1800 h in SPN, MPN, AHA, RCA, and ME. No such pattern of change occurred on diestrous day 1. Phenobarbital failed to prevent the afternoon decline in LHRH between 1200 and 1500 h in any of the brain tissue examined, although plasma LH and FSH levels remained basal at least to 1800 h proestrus. In other rats, ME-LHRH, plasma LH, FSH, prolactin, E$_2$, P$_4$ (RIA) and turnover rates of norepinephrine (NE) and dopamine (DA) were measured (radioenzymatic method) in the same animal. CA turnover rates at 0900 – 1100 h, 1200 – 1400 h and 1500 – 1700 h were examined in proestrous rats by measuring the decline in NE and DA at 0, 60, and 120 min after the ip injection of 400 mg/kgαMpT. Protein concentrations were measured by the Bradford dye-binding assay. NE turnover rates were significantly elevated in ME and SCN at 1200 and 1500 h and in MPN at 1500 h as compared to 0900 h. DA turnover in ME was significantly reduced at 1500 h but there was no

333

rate change in MPN–DA. In the same ME samples, LHRH concentrations increased between 0900 and 1200 h and then declined between 1200 and 1500 h. Plasma LH levels rose between 1200 – 1500 h but plasma E_2 was unchanged and P_4 increased with plasma LH. Phenobarbital completely blocked ME–NE turnover between 1500 – 1700 h but not 1200 – 1400 h rates when given at 1200 h. No changes in LHRH, CA turnovers or plasma gonadotropins or E_2 occurred on diestrous day 1.

To determine the role of E_2 and P_4 in changing hypothalamic LHRH concentrations and CA turnover rates, rats were ovariectomized and 7 days later (day 0, 0900 h) a Silastic E_2 capsule was inserted sc; 2 days later (day 2, 0900 h) Silastic capsules of oil or P_4 in oil were implanted sc. Plasma E_2 and P_4 levels in such rats were 15.7 ± 1.3 pg/ml and 15.0 ± 1.1 ng/ml, respectively. Rats were killed at 1000, 1200 and 1500 h day 2. Peak serum LH concentrations (1500 h) were 4-fold greater in E_2P_4-treated (5446 ± 709 ng/ml) than E_2-treated (1304 ± 309 ng/ml) rats. LHRH concentrations changed only in ME of E_2P_4-treated but not E_2-treated rats; LHRH levels increased between 1000 and 1200 h and decreased between 1200 – 1500 h. E_2-treated rats had elevated NE turnover rates in the SCN, MPN, and ME in the afternoon compared to morning values. ME–NE turnover rates already were elevated in the morning of E_2P_4-treated rats; however, no increase in NE turnover was observed in the SCN. DA turnover rates did not change in brain areas of any experimental group between morning and afternoon. These combined data suggest that in normal cyclic rats LHRH increases in all component parts of the preoptico–suprachiasmatic–tuberal system (PSTS) during the morning of proestrus and it may be this newly synthesized material which is released on the afternoon of proestrous to induce preovulatory LH, FSH surges. Concomitant with the decline in ME–LHRH, NE turnover rates increase and DA declines on proestrus betwen 1200 – 1500 h. Further, steroid-induced gonadotropin surges also are accompanied by increased NE turnover rates but a decline in DA turnover rates does not necessarily accompany this event. P_4 may augment and advance the LH surge both by increasing ME–LHRH concentrations and increasing and advancing the time that NE turnovers occur. Seemingly, two central systems are operative on proestrus; increased LHRH synthesis (within PSTS) and

334

increased NE turnover to evoke release of the newly synthesized LHRH. When both events occur, LH and FSH preovulatory surges result.

Supported by USPHS Grant HD-02138.

335

Mechanisms Involved in Selective FSH Release During Estrus in the Cyclic Rat

C.A. Blake, K.A. Elias, O.A. Ashiru, M.E. Rush, R.P. Kelch and R. Sridaran, Omaha and Ann Arbor

Serum FSH concentration is elevated during the afternoon and early evening of proestrus (the first phase of FSH release which accompanies the preovulatory LH surge) and during the late evening of proestrus and the morning of estrus (the second or selective phase of FSH release which occurs when LH is low in serum) during the rat 4-day estrous cycle. We conducted a series of experiments to identifiy the mechanisms responsible for the second phase of FSH release. Injection of phenobarbital or anti-LHRH sera on the early afternoon of proestrus blocked both phases of increased plasma FSH. Injection of LHRH, low or high doses of rat FSH, or high doses of rat LH on the afternoon of proestrus to phenobarbital-blocked rats or rat FSH to anti-LHRH sera-blocked rats stimulated endogenous FSH release during the evening of proestrus and the morning of estrus. Administration of phenobarbital or anti-LHRH sera during the evening of proestrus (at doses which are effective in blocking the first phase of FSH relase when administered on the early afternoon of proestrus) had no effect on the second phase of FSH release. Similarly, complete surgical deafferentation of the medial basal hypothalamus or aspiration of the medial basal hypothalamus during the evening of proestrus did not alter the second phase of FSH release. Anterior pituitary gland FSH concentration did not change during the time of heightened periovulatory FSH secretion. Yet, in vitro incubation of anterior pituitary glands removed from rats at different times during the estrous cycle for a 2 h period revealed that the basal FSH secretion rate increased markedly during the late evening of pro-estrus and decreased markedly during the morning of estrus. We feel it unlikely that elevations in plasma gonadotrophins during pro-

336

estrous afternoon mediate this increase in the basal FSH secretory rate by a direct action on the pituitary gland since small (2-fold) elevations in peripheral plasma FSH stimulate endogenous FSH release in the phenobarbital-blocked, proestrous rat and such a small peripheral elevation would likely not be recognized by the FSH gonadotrophs. Similarly, the gonadotrophins cannot mediate the second phase of FSH release be an action on the adrenal glands. In long-term (3 week) adrenalectomized rats, the periovulatory increases in serum FSH are not different from those of controls. As ovariectomy on the early afternoon of proestrus does not alter either phase of FSH relase, it is possible that a decrease in ovarian secretions is involved in causing the second phase. A decrease in plasma estrogen alone cannot be involved since sc implanation of E_2-silastic capsules on the early afternoon of proestrus had no effect on the periovulatory FSH surges in intact rats. In contrast, administration of porcine follicular fluid was effective in blocking either or both phases of FSH release. These results suggest that 1) the brain is likely not involved in the second phase of FSH release after the first phase of FSH release has occurred, 2) increases in plasma gonadotrophins during the afternoon of proestrus likely mediate the second phase of FSH release by an action exerted at the level of the ovary, 3) the elevated plasma gonadotrophins may act to decrease ovarian secretion(s), possibly the secretion of "inhibin", and 4) ultimately changes occur at the level of the anterior pituitary gland which result in a selective increase in the basal FSH secretion rate which we suggest is responsible for the second phase of elevated FSH in plasma.

Supported by grants from the NIH (HD 11011, HD 07097, HD 08333).

A Dual Effect of Dopamine on Both Release and Degradation of LH-RH by Hypothalamic Synaptosomes

D.M. de Cotte and J.A. Edwardson, London and Newcastle

Relatively high levels of monoamines and other neurotransmitters occur in the hypothalamus and there is evidence that these substances may regulate release of the peptide hormones which control anterior pituitary function.   Immuno-histochemical studies have shown the existence of synapses between nerve endings containing dopamine (DA) and gonadotrophin releasing hormone (LH-RH) respectively in the hypothalamic median eminence (Ajika, 1979).   It is generally accepted that this transmitter is involved in the regulation of gonadotrophin secretion as a modulator of LH-RH release, although the evidence is conflicting and both inhibitory and excitatory actions of DA have been reported.

Low concentrations of DA have been shown to release LH-RH from hypothalamic synaptosomes (Bennett et al., 1975).   Recently, we have shown that DA at high concentrations stimulates the disposal of LH-RH by female rat hypothalamic synaptosomes but not from male rat hypothalamic synaptosomes (Marcano de Cotte et al., 1980).   Further studies have revealed a complex synaptosomal mechanism by which DA stimulates either the release or the degradation of LH-RH depending on the stage of the reproductive cycle or the dose of dopamine involved.

Synaptosomes isolated from the hypothalamus of adult female rats killed at known stages of the oestrous cycle were suspended in Krebs-Ringer Bicarbonate medium at a tissue concentration of 1 hypothalamic equivalent ml^{-1} and incubated at $37^{o}C$.   After 15 min preincubation, DA in ascorbic acid was added to give a range of concentrations from 10^{-8} to $10^{-4}M$ and incubated for 5 min.

Lower concentrations of DA (10^{-8} – 10^{-6}M) stimulated the release of LH–RH from synaptosomes isolated from rats in oestrus and diestrus. No effect was observed with proestrous preparations. However, at higher concentrations (10^{-4}), DA was shown to stimulate the disposal of LH–RH from synaptosomes at every stage of the reproductive cycle, the effect being most marked in proestrous preparations.

It is evident that both the dose of DA employed and the stage of the oestrous cycle determine the responses of synaptosomes to exogenous dopamine. Thus, a dual type of control of LH–RH could be brought about by dopamine, either by steroid hormone-dependent changes in the responsiveness of the DA receptor(s) or by concentration-dependent effects on the regulation of the disposal of the LH–RH.

DMC is supported by a grant from CDCH, Universidad Central de Venezuela.

Ajika K (1979) Simultaneous localization of LH–RH and catecholamines in the rat hypothalamus. J Anat 128:331–347.
Bennett GW, Edwardson JA, Holland D, Jeffcoate SL, White N (1975) Release of immunoreactive luteinising hormone-releasing hormone and thyrotropin-releasing hormone from hypothalamic synaptosomes. Nature 257:323–325.
Marcano de Cotte D, De Menezes CEL, Bennett GW, Edwardson JA (1980) Dopamine stimulates the degradation of gonadotropin releasing hormone by rat synaptosomes. Nature 283:487–489.

Serotonin: Possible Function in Diurnal Regulation of LH and Prolactin Release

E. Düker, W. Hilgendorf and W. Wuttke, Göttingen

Serotonin concentrations in various CNS-structures are subject to a diurnal rhythm. They are low in the morning and high in the afternoon. Since the major 5-HT metabolite 5-HIAA shows an opposite pattern, we feel safe to conclude that the 5-HT release is high in the morning and low in the afternoon. Hence, 5-HT concentrations seem to correlate inversely with the state of release of this amine.

We measured serotonin concentrations by a radioenzymatic assay in micropunches from rat brain slices under different endocrine situations: diestrous (D), proestrous (P), ovariectomized (ovx), ovx and estradiol-primed (ovxE2), and ovxE2 plus an additional pro-gesterone treatment (ovxE2+Pr).

In the two limbic structures, the nucleus accumbens and the mediocortical amygdala, which are known to be involved in the regulation of behaviour, the diurnal rhythm has a small amplitude and is not affected by the endocrine situation.

In the anterior and posterior mediobasal hypothalamus (AMBH and PMBH) and in the medial preoptic area (MPO) steroids feedback on LHRH and prolactin controlling neurons. In these structures however, the diurnal rhythm with low morning and high afternoon concentrations is expressed more clearly, as shown in the figure for the AMBH.

Since serum prolactin and LH levels are lower in the morning than in the afternoon, and since 5-HT has been shown to stimulate prolactin release, the higher 5-HT release in the morning as compared to the afternoon suggests that 5-HT is not involved in the regulation of the diurnal rhythm of serum prolactin levels. In P rats, however, the diurnal pattern of 5-HT release is abolished; the

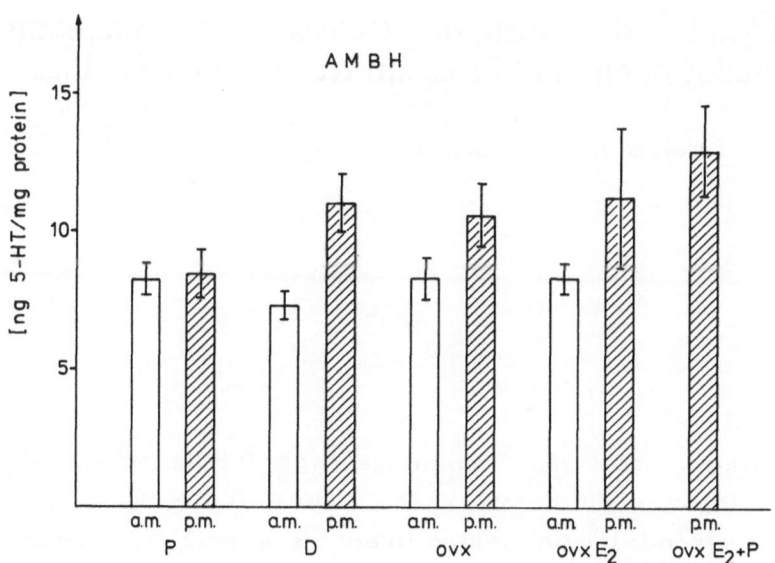

Serotonin concentrations in the anterior mediobasal hypothalamus (AMBH) of the rat under different endocrine situations

concentrations are as low in the afternoon as in the morning. The low 5-HT concentration in the afternoon at the time of the pre-ovulatory prolactin peak suggests a stimulation of prolactin by 5-HT at this time.

Effect of ACTH-induced Testosterone Release on the Secretion of Pituitary Gonadotrophin and Prolactin Release in Male Pigs

M. Fenske, W. Holtz, L. Pitzel and A. König, Göttingen

Chronically cannulated adult male miniature pigs (Göttingen strain) following an i.m. injection of depot-$^{1-24}$ACTH (10 µg/kg body weight, Synacthen, CIBA) responded with a significant release of testosterone (T) within 30 min. T levels remained elevated for 3 h, however at 6 to 12 h after injection they were significantly decreased. Plasma corticosteroid levels were significantly elevated at 1 – 20 h after ACTH administration. Plasma LH concentrations ranging from 7.9 – 8.1 ng/ml during the pretreatment period dropped gradually to 3.1 – 3.6 ng/ml between 1 – 12 h after ACTH injection and recovered to pretreatment levels at 20 h p.i. The LH decrease was significant between 3 – 13 h p.i. Plasma prolactin levels remained uneffected by ACTH administration.

To test whether the ACTH-induced increase of plasma T levels is due to a stimulation of testicular or adrenal T secretion, pigs that were either intact, castrated or castrated + adrenalectomized were injected intravenously with 10.0 µg/kg body weight $^{1-24}$ACTH (Synacthen). While in intact animals ACTH induced a mean T increase from 314 to 1036 ng/100 ml plasma, in castrates plasma T levels were only slightly increased (pretreatment: 40 ng/100 ml, post-treatment: 61 ng/100 ml) and in castrated + adrenalectomized pigs, T levels remained constant.

Our data show that ACTH, administered either i.m. or i.v., strongly stimulates testicular T secretion. This effect that is apparently not mediated by LH or prolactin, may be due to a direct action of ACTH on Leydig cells, as suggested from human studies by Beitins et al. (1973). The decline of plasma LH after injection of depot-ACTH may result from a negative feedback effect exerted by T.

Further studies are in progress to test whether a similar stimulatory effect of endogenous ACTH, released under stress, will stimulate T release and thereby influence LH secretion.

Beitins IZ, Bayard F, Kowarski A, Migeon CJ (1973) Steroids 21:553.

Influence of 4-Hydroxyestradiol, Ethynylestradiol, Estradiol and Danazol on the LH-RH-induced Gonadotrophin Release in Ovariectomized Rats

U. Gethmann, P. Ball and R. Knuppen, Lübeck

Recently it was shown by several investigators that catecholestrogens are involved in the regulation of pituitary LH and/or hypothalamic LH–RH release (Naftolin et al., 1975; Gethmann et al., 1978; Ball et al., 1979; Martucci and Fishman, 1979). These effects of catechol estrogens on central target organs are, however, equivocal. To obtain further information on the mode of action of catechol and parent estrogens the LH response to endogenous and exogenous LH–RH was monitored after pretreatment with different steroids.

To this end ovariectomized (ovx) Wistar rats housed under controlled conditions ($22^{\circ}C$, lights on 5 am, lights off 7 pm), 6 weeks after castration, weighing 200–250 g, were treated daily for 5 days with vehicle or different steroids either alone or in combination. Part of the animals received an additional LH–RH injection on day 6. Blood samples were collected by decapitation and serum luteinizing hormone (LH) levels measured in duplicate by radioimmunoassay (NIAMD–RP–1 standard). Statistical analysis was performed using Student's t-test for paired samples.

The following results were obtained (Fig. 1 and 2):

1. Former experiments had shown that regular administration of relatively low doses of estradiolbenzoate (E_2B), 4-hydroxyestradiol ($4-OHE_2$) or ethynylestradiol (EE) suppressed LH levels in ovx rats when blood sampling was performed in the morning, whereas – beginning 2–3 days after starting the treatment – a rhythmical LH–surge (positive feedback effect) was observed in the afternoon. Accordingly the E_2B, $4-OHE_2$ or EE treated groups (#1–3) had afternoon LH–Levels in the range of more than three times the morning levels.

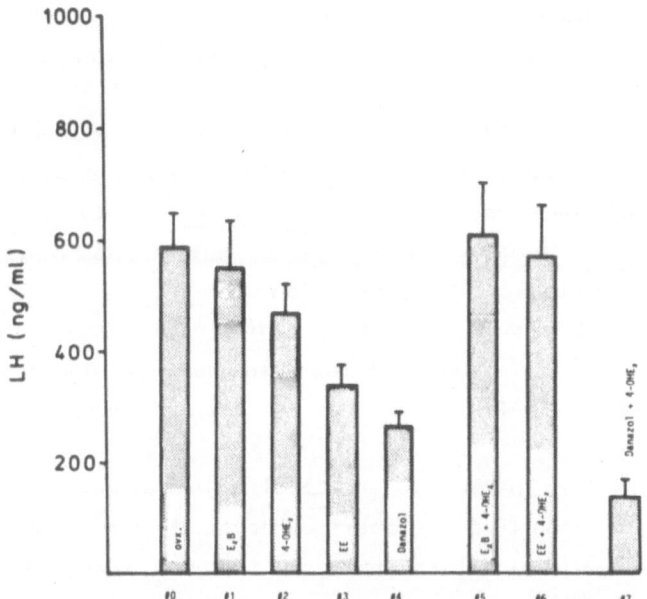

Fig. 1. Effect of different pretreatments on LH-levels (mean ± SEM) in
ovariectomized rats, groups (#) of 8 animals each received daily for 5 days
either vehicle (0.1% ascorbic acid in propylene glycol) (#0), 1µg E_2B (# 1),
10 µg 4-OHE$_2$ (# 2) or 4 µg EE (# 3) i.m. or 40 mg Danazol dissolved in 10%
ethanol in corn-oil (# 4) orally or a combination of these regiments (# 5-7),
blood was collected at 5 p.m. on day 6

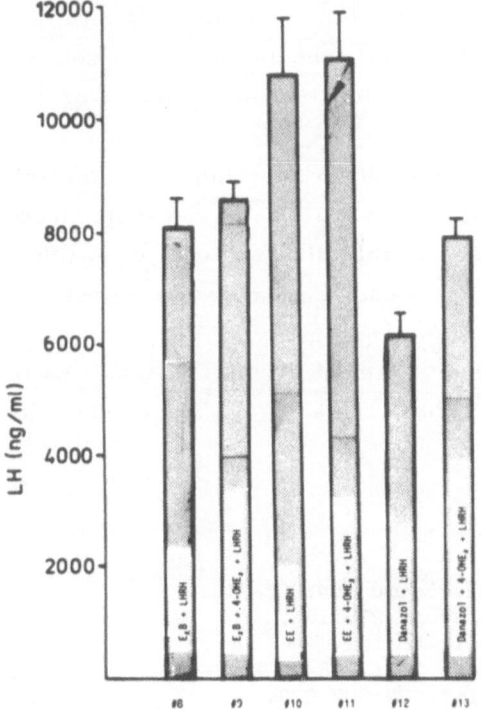

Fig. 2. Effect of LH-RH on
LH-levels (mean ± SEM) in the
different pretreatment groups.
In addition to the pretreatment (see legend Fig. 1) these
animals received a single i.p.
injection of 10 µg of LH-RH
at 8 a.m. on day 6 (# 8-13).
Blood was collected at 9 a.m.
of the same day

2. The E_2B and EE induced high LH afternoon levels may be further augmented by $4-OHE_2$ (#5,6); this effect was , however, statistical significant only for EE (#6).

3. Danazol (17 -pregn-4-en-20-yno(2,3-d)isoxazol-17-ol) lowered the serum LH levels in female castrated rats by 65% as compared to controls. With regard to the results of Shane et al (1978) the hypothesis is forwarded that Danazol lowers serum LH levels primarily by inhibition of hypothalamic LH-RH secretion.

4. $4-OHE_2$ increased this inhibitory effect of Danazol significantly by further 20%. It is assumed that this may be due to the direct inhibitory action of $4-OHE_2$ on the LH release from the pituitary LH depots.

5. The increase in LH levels after LHRH stimulation was inversely correlated to the positive feedback effect of the test-substances. So, E_2B pretreatment which lead to highest basal LH levels in the afternoon (#1) was less effective in LH-RH induced increase in LH (#8) than EE (#10), which in turn was less effective with respect to basal LH afternoon levels (#3). Additional pretreatment with $4-OHE_2$ had no measurable effect.

6. After Danazol pretreatment the LH-RH induced increase in LH levels (#12) was lower than in all other groups (#8-11). Following Danazol treatment the pituitary LH depots are supposed to be smaller (s.a.) and consequently the LH-RH induced release of LH is lower.

7. The depressed pituitary responsiveness to LHRH by Danazol could be reversed by $4-OHE_2$ administration. This may result from greater pituitary LH depots partly due to the direct effect of $4-OHE_2$ on the pituitary, and partly due to a possible stimulative effect on LH-RH production.

In summary, these findings make it evident that $4-OHE_2$ with regard to the modulation of gonadotrophin release is an estrogenic acting steroid.

Naftolin et al. (1975) Biochem Biophys Res Commun 64:905-910.
Gethmann U et al. (1978) Acta Endocrinol Suupl 215:102.
Ball P et al. (1979) Acta Endocrinol Suppl 225:102.
Martucci CH, Fishman J (1979) Endocrinology 105:1288-1292.
Shane JM et al. (1978) Fertility & Sterility 29:637-639.

Dihydrotestosterone and Estradiol Regulating the Activity of 3α-Hydroxysteroid Dehydrogenase in the Pituitary Gland of the Rat: Action of Antiestrogens

R. Ghraf, K. Schneider, J. Kirchhoff and C. Hiemke, Essen

3α–Hydroxysteroid dehydrogenase (3α–HSDH) which catalyzes the inter-conversion of 5α–dihydrotestosterone (DHT) and 5α–androstane–3α,17β–diol (3α–DIOL), and of 5α–dihydroprogesterone (DHP) and 3α–hydroxy-5α–pregnan–20–one respectively, is widely distributed in the central nervous system of the rat. It might be expected that in neuro-endocrine tissues changes in enzyme activity could determine the effectiveness of DHT and DHP in initiating neuroendocrine events (for reviews see Karavolas and Nuti, 1976; McEwen, 1978).

Recently we have demonstrated that the activity of 3α–HSDH in the pituitary gland, but not the cerebral cortex or the mediobasal hypothalamus of the rat is regulated by gonadal steroids (Ghraf et al., 1980). Gonadectomy of rats of either sex led to a considerable increase in 3α–enzyme activity (2.5– to 4–fold) which could be completely reversed by chronic s.c. administration of estradiol (E_2, 15 µg/day/14 days) or DHT (1 mg/day/14 days).

In the present investigation we have studied the effect of chronic s.c. administration (0.5 mg/day/14 days) of antiestrogens (tamoxifen, enclomiphene, nitromifene, nafoxidine) on the activity of hypophyseal 3α–HSDH. All the antiestrogens investigated, when administered alone, had strong estrogenic effects on the 3α–enzyme activity in the gonadectomized female rat. In the gonadectomized male rat, however, only nitromifene was estrogenic, though to a lesser degree than in the female. When administered simultaneously with E_2 (15 µg/day/14 days) the antiestrogens did in no case block or significantly diminish the repressive effects of E_2 on 3α–HSDH activity. In the gonadectomized female rat they even enhanced the suppressive effect of E_2. Under the various treatments serum levels

347

of LH, and especially of FSH, did not always covariate with the hypophyseal 3α-enzyme activity. In some cases stimulated FSH secretion was accompanied by highly suppressed 3α-enzyme activity.

It is concluded that chronic administration of antiestrogens to gonadectomized rats can lead to divergent effects on gonadotropin secretion and hypophyseal 3α-HSDH activity. In addition, a marked sex difference exists concerning the sensitivity to estrogen-agonistic action of antiestrogens.

Supported by Forschungsförderung des Ministeriums für Wissenschaft und Forschung des Landes Nordrhein-Westfalen.

Ghraf R, Schneider K, Kirchhoff J, Niemke C (1980) Subcellular distribution and gonadal regulation of 3α-hydroxysteroid dehydrogenase in rat pituitary. Proceedings of the Third Meeting of the European Society for Neurochemistry, Abstract 657.
Karavolas HJ, Nuti KM (1976) Progesterone metabolism by neuroendocrine tissues. In: Naftolin F, Ryan KJ, Davies J (eds) Subcellular Mechanisms in Reproductive Neuroendocrinology. Elsevier Scientific Publishing Company, Amsterdam, pp.305-326.
McEwen BS (1978) Gonadal Steroid Receptors in Neuroendocrine Tissues. In: O'Malley BW, Birnbaumer L (eds) Receptors and Hormone Action. Academic Press, New York, Vol. 2, pp.353-400.

Circulating Steroid Levels and Brain Neurotransmitter Concentrations in the Midterm Human Fetus

D.P. Gilmore, N.A. Masudi and C.A. Wilson, Glasgow and London

The critical period for male differentiation of the human hypothalamus is known to be around mid gestation, at the time when fetal plasma testosterone levels are elevated.

In order to investigate whether the differentiation might be influenced by various neurotransmitters in the central nervous system we have measured their concentrations by fluorometric assays, in the hypothalamus, cortex and cerebrospinal fluid (CSF) of fetuses aged from 10–23 weeks.

Twentyone male and 11 female fetuses were collected within 5–10 minutes of their removal from the uterus by hysterotomy. Cord blood was taken and the plasma separated and frozen. CSF was aspirated by lumbar puncture and frozen in liquid nitrogen as were the hypothalamus and a portion of cortex.

At a later date the frozen tissue was thawed. Concentrations of 5–hydroxy–tryptamine (5HT) and 5–hydroxyindoleacetic acid (5HIAA) were measured by a modification of the method of Curzon and Green (1970) and those of noradrenaline (NA) and dopamine (DA) by the method of Shellenberger and Gordon (1971). The results obtained are summarized in the attached table. Group means were compared by Student's t test. Levels of testosterone were measured by radioimmunoassay and in male fetuses ranged from 150 to almost 800 ng/100 ml, significantly higher than in the females. These results are in close agreement with those of Reyes, Boroditsky, Winter and Faiman (1974).

In the male fetuses concentrations of 5HT and 5HIAA were found to be significantly higher in the hypothalamus and CSF than in the cortex. Concentrations of NA were also significantly higher in the

Table 1: Concentration (ng/100 mg) of 5HT, 5HIAA, NA and DA in the Midterm Fetus (M + SEM)

	5HT		5HIAA		NA		DA	
Cortex	♂23.8 ± 2.1	(20)	11.3 ± 2.3	(18)	12.6 ± 1.9	(15)	30.8 ± 4,2	(12)
	♀20.1 ± 4.4	(7)	6.1 ± 2.4	(7)	28.7 ± 9.8	(6)	26.0 ± 7.4	(6)
Hypothalamus	♂37.7 ± 5.6**	(15)	20.4 ± 3.8*	(14)	45.4 ± 10.5***	(14)	44.9 ± 9.6	(21)
	♀23.7 ± 6.6	(7)	21.3 ± 2.2***	(7)	42.6 ± 12.0	(5)	5.0	(1)
CSF	♂38.9 ± 5.7**	(16)	41.3 ± 6.4***	(15)	21.3 ± 4.9	(15)	192.8 ± 38.7***	(17)
	♀26.5 ± 9.7	(6)	46.2 ± 12.0***	(57	10.8 ± 3.4	(4)	291.4 ±146.4***	(4)

* p < 0.05
** p < 0.02
*** p < 0.001

hypothalamus whereas DA levels are greatly raised in the CSF from fetuses of all ages.

Because the number of female fetuses collected was small, the results were less meaningful. However, 5 HIAA concentrations were found to be significantly higher in the hypothalamus and CSF when compared to the cortex, and DA levels in the CSF were also greatly elevated.

When the male fetuses were placed in 3 different age groups (10-13, 14-16 and 17-23 weeks) hypothalamic concentrations of NA were found to be greatest in the middle age class where they were significantly higher than in the 2 other groups. Plasma testosterone levels were also elevated at this time.

Curzon G, Green AR (1970) Rapid method for the determination of 5-hydroxy-tryptamine and 5-hydroxyindoleacetic acid in small regions of rat brain. British Journal of Pharmacology 39:653-655.

Shellenberger MK, Gordon JH (1971) A rapid simplified procedure for simultaneous assay of norepinephrine, dopamine and 5-hydroxy-tryptamine from discrete brain areas. Analytical Biochemistry 39:356-372.

Reyer FI, Boroditsky RS, Winter JSD, Faiman C (1974) Studies on human sexual development. II Fetal and maternal gonadotropin and sex steroid concentrations. Journal of Clinical Endocrinology and Metabolism 38:612-617.

Comparison of Estrogenic Versus Anti-estrogenic Influences on Postnatal Defeminization and Masculinization of the Rat-brain

J.L. Hancke and K.-D. Döhler, Hannover

Postnatal treatment of female rats with estrogens or with aromatizable androgens leads to defeminization and to masculinization of the brain. Paradoxically, postnatal treatment of female rats with estrogen antagonists leads to defeminiziation as well. In the subsequent studies we investigated whether estrogenic or anti-estrogenic activity of these compounds may be responsible for their defeminizing action.

Experiment 1: Newborn female rats were treated daily for 5 days either with 0, 0.5, 1, 2, 4 or 20 µg of tamoxifen, an estrogen antagonist with low estrogenic activity in rats, or with 0, 0.5, 1, 2 or 4 µg of ICI 47699, the cis-isomer of tamoxifen, which possesses not only anti-estrogenic but also estrogenic activity in rats. In case permanent defeminization and masculinization is caused by postnatal estrogenic activity alone, ICI 47699 should be expected to be more potent to induce permanent anovulatory sterility (PAS), than the less estrogenic isomer tamoxifen. In addition, defeminization should always be accompanied by masculinization.

PAS was induced in 100% of the animals treated with 1, 4 or 20 µg tamoxifen daily, but in none of the animals treated with 0 or 0.5 µg. Treatment with ICI 47699 was less effective (no PAS at 1 or 2 µg; 80% PAS at 4 µg per day). After ovariectomy, all animals were treated for 2 weeks with daily 1 mg testosterone propionate and the frequency of male type of intromission behavior was recorded during a 20 min period of confrontation with an estric female. Intromission frequency was increased from 0.61/min (mean of controls) to maximally 0.96/min in animals postnatally treated with ICI 47699 (2 µg/day). Intromission frequency was reduced in all animals treated postnatally with tamoxifen (i.e. 0.02 intromissions/min at 20 μg tamoxifen/day).

Experiment 2: Newborn female rats were treated for 5 days with either 1 μg tamoxifen, 0.1 μg estradiol or with 0.1 μg estradiol in addition to 1 μg tamoxifen daily. Postnatal treatment with 1 μg tamoxifen daily caused PAS in all animals (n=7). This effect was prevented in 6 out of 10 animals by simultaneous treatment with 0.1 μg estradiol daily. One out of nine rats became anovulatory after daily postnatal treatment with 0.1 μg estradiol only.

The results of both experiments demonstrate that compounds with high estrogenic activity are not necessarily more potent to induce permanent defeminization, than compounds with low estrogenic activity. They further demonstrate that postnatal treatment with tamoxifen induces defeminization but not masculinization, and that tamoxifen-induced defeminization can be attenuated by concomitant treatment with estradiol. The results favor the proposal that not only male, but also female sexual brain differentiation is estrogen dependent (Döhler, 1978).

Döhler K-D (1978) Is female sexual differentiation hormone-mediated? Trends in Neurosciences 1:138-140.

Effect of Estradiol on Catecholamine Turnover and on the Activities of Catecholamine Degrading Enzymes in Brain Areas of Ovariectomized Rats

C. Hiemke, C. Becker, M. Becker and R. Ghraf, Essen

There is increasing evidence that in the rat the neuronal substrate mediating the effect of ovarian hormones on gonadotropin secretion consists of, at least in part, the catecholaminergic system. Estradiol administration was found to affect the turnover rate of catecholamines and the activities of monoamine oxidase (MAO) and catechol-O-methyltransferase (COMT), both of which are involved in the degradation of catecholamines in discrete brain areas. The hormone induced effects were obtained under different experimental conditions. We therefore have studied the effects of chronic administration of estradiol benzoate (EB) on serum gonadotropins, on the turnover rates and concentrations of dopamine (DA), noradrenaline (NA) and adrenaline (A) as well as activities of COMT, MAO-A and MAO-B in identical brain area preparations of adult ovariectomized rats.

The animals received daily injections of 15 µg EB for 7 days starting 7 weeks after castration. In order to measure catecholamine turnover one half of the animals were treated with α-methyl-p-tyrosine. The preoptic area (POA), the mediobasal hypothalamus (MBH), the corticomedial amygdala (CMA) and the frontal cortex (COR) were prepared according to the method of Luine et al. (1974). DA, NA and A were determined radioenzymatically. The activities of MAO-A (substrate, 0.2 mM serotonin), MAO-B (substrate, 0.01 mM phenylethylamine) and COMT (substrate, 1.0 mM 3,4-dihydroxybenzoic acid) were determined radiochemically in Tris-buffered homogenates containing 0.1% Triton X-100. EB administration, which lowered serum LH and FSH levels significantly, reduced the concentration of DA in the MBH without affecting the turnover rate and reduced the NA and

A turnover rates in the POA without affecting the steady state levels. In the CMA and COR significant alterations were not observed. The activities of COMT, MAO-A and MAO-B remained unaffected in all areas studied.

Another approach will be required to elucidate the mechanisms underlying the estradiol-induced changes in catecholaminergic neuro-transmission.

Supported by Deutsche Forschungsgemeinschaft (SPP Neuroendo-krinologie).

Luine VN, Khylchevskaya RI, McEwen BS (1974) Oestrogen effects on brain and pituitary enzyme activities. J Neurochem 23:925-934.

Chinning in Male Tupaia Belangeri and its Hormonal Modification in Short- and Long-term Castrates

D. v. Holst, Bayreuth

As part of a program of experiments on social behavior and social stress in tree-shrews (tupaia belangeri), we have studied the marking behavior of this species.

Males have a clearly demarcated gland in the sternal region of the skin which produces a yellowish-brown, strong smelling secretion. This secretion is distributed in the animal's surrounding by a specific sequence of movements which has been given the descriptive name "chinning".

Chinning of males was measured during ten-minute periods in experimental cages (floor area 70 x 50 cm, hight 50 cm) which contained the scent marks of fertile unknown male conspecifics which had spent ten minutes in the cage less than one hour prior to the beginning of the experiment. The number of chinning actions during ten-minute periods differed considerably between animals, but for a given individual was quite constant in repeated experiments. The average number of chinnings per 10-minute-experiment for each animals is called its chinning value.

Results

1. Male tree-shrews show no chinning activity before puberty (11 animals). With the onset of puberty (at an age of about 50 days) they begin to mark with their sternal glands and reach within about 60 days a level that does not change over years as long as the situation remains constant.

356

2. The chinning values of individual adult males vary over a wide range (from less than 3 to more than 50; 80 animals). The concentrations of androgens in the serum vary, dependent on the individual, between 20 and 80 ng/ml testosterone (and dihydroxy-testosterone) resp. between 1,5 and 20 ng/ml for androstenedione but there is no correlation at all between marking behavior of the animals and their blood androgen concentrations (26 animals).

3. Castration results in all animals in a highly significant decrease of marking activity (21 animals). The amount of this decrease and its course varies greatly from animal to animal: In some individuals, marking activity is reduced within one day to its lowest level, in others, the reduction comes about during the course of up to 4 weeks. Adult castrates, however, in all cases retain a certain degree of "residual marking activity", which varies between less than 1 and more than 30 chinnings per 10-minute periods. The marking activity of the castrates is greater the greater the activity measured before castration ($r > 0.9$; $p < 0.001$).
The testosterone concentration in the serum of all individuals is less than 1.0 ng/ml the day after castration.

4. When castrates are injected with testosterone propionate at doses between 0.5 and 2.0 mg twice a week, their marking activity rises roughly linearly with the logarithm of the dose; higher doses of testosterone have no additional effect on chinning values which are more than 10 times higher than before castration. The response to the hormone is present always one day after hormone injection.

   Each individual responds in different degrees to the testosterone injection, the response being greater the more the animal had marked before castration or as a castrate ($r \gg 0.9$; $p < 0.001$).

   However, although the absolute chinning values of the individuals at a given hormone level differ widely, the percentage changes – with respect to initial rates for each animal – are very nearly the same and entirely reproducible. The behavior of a particular individual thus reflects its hormonal state quite precisely; but the comparison of individuals is unhelpful unless their respective androgen sensitivities are known.

5. Contrary to our expectations the marking activity increased in the course of month following castration progressively in all castrates (13 animals) observed over years. After about 2 years the chinning values reached precastration levels, and after 4 years their values were more than 100% above precastration values (p < 0.001). The cause of this increase is not understood. An age-dependent increase has not been observed in fertile control animals and we exclude this possibility for castrates.

6. If long-term castrates are injected with testosterone more than 200 days after castration no response is shown to a single 2 mg dose. In castrates within the first 100 days after castration this dose, however, results within 24 hours in a highly significant increase of marking activity.

   If the testosterone levels in the blood of long-term castrates are increased by repeated high doses over more than 10 days (leading to testosterone levels 2 – 5 times of the precastration values) then their marking activity decreases after about 2 days to a level about 23% below initial values and increases with a mean of 21 days to a level of 25% above the initial values (13 experiments with 8 animals; decrease and increase statistically different from initial value, p < 0.001). We have no explanation for this bimodal reaction which runs counter to all present day understanding of the hormonal control of behavior.

Interactions of Catecholoestrogens with Oestrogen Receptors of Rat Pituitary and Hypothalamus

J. Kirchhoff, E. Hornung and R. Ghraf, Essen

It has recently been established that catecholoestrogens in the CNS are not merely metabolic endproducts of primary oestrogens, but have both oestrogenic (Ball et al., 1980; Gethmann and Knuppen, 1976) and antioestrogenic activities (Paul and Skolnick, 1977) of their own. It was therefore of interest to establish whether these neuroendocrine activities are mediated by a steroid receptor mechanism involving the binding of catecholoestrogens to cytoplasmic receptors and subsequent translocation of the steroid – receptor complex into the nucleus.

To this end the affinity of several highly purified catecholoestrogens (kindly supplied by Professor Knuppen, Lübeck, FRG) for oestrogen receptors in the hypothalamic and pituitary cytosol from ovariectomized adult rats was assessed by a competitive equilibrium binding assay at $4^{\circ}C$ (Kirchhoff et al., 1980). The Lineweaver – Burk plots of the specific binding data demonstrated a competition of catecholoestrogens for specific oestradiol binding sites. The affinities of 2- and 4-hydroxyoestradiol, 2-hydroxyethinyloestradiol and 4-hydroxyoestrone for these receptors was only slightly lower (K_i = 0.3 - 0.7 nM) than that of their parent compounds. However, hydroxylation of oestrone at C_2 or methylation of the 2-OH group led to a great loss in binding affinity in both tissues.

The nuclear translocation of catecholoestrogen-recepetor complexes was studied following the injection of 75 µCi ($\approx$400 ng) ^{3}H-2-hydroxyoestradiol or ^{3}H-4-hydroxyoestradiol into the jugular vein. 1 h after the injection, highly purified nuclear fractions were prepared from pooled tissue (n=5) and extracted with Tris – KCl buffer containing bacitracin (Roy and McEwen, 1977). Aliquots of the KCL-extracts, were analysed by sedimentation through linear sucrose gradients (5 - 20%, w/v). The sedimentation profiles demonstrated the uptake of ^{3}H-catecholoestrogens into the nuclei of hypothalamus and pituitary, where they were bound to macromolecules sedimenting at 5 - 6 S in high salt (0.4 M KCl) sucrose gradients. The injection (i.p.) of a large dose (0.1 mg) of unlabeled 4-hydroxy-oestradiol 30 min prior to the application of radioactive label led to a considerable reduction of the radioactive peak in the sedimentation profiles of nuclear KCl-extracts suggesting a substantial depletion of cytoplasmic binding sites at 30 min, due to the previous trans-location of receptors into the nuclei by unlabeled 4-hydroxyoestradiol.

The receptor translocation capacity of catecholoestrogens was further investigated using a modified nuclear exchange assay (Roy and McEwen, 1977) 1 h after the injection (i.p.) of 0.1 mg ethinyl-oestradiol or catecholoestrogen. A comparison of the increase in nuclear oestrogen receptor concentration measured by in vitro exchange with ^{3}H-oestradiol showed that the catecholoestrogens, with high affinity for the cytosol receptor, possess 60 - 70% of the translocation capacitiy of ethinyloestradiol.

Our results suggest that at least some of the reported neuro-endocrine activities of catecholoestrogens in the rat could be mediated via a classical steroid receptor mechanism in specific brain areas and the pituitary.

Supported by Forschungsförderung des Ministeriums für Wissenschaft und Forschung des Landes Nordrhein-Westfalen.

Ball P, Naish SJ, Naftolin F (1980) Catecholoestrogens and the induction of sexual receptivity in the ovariectomized rat. Acta Endocr (Kbh) 94, Suppl 234:103-104.
Gethmann U, Knuppen R (1976) Effect of 2-hydroxyoestrone on lutropin (LH) and follitropin (FSH) secretion in the ovariectomized primed rat. Hoppe-Seyler's Z Physiol Chem 357:1011-1013.
Kirchhoff J, Hornung E, Ghraf R (1980) Oestrogen receptors of rat pituitary and hypothalamus: in vitro competition studies using non-steroidal anti-oestrogens. Acta Endocr (KbH) 94, Suppl 234:93-94.
Paul SM, Skolnick P (1977) Catecholoestrogens inhibit oestrogen elicited accumulation of hypothalamic cyclic AMP suggesting role as endogenous anti-oestrogens. Nature 266:559-561.
Roy EJ, McEwen BS (1977) An exchange assay for oestrogen receptors in cell nuclei of the adult rat brain. Steroids 30:657-669.

Direct Effect of 2-Hydroxy-oestradiol-17β on the Hypothalamus and the Control of LH-secretion

W. Ladosky, H.T. Schneider, H. Azambuja and M.L.M. Alessio, Recife and Bonn

Results from our laboratories show that 2-hydroxy-oestradiol-17β as well as oestradiol-17β is able to decrease LH concentration in plasma of ovariectomized rats after systemical administration (Breuer et al., 1980). The present study was undertaken to further elucidate the hypothalamic sites of action of 2-hydroxy-oestradiol-17β and to compare its activity with oestradiol-17β.

Female virgin rats weighing 200 to 220 g were kept under controlled light conditions (lights on from 6 am to 8 pm). Vaginal smears were taken daily between 9 to 10 am. Only animals showing three consecutive 4 day cycles were used for the experiment. Animals were placed in a David Kopf #900 stereotaxic apparatus and injected at 10 am on dioestrus or proestrus with: a) oil (control group), b) 2-hydroxy-oestradiol-17β (0.05 µg/1 µl) or c) oestradiol-17β (0.05 µg/1µl). For LH determination, 1 ml blood was taken from the jugular vein just before steroid or oil injection and at 4 pm on the same day, as well as 10 am and 4 pm on the following two days. LH was measured by double antibody RIA (Anti Rat-LH S4 obtained from NIAMDD and goat anti-rabbit from Faculdade de Medicina, Ribeirão Preto). After the last collection, animals were sacrificed by deep ether narcose, the brain was rapidly removed, fixed in formalin and sliced in a freezing microtome for control of injection placement.

After the injection of oestradiol-17β as well as 2-hydroxy-estradiol-17β into the preoptic area on the day of proestrus a statistically significant increase in plasma LH above the control was observed in the afternoon of the same day. Oestradiol-17β was more potent than 2-hydroxy-oestradiol-17β in inducing this increase. When injected at dioestrus in the arcuate nucleus, both substances blocked the ovulatory peak which normally occurs in the afternoon of the next day. When the same nucleus was injected at proestrus only 2-hydroxy-oestradiol-17β induced a significant increase in plasma LH on the afternoon of the same day.

The preoptic area in rats has been reported to be the site for positive feedback action of oestrogens (Ladosky and Wandscheer, 1975; Saywer, 1975), and the above findings confirmed this. Although 2-hydroxy-oestradiol-17β is less active than oestradiol-17β, it still induces a significant increase in plasma LH above control values, suggesting that both substances are acting through the same mechanism, with oestradiol-17β being the more active hormone.

The negative feedback action of oestrogens when injected on the dioestrus, as already reported (Blake et al., 1974) was also confirmed. 2-hydroxy-oestradiol-17β has the same activity as oestradiol-17β and no significant difference was observed. However, when these steroids were injected on proestrus, oestradiol-17β induced no change when compared to control, although 2-hydroxy-oestradiol-17β caused a sharp and significant increase in LH release on the afternoon of the same day.

The arcuate nucleus is not only considered the region for the direct negative feedback action of oestrogen (Blake et al., 1974; Ladosky and Wandscheer, 1975) but also the nucleus where catecholaminergic terminals coming from the preoptic or suprachiasmatic areas induce the ovulatory surge in LH (Kordon and Ramirez, 1975; Ladosky and Wandscheer, 1975). The inhibitory action of oestrogens injected in the morning of dioestrus is being interpreted as a consequence of the increase of threshold to the impulses coming from other regions (Blake et al., 1974; Ladosky and Wanscheer, 1975; Nagle and Rosner, 1976). According to our results 2-hydroxy-oestradiol-17β would have the same activity as oestradiol-17β. When injected on proestrus however, oestradiol-17β would be unable to impede the ovulatory peak due to the fact that the impulses have already been given and the LH releasing mechanism is under way. Since 2-hydroxy-oestradiol-17 has been reported to inhibit the inactivation of noradrenaline by COMT (Breuer and Köster, 1974), the increase in plasma LH after this oestrogen has been injected, may be interpreted as a consequence of a longer activity of noradrenaline

which is normally liberated before the afternoon discharge of LH
(Ladosky and Wandscheer, 1975; Nagle and Rosner, 1976).

Blake CA, Norman RL, Sawyer CH (1974) Localization of the Inhibitory Actions of Estrogen and Nicotine on Release of Luteinizing Hormone in Rats. Neuroendocrinology 16:22-35.

Breuer H, Köster G (1974) Interaction between oestrogens and neurotransmitters at the hypophysial-hypothalamic level. J Steroid Biochem 5:961-967.

Breuer H, Schneider HT, Doberauer C, Grüter S, Ladosky W (1980) Effects of oestradiol-17β and 2-hydroxy-oestradiol-17β on LH concentrations in plasma and COMT activities in hypothalamic nuclei of rats. Experimental Brain Res, in press.

Kordon C, Ramirez VD (1975) Recent Developments in Neurotransmitter Hormone Interactions. Anatomical Neuroendocrinology Intern Conf Neurobiology of CNS-Hormone Interactions, Chapel Hill 1974, pp.409-419.

Ladosky W, Wandscheer DE (1975) Interactions between Estrogen and Biogenic Amines in the Control of LH Secretion. J Steroid Biochem, Vol. 6:1013-1020.

Legan SJ, Allyn Coon G, Karsch FJ (1975) Role of Estrogen as Initiator of Daily LH Surges in the Ovariectomized Rat. Endocrinology 96:50-56.

Nagle CA, Rosner JM (1976) Plasma Norepinephrine during the Rat Estrous Cycle and after Progesterone Treatment to the Ovariectomized Estrogen-Primed Rat. Neuroendocrinology 22:89-96.

Sawyer CH (1975) Some recent developments in brain-pituitary-ovarian physiology. Neuroendocrinology 17:97-124.

Effects of 2-hydroxyoestradiol and Dopamine on the Release of Prolactin and Luteinising Hormone From Rat Pituitary Glands in Vitro

E.A. Linton, N. White, O.L. de Tineo and S.L. Jeffcoate, London

It has been proposed that 2-hydroxyoestradiol (2 OH-E$_2$) may play a role in the regulation of prolactin (Prl) secretion by competition for dopamine (DA) receptors in the anterior pituitary (Schaeffer, 1979), and it has also been shown to increase luteinising hormone (LH) secretion by pituitary cells in culture (Franks et al., 1979). Since relatively little is known about the effects of catecholoestrogens on Prl and LH secretion and their interaction with catecholamines in vitro, we have investigated this using male rat pituitaries in a continuous superfusion system.

Pituitaries from adult male Sprague-Dawley rats were placed in individual superfusion chambers and perfused with Krebs bicarbonate buffer. After a one hour pre-incubation period, 6-minute fractions were collected for two hours, during which each pituitary was exposed to 2 OH-E$_2$ (10^{-7}M or 10^{-10}M) and/or DA (5×10^{-7}) on two occasions, allowing an intervening recovery period. The fractions were stored at -20°C until assayed for Prl and LH using radioimmunoassay reagents supplied by NIAMDD.

The findings were as follows:

1. DA alone produced the expected reduction in Prl release, 58% at 5×10^{-7}M.

2. 2 OH-E$_2$ alone decreased Prl release by 46% at 10^{-10}M and by 30% at 10^{-7}M.

3. Pre-treatment with 2 OH-E$_2$ (10^{-7}M) did not inhibit the DA effect. The two together produced a 60% reduction.

4. In all experiments except one, levels of LH release were unaffected. In one experiment 4 out of 5 pituitaries showed

increased levels of LH release immediately following exposure to 2 OH-E$_2$ (10^{-7}M).

5.   DA (5×10^{-7}) had no effect on LH release.

These results, using a continuous superfusion system, show that both 2 OH-E$_2$ and DA decrease Prl release, and so do not support Schaeffer's proposal that 2 OH-E$_2$ antagonises DA action on Prl. We have also been unable to confirm the observation that 2 OH-E$_2$ will increase LH secretion (Franks et al., 1979). It is possible that these conflicting results may be attributed to the different types of in vitro preparation used.

Franks S, Merriam G, Goodyer CB, Naftolin F (1979) Catecholoestrogens stimulate LH secretion by dispersed rat pituitary cells in culture. Abstracts book "The Endocrine Society 61st Annual Meeting", Anaheim, California, USA, p.302.

Schaeffer JM (1979) Dopamine receptors in the anterior pituitary: Inhibition of ^{3}H-spiroperidol binding by 2-hydroxyoestradiol. Abstracts book "The Endocrine Society 61st Annual Meeting", Anaheim, California, USA, p.138.

Involvement of GABA in Negative Feedback Action of Estradiol

T. Mansky and W. Wuttke, Göttingen

It has often been suggested that GABA plays an important role as neurotransmitter in the hypothalamus. Nevertheless in neuroendocrine research mainly pharmacological investigations have been reported so far. It is difficult, however, to conclude about physiological functions on the basis of pharmacological experiments, because GABA receptors are widespread in the CNS (Krnjevic, 1976) and unspecific actions of GABAergic drugs cannot be excluded. Furthermore it has been shown (Perez de la Mora, 1979) that different GABAergic drugs such as GABA transaminase inhibitors (γ-acetylenic GABA etc.) and GABA receptor agonists (muscimol) can exert opposite effects on the same system (GABA-T inhibitors reduce, muscimol increases dopamine turnover). We therefore tried to investigate the physiological role of GABA by determining GABA concentrations and turnoverrates under different endocrine situations in diestrous (D), proestrous (P) and ovariectomized (OVX) and OVX animals treated with estradiol-benzoate (OE) 12 h or 24 h before decapitation.

There are at least two commonly used methods for determination of the GABA turnover, which both act by blocking degradation of GABA. The pharmacological method blocks GABA-transaminase with amino-oxy-acetic-acid (AOAA). The other method, which we used, utilizes the fact that degradation of GABA, which is oxygen dependent, stops immediately after decapitation, whereas synthesis continues for the first five min post mortem and leads to a linear increase in GABA concentrations. This is schematically demonstrated in Fig. 1.

Patel and coworkers (1974) showed that the linear increase of GABA within the first 5 postmortal minutes is a reliable parameter

TURNOVER OF GABA IS
MEASURED AFTER BLOCKING
METABOLISM BY DECAPITATION

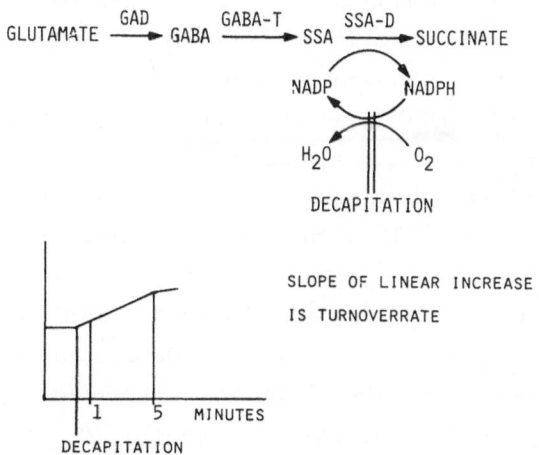

Figure 1: GABA is metabolized to succinate via succinic-semialdehyde
(SSA) by the enzymes GABA-transaminase (GABA-T) and SSA-dehydrogenase
(SSA-D). The oxidation by SSA-D requires NADP and thus oxygen.
Decapitation blocks this step by interrupting oxygen supply and leads to
a linear increase in GABA concentrations reflecting the in vivo turnover

for GABA turnover. This postmortem increase of GABA is not only
dependent on GAD activity but also on the compartmentation and
availability of glutamic-acid decarboxylase (GAD), its coenzyme and
the GABA precursor glutamate. Measurement of turnoverrates with
this method has the advantage of being more specific and selective
than turnover determination by use of AOAA. Although the measured
turnover of GABA does not only reflect the neuronal but also the
metabolic turnover of GABA which may be up to 50% of the total
(postmortem) turnover, we think that this interference should not
contribute to the specific hormone dependent changes of turnoverrates
but only provide a constant background noise increasing the
standarddeviation of turnoverrates.

After decapitation the brains are cut sagitally with a sharp
razor blade. The first half is then frozen 1 min the other half
5 min after decapitation on dry ice. Both halves are cut on a
freezing microtome and punches of the different regions are taken

according to the method of Palkovits et al. (1974). The concentrations of GABA are measured with the very sensitive and precise enzymatic-fluorometric assay (Collins, 1972).

Using the brain splitting the turnover can be measured in individual animals and the interindividual variations of GABA concentrations are eliminated from the turnover determination.

In the medial preoptic area (MPO) we measured the highest concentrations of GABA compared to the other nuclei investigated so far. Only for the substantia nigra comparably high concentrations have been reported in the literature. This high concentration may support our view that GABA plays an important role as neurotransmitter in the MPO were estrogen receptive neurons and the perikarya of the LHRH producing cells are located. Details about the results obtained for the MPO and the AMBH are reported by Wuttke and Mansky (this volume). It can be concluded that GABAergic mechanisms in the MPO mediate the negative feedback action of estrogens on LHRH.

In the anterior mediobasal hypothalamus (AMBH) a slight correlation of GABA-turnover and prolactin levels can be shown. The differences between groups, however, are not significant.

In the posterior part of the mediobasal hypothalamus (PMBH) we find a significant decrease of GABA concentrations in all OVX animals but no significant changes in turnover rates (Fig. 2).

In the mediocortical amygdala (AMY) there are no significant changes in concentrations and turnover (Fig. 3).

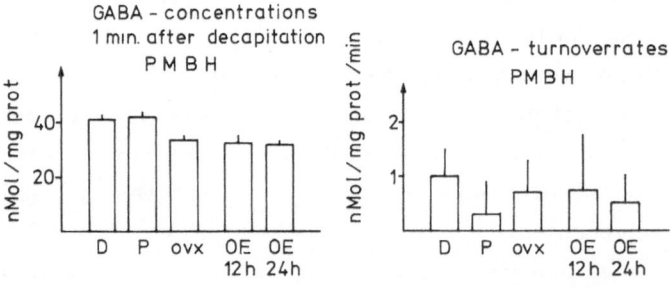

Figure 2: GABA concentrations in the posterior part of the mediobasal hypothalamus show a decrease in ovariectomized rats but no significant changes in turnoverrates. Means ± SEM are shown

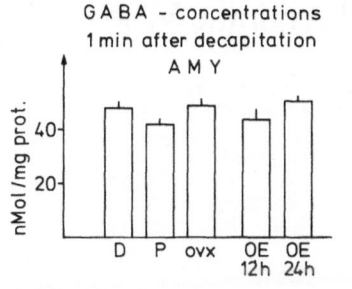

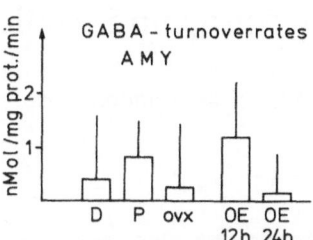

Figure 3: No significant changes of GABA concentrations and turnover-rates can be observed in the mediocortical amygdala under different endocrine states

Results are suggestive that GABA may be the transmitter of estrogen-receptive neurons in the MPO but not in the other regions investigated mediating the negative feedback of estrogens on LH. In the AMBH GABA shows a slight positive correlation with prolactin while in the PMBH and AMY no relation of GABA to the different endocrine states can be shown.

Collins GGS (1972) GABA-2-oxoglutarate transaminase, glutamate decarboxylase and the half-life of GABA in different areas of the rat brain. Biochem Pharmacol 21:2849-2858.
Krnjevic K (1976) Inhibitory action of GABA and GABA-mimetics on vertebrate neurons. In: Roberts E, Chase TN, Tower DB (eds) GABA in nervous system function. Raven Press, New Yor.
Palkovits M, Brownstein M, Saavedra JM, Axelrod J (1974) Norepinephrine and dopamine content of hypothalamuc nuclei of the rat. Brain Res. 77:137-149.
Patel AJ, Johnson AL, Balazs R (1974) Metabolic compartmentation of glutamate associated with the formation of -aminobutyrate. J Neurochem 23:1271-1279.
Perez de la Mora M, Fuxe K, Andersson K, Hökfelt T, Ljungdal A, Possani L, Tapia R (1974) Studies on GABA-monoamine and GABA-endorphin interaction. In: Usdin E, Kopin IJ, Barchas J (eds) Catecholamines: Basic and clinical Frontiers. Pergamon Press, New York, vol. 2, pp.1032-1034.

The Role of Substance P, Neurotensin and Arginine Vasotocin in the Control of Gonadotrophin Secretion

K. Nesbitt, K. Selby and S.A. Whitehead, London

The growing interest in possible peptide-peptide interactions in the central nervous system has prompted numerous investigations into the actions of neuropeptides in modulating anterior pituitary secretions. Substance P (SP) and Neurotensin (NT) are two neuropeptides which have been shown to alter luteinizing hormone (LH) secretion (Vijayan and McCann, 1979) and results implicate a central action of these peptides on the release of gonadotrophin releasing hormone (GnRH). Another peptide, arginine vasotocin (AVT), which differs in structure from oxytocin and arginine vasopressin by only one amino acid, has also been shown to affect LH secretion (Pavel et al., 1979) although the presence of AVT in the mammalian hypothalamus has not been demonstrated. However, to date there have been no reported studies on the direct effect of such peptides on GnRH secretion.

In present experiments, an in vitro system was adopted to investigate the action of SP, NT and AVT on the basal and electrically stimulated secretion of GnRH from whole incubated medio-basal hypothalami obtained from normal cycling, intact female rats. Aliquots of the krebs bicarbonate incubating medium (200 μl) were taken every fifteen minutes throughout the 2 h incubation period and were replaced by an equal volume of the medium. The tissue was subjected to two fifteen minute stimulation periods (square wave pulses, 1 msec, 40 Hz, 15 mA) during the course of the experiment and this resulted in a highly significant increase in GnRH secretion, which was shown to be CA^{++}-dependent. At the end of the experiment, the remaining GnRH was extracted from the hypothalami so that the amount of GnRH measured in the aliquots, by radioimmunoassay, could be expressed as a percentage release of the total GnRH originally present in the tissue.

SP (10^{-6}M) had no effect on the basal and electrically stimulated release of GnRH compared to the controls, whereas the same dose of NT and AVT inhibited GnRH release. AVT was a more potent inhibitor than NT and it completely abolished the ability of the tissue to respond to electrical stimulation. Even at a lower concentration of 10^{-9}M AVT produced similar inhibition of GnRH secretion, whereas 10^{-8}M NT had no effect when compared to the controls. Oxytocin and arginine vasopressin (10^{-6}M) did not alter GnRH release suggesting the action of AVT is selective.

As a parallel study, the effect of these peptides on the <u>in</u> <u>vitro</u> release of LH from perifused pituitary glands was investigated. Preliminary studies showed they have no effect on basal LH release nor on the responsiveness of the pituitary gland to five minute pulses of GnRH at a concentration of 10 ng ml^{-1}.

The results, in agreement with other studies, show that AVT and NT can inhibit LH secretion via a hypothalamic site of action, whereas SP, which has been shown to raise plasma LH levels, <u>in</u> <u>vivo</u> (Vijayan and McCann, 1979) does not appear to alter GnRH release.

Pavel S, Luca N, Calb M, Goldstein R (1979) Inhibition of release of luteinizing hormone in the male rat by extremely small amounts of AVT. Further evidence for the involvement of 5-hydroxytryptamine – containing neurones in the mechanism of action of arginine vasotocin. J Endocrinology 84:159–162.

Vijayan E, McCann S (1979) <u>In</u> <u>vivo</u> and <u>in</u> <u>vitro</u> effectsof Substance P and Neurotensin on Gonadotrophin and Prolactin Release. Neuroendocrinology 25:64–68.

Gonadal Steroids in the Amygdala – Differential Effects on LH

N. Parvizi and F. Ellendorff, Neustadt

With the aid of a new approach combining electrical stimulation with microinjection in a chronic preparation, we tested the hypothesis that (a) gonadal steroids alter the sensitivity of the amygdala (AMY) to electrical stimulation, resulting in changes in plasma LH levels and (b) the amygdala is able to discriminate between various gonadal steroids.

Adult castrated male miniature pigs with bilateral "electro-tubes" chronically implanted into the AMY were used. Electrical stimulation (10 Hz, 200 μA – shorter wire cathode – 0.1 msec, 30 sec on/off, 60 min) of the AMY without any pretreatment or microinjection with solvent (1 μl of a solution containing 2 ml 10% ethanol plus 8 ml 0.9% saline) followed 210 min later by electrical stimulation resulted in decreased plasma LH-levels in all animals (n=7). In contrast, microinjection of 60 ng testosterone 210 min prior to electrical stimulation caused LH levels (in 5 out of 6 animals) to increase upon stimulation. However, prior microinjection of estradiol-17β (6 ng) or 5α-dihydrotestosterone (60 ng) abolished the effects of electrical stimulation obtained after no treatment. Four out of 7 animals responded to microinjection of 2-hydroxy-estradiol-17β (60 ng, solvent contained 0.01% ascorbic acid) with a fall in plasma-LH-levels. Electrical stimulation increased LH-levels up to those seen before microinjection in these animals. In the other three animals, with no response to catecholestrogen microinjection, the response to electrical stimulation was a depression in LH-levels. Control blood sampling over 30 min (in 10 min intervals) had no significant effects on LH-levels.

The results suggest a direct and differentiated effect of steroids on the AMY; the action of testosterone is independent of its aromatization or reduction and steroids act on the AMY to inhibit or stimulate the inhibitory role of the amygdala in the control of pituitary LH secretion.

This work was supported by the Deutsche Forschungsgemeinschaft. This paper is published in full length in BRAIN RESEARCH (1980 in press).

Experimental Brain Research/
Supplementum 1

Afferent and Intrinsic Organization of Laminated Structures in the Brain

(7th International Neurobiology Meeting)
Editor: O. Creutzfeldt

1976. 127 figures. XXIII, 579 pages
ISBN 3-540-07923-8

Contents: Cerebellum. – Allocortex: Anatomy. Physio-
logy. – Neocortex: Development Cortical Circuitry.
Functional Organization. – Subcortical Laminated
Structures: Medial and Lateral Geniculate Body. The
Optic Tectum. – Electric Lobe.

Experimental Brain Research/
Supplementum 2

Hearing Mechanisms and Speech

EBBS-Workshop, Göttingen, April 26–28, 1979
Editors: O. Creutzfeldt, H. Scheich, C. Schreiner

1979. 85 figures, 12 tables. XXIII, 413 pages
ISBN 3-540-09655-8

Contents: Functional and Structural Conditions for
Transmission of Auditory Signals in the Nervous
System. – The Representation of Complex Natural
Sounds in the Auditory System. – Brain Mechanisms of
Speech Perception and Production. – Psychoacoustic
Elements in Language. – Linquistic Elements in Speech
Perception. – Receptive Defects of Linguistic Elements
in Aphasia.

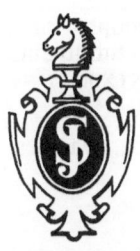

Springer-Verlag
Berlin
Heidelberg
New York

Brain and Heart Infarct II

Editors: K.J.Zülch, W.Kaufmann,
K.-A.Hossmann, V.Hossmann
With contributions by numerous experts

1979. 114 figures, 22 tables. XII, 330 pages
ISBN 3-540-09401-6

Current Topics in Extra-pyramidal Disorders

Editors: A.Carlsson, K.Jellinger and
P.Riederer

1980. 1 portrait, 31 figures, 37 tables.
X, 241 pages. (Journal of Neural Trans-
mission/Supplementum 16)
Wien–New York: Springer-Verlag
ISBN 3-211-81570-8

R.Hassler, F.Mundinger, T.Riechert
Stereotaxis in Parkinson Syndrome

Clinical-Anatomical Contributions to Its
Pathophysiology

With an Atlas of the Basal Ganglia in
Parkinsonism by R.Hassler
Foreword by E.A.Spiegel
1979. 163 figures in 235 separate illustrations,
11 tables. XII, 315 pages
ISBN 3-540-08005-8

Neural Mechanisms in Behavior

A Texas Symposium

Editor: D.McFadden
With contributions by numerous experts

1980. 151 figures, 1 table. XI, 308 pages
ISBN 3-540-90468-9

D. W. Pfaff
Estrogens and Brain Function

Neural Analysis of a Hormone-Controlled
Mammilian Reproductive Behavior

1980. 109 figures, 1 in color, 20 tables.
X, 281 pages
ISBN 3-540-90487-5

Psychotropic Agents

(Handbook of Experimental Pharmacology,
Vol. 55 in 3 parts)

Part 1: Antipsychotics and Antidepressants
With contributions by numerous experts
Editors: F.Hoffmeister, G.Stille

1980. 82 figures, 74 tables. XXIV, 734 pages
ISBN 3-540-09838-5

Part 2: Anxiolytics, Gerontopsychopharmaco-
logical Agents, and Psychomotor Stimulants
With contributions by numerous experts
Editors: F.Hoffmeister, G.Stille

1981. Approx. 100 figures, approx. 50 tables.
Approx. 830 pages
ISBN 3-540-10300-7

Part 3: Alcohol and Psychotomimetics,
Psychotropic Effects of Central Acting Drugs
With contributions by numerous experts
Editors: F.Hoffmeister, G.Stille

1981. Approx. 500–600 pages
ISBN 3-540-10301-5

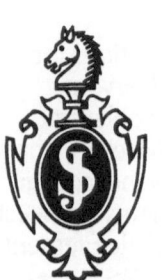

Springer-Verlag
Berlin
Heidelberg
New York